T0235980

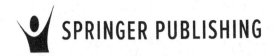

GET THE MOST FROM YOUR BOOK

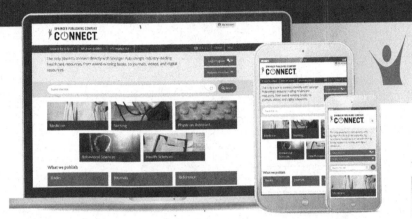

SPRINGER PUBLISHING
C🜚NNECT™

VOUCHER CODE:

XSM7GYG2

Online Access

Your print purchase of *Writing for Publication in Nursing, Fourth Edition*, includes **online access via Springer Publishing Connect**™ to increase accessibility, portability, and searchability.

Insert the code at http://connect.springerpub.com/content/book/978-0-8261-4721-9 today!

Having trouble? Contact our customer service department at cs@springerpub.com

Instructor Resource Access for Adopters

Let us do some of the heavy lifting to create an engaging classroom experience with a variety of instructor resources included in most textbooks SUCH AS:

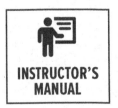

INSTRUCTOR'S MANUAL

POWERPOINTS

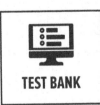

TEST BANK

Visit **https://connect.springerpub.com/** and look for the **"Show Supplementary"** button on your **book homepage** to see what is available to instructors! First time using Springer Publishing Connect?

Email **textbook@springerpub.com** to create an account and start unlocking valuable resources.

WRITING FOR PUBLICATION IN NURSING

MARILYN H. OERMANN, PhD, RN, ANEF, FAAN, is the Thelma M. Ingles Professor of Nursing and Director of Evaluation and Educational Research at Duke University School of Nursing, Durham, North Carolina. She is author/coauthor of 21 books and many articles on evaluation, teaching in nursing, and writing for publication. She is the editor of *Nurse Educator* and the *Journal of Nursing Care Quality*. She lectures widely on teaching and evaluation in nursing and on writing for publication. Dr. Oermann received the Margaret Comerford Freda Award for Editorial Leadership in Nursing from the International Academy of Nursing Editors.

JUDITH C. HAYS, PhD, RN, FGSA, is Associate Professor Emerita at Duke University School of Nursing, Durham, North Carolina. She is author/coauthor of a psychiatric epidemiology textbook and more than 70 scientific articles on late-life living arrangements, religiousness, depression, palliative care and bereavement, and nursing history. She is coeditor emeritus of the journal *Public Health Nursing*. Dr. Hays edits the scientific writing of faculty in baccalaureate, master's, and doctor of nursing practice (DNP) programs.

WRITING FOR PUBLICATION IN NURSING

FOURTH EDITION

Marilyn H. Oermann, PhD, RN, ANEF, FAAN

Judith C. Hays, PhD, RN, FGSA

SPRINGER PUBLISHING COMPANY

Springer Publishing Company, LLC
11 West 42nd Street
New York, NY 10036
www.springerpub.com

Acquisitions Editor: Adrianne Brigido
Compositor: diacriTech, Chennai

ISBN: 978-0-8261-4701-1
ebook ISBN: 978-0-8261-4721-9
Instructor's Manual ISBN: 978-0-8261-4702-8
Instructor's PowerPoint ISBN: 978-0-8261-4703-5

Instructor's Materials: Qualified instructors may request supplements by emailing textbook@springerpub.com

18 19 20 21 22 / 5 4 3 2 1

Library of Congress Cataloging-in-Publication Data
Names: Oermann, Marilyn H., author. | Hays, Judith C., author.
Title: Writing for publication in nursing / Marilyn H. Oermann, Judith C.
  Hays.
Description: Fourth edition. | New York, NY : Springer Publishing Company,
  LLC, [2018] | Includes bibliographical references and index.
Identifiers: LCCN 2018013503 | ISBN 9780826147011
Subjects: | MESH: Medical Writing | Periodicals as Topic | Publishing |
  Nurses' Instruction
Classification: LCC RT24 | NLM WZ 345 | DDC 808/.06661—dc23
LC record available at https://lccn.loc.gov/2018013503

Contact us to receive discount rates on bulk purchases.
We can also customize our books to meet your needs.
For more information please contact: sales@springerpub.com

Printed in the United States of America.

CONTENTS

APPENDICES

CONTRIBUTOR TO THE THIRD EDITION

Jeffrey Beall, MA, MSLS
Scholarly Communications Librarian, Auraria Library
Associate Professor, University of Colorado Denver
Denver, Colorado

PREFACE

Writing for publication in nursing is essential to disseminate evidence, share initiatives and innovations with others, provide new information to keep nurses up to date, communicate the findings of research studies, and develop the science base of the profession. Writing manuscripts is hard work, but the process can be simplified by understanding how to develop a manuscript and submit it for publication. *Writing for Publication in Nursing*, now in its fourth edition, was prepared for beginning and experienced authors, for nurses, and for graduate students in nursing to guide them in writing literature reviews, research reports, quality improvement and clinical articles, and other types of papers.

This book describes the process of writing, beginning with an idea, searching the literature, preparing an outline, writing a draft and revising it, and developing the final paper. How to select a journal and gear the writing to the intended audience, submit a manuscript to a journal, revise a paper and respond to reviewers, and carry out other steps to facilitate publication are discussed in the book. A chapter is devoted to writing research articles to assist nurses in preparing their work for publication; strategies are included for developing manuscripts from theses and dissertations. Other chapters describe principles for writing quality improvement articles and preparing articles that disseminate the outcomes of reviews of research evidence, articles on clinical practice topics and evidence-based practice (EBP), case reports, and chapters and books. The book serves as a reference for students at all levels of nursing education to guide them in writing papers for courses. Many nursing programs expect students to demonstrate competency in writing as an outcome of the program. *Writing for Publication in Nursing* is a good resource for that purpose. Graduate students in particular can use the book to learn how to write for publication—an essential skill for advanced practice nurses, researchers, educators, administrators, and nurses in other roles to disseminate their work and for their career advancement.

Writing for Publication in Nursing can be used in conjunction with the style manual in the nursing program. While style manuals direct students in preparing citations, references, tables, and figures, and guide them on other aspects of style, these manuals do not teach students the process of writing or how to prepare a paper for publication in nursing.

This book contains many examples and resources for writing in nursing and other healthcare professions. These resources make writing easier for both novice and experienced authors.

SECTION I: PREPARING TO WRITE

Writing for publication is essential to disseminate the findings of research and evidence for practice, communicate knowledge and share expertise with other nurses, inform nurses of initiatives and innovations developed for patient populations and settings, and advance the profession. Chapter 1 introduces the steps the author follows in planning, writing, and publishing manuscripts in nursing. The focus is on early writing decisions, such as generating ideas, selecting a topic, and deciding on the type of article to be written. The author evaluates if the ideas to be presented are new, are worth writing about, and are important enough to be published.

The next steps are to identify the audience to whom the manuscript will be directed and to select a journal that might be interested in publishing it. The purpose of the manuscript and how it will be developed guide the author in deciding on possible journals. The goal is to match the topic and type of manuscript with an appropriate journal and readers who would be interested in it. Chapter 2 discusses how to evaluate possible journals, select an appropriate one, and write a query email to gauge the interest of the editor of the journal. Valuable resources in this chapter include a description of online directories of journals for searching for a potential journal and a sample query email.

Decisions about the focus of the manuscript, audience, and journal are important early in the writing process. Other decisions pertain to authorship; if these are not made before beginning the writing project, they may create problems and conflict among the authors later on. Each individual designated as an author on a manuscript or other type of paper should have contributed sufficiently to it. Chapter 3 addresses authorship and author responsibilities in preparing to write. Because many papers are written in groups, strategies are provided to facilitate this process.

Chapter 4 prepares the author for reviewing the literature and writing a literature review for a manuscript and other types of papers. Although literature reviews for research studies, academic papers, evidence syntheses, and other purposes vary in the types of literature used, their comprehensiveness, and how they are summarized for the reader, the process of reviewing the literature is the same. Chapter 4 describes bibliographic databases useful for literature reviews in nursing, selecting databases to use, search strategies, analyzing and synthesizing the literature, and writing the literature review. This chapter provides many resources to help nurse authors with their literature reviews. Strategies to avoid plagiarism and information about obtaining permission to reproduce copyrighted material in a manuscript are included in the chapter.

SECTION II: WRITING RESEARCH, EPB, QUALITY IMPROVEMENT, AND CLINICAL PRACTICE ARTICLES

Research projects are not complete until the findings are communicated to others. All too often nurses conduct important research studies but fail to disseminate the results of their work. Some nurses are not prepared for their role as an author and are unsure how to proceed; others may believe that their work does not warrant publication. However, rigorous research is important to communicate to others, regardless of whether the findings were anticipated or not. Research papers present the findings of quantitative and qualitative research based on original data. Chapter 5 begins with a discussion of how to report research using the conventional format of an introduction and literature review; a methods section, including design and sample, measurements, and analytic strategy; a results section; and a discussion. This basic structure of research articles is known as IMRAD, that is, Introduction, Methods, Results, and Discussion. Examples are provided of quantitative, qualitative, and mixed-methods research articles for authors to learn how to write different sections of these manuscripts, as well as reporting guidelines such as the Consolidated Standards of Reporting Trials (CONSORT). Ethical considerations when writing research papers include deciding the appropriate number of articles to write from a single study and avoidance of redundant or duplicate publications. Authors should take care to protect the privacy rights of their subjects. The chapter concludes by describing pitfalls to avoid when reporting research findings and revising academic papers as research manuscripts.

Nurses in all clinical settings require the most current and complete evidence of effective approaches to guide their decision making and practice. The evidence should be based on a critical appraisal of studies that answer a specific clinical question or examine best practices and the synthesis of findings from across these studies. In EBP, nurses rely on the synthesis of evidence from multiple studies rather than the report of one original research study. Methods are available to nurse authors for reviewing and integrating individual studies and summarizing the evidence from them to answer a clinical question or explore a topic of interest. These review methods include integrative reviews, systematic reviews, meta-analyses, qualitative syntheses, and others. Chapter 6 describes these methods and presents guidelines for developing manuscripts on different types of reviews. This chapter includes an explanation and examples of the Preferred Reporting Items for Systematic Reviews and Meta-Analyses (PRISMA), which are the recommended guidelines for reporting these reviews; PRISMA also can be used for literature reviews, as discussed in this chapter. Nurses also write about changes in practice, the effectiveness of new approaches to care, and the process used in a clinical setting to engage in EBP. Chapter 6 presents guidelines for preparing articles related to EBP in nursing.

With the focus on quality and safety in healthcare, it is important for nurse authors to learn about guidelines for reporting quality improvement (QI) studies. Good reporting of QI is critical for readers to understand the problem, context of the study, interventions, and if they made a difference in outcomes. Chapter 7 describes how to write manuscripts that report QI. The Standards for Quality Improvement Reporting Excellence (SQUIRE) are presented as guidelines for preparing these manuscripts.

Chapter 8 presents strategies for writing articles about clinical practice. There are many opportunities for preparing these manuscripts. Nurses can write about their innovations in practice, new initiatives and projects in their clinical setting, updates on clinical topics, and new directions in patient care. Considering the wealth of clinical journals in nursing, these publications provide a venue for nurses to share their work with others. General guidelines for writing clinical articles are presented in the chapter, including writing research reports for clinical journals.

SECTION III: CHAPTERS, BOOKS, AND OTHER FORMS OF WRITING

Although research and clinical practice articles are primary formats for nurses to present knowledge to readers, other forms of writing are equally important. Some articles address emerging issues that affect nursing practice, education, or research. These articles may include case reports; descriptions of theory development; commentaries on policies, ethics, or legal aspects of nursing; innovative research methods; historical studies; editorials; and letters to the editor. Nurses also write book reviews and articles for consumer and nonprofessional audiences. These other types of writing differ in the purposes they are trying to achieve, their format, and often their writing style. Yet all are similar because they address nontrivial topics, provide original insight, and have implications for advancing health and well-being. Chapter 9 describes these other types of papers and provides many examples to guide these forms of writing.

Writing a book or book chapter is different from writing an article because the author has more opportunity to provide background information and discuss related content, with more pages allowed, than in a manuscript for a journal. Whereas articles generally focus on one topic, books address multiple but related content areas and also require a significant time commitment. Chapter 10 provides information for nurse authors who are interested in writing a book, including contacting a publisher, developing the prospectus, outlining the responsibilities of the author and publisher, detailing the process of writing the book, and working with contributors in an edited book. There also is a section on writing a book chapter.

SECTION IV: THE WRITING PROCESS

At this point in the process of writing, the author has identified the type of manuscript, the purpose of the paper, potential journals, and the audience toward
which the paper will be geared. The author has obtained author guidelines
from the target journal, has conducted or updated the literature review, has
completed other preparations for writing, and is now ready to begin writing
the manuscript. Chapter 11 focuses first on preliminary questions to ask before
starting to write and on organizing the content into an outline. Next, the chapter describes how to write the first draft of the manuscript. Finally, the chapter
describes the steps in revising the content and organization of the paper and
then revising the writing structure and style. Some principles are provided for
improving how the paper is written.

Most papers written for publication in nursing include references. The references in the manuscript document the literature reviewed by the author who
prepared the paper and provide support for the ideas in it. In Chapter 12, the
focus is on citing the references in the manuscript and preparing the reference
list. Journals use different reference formats, and the author must prepare the
references according to the journal guidelines. Examples are provided of how to
cite references in the text and in the reference list using different reference styles.

Tables are essential when the author needs to report detailed information
and numeric values. It is often clearer and more efficient to develop a table
than to present the information in the text. Figures are valuable for demonstrating trends and patterns, and for some manuscripts the author may include
an illustration of a new procedure or a photograph of a patient. Not every
manuscript, though, needs tables and figures, and whether to include them
is a decision made during the drafting phase of writing the paper. Chapter 13
provides guidelines for deciding when to prepare tables and figures and how
to develop them. Examples are included of different types of tables, presenting
information in a table or as text, and developing figures for a manuscript.

SECTION V: FINAL PAPER THROUGH PUBLICATION

When the author has completed the revisions of the content and format of the
paper and prepared the references, tables, and figures, the author is ready to
submit the paper to the journal. Prior to submission, the author has some final
responsibilities to ensure that the manuscript is consistent with the journal
requirements and contains all the required parts for submission. The manuscript is then ready to submit to the journal for review. Chapter 14 describes
the steps in preparing all elements of the final paper to submit to the journal
and details associated with this submission. Examples of these elements are

provided in the chapter, and a checklist is included for authors to ensure that all items are submitted with the manuscript to avoid delays in its review.

Chapter 15 presents the editorial review process from the point at which the paper is received in the journal office through the final editorial decision. The roles and responsibilities of the editor, editorial board, and peer reviewers are discussed, and examples are provided of criteria used by reviewers when asked to critique a manuscript for publication. Manuscripts submitted to a journal may be accepted without revision or accepted provisionally pending revision, may be returned to the author for a major revision and resubmission, or may be rejected. Each of these editorial decisions has implications for the author and how the author responds to the editor: These are presented in the chapter. Resources for readers include a sample peer-review form and sample letters, which document changes made in the manuscript in response to the reviewers' comments, to submit with the revised manuscript.

When the manuscript is accepted for publication, the paper moves into the publishing phase. The author has some responsibilities here, such as answering queries and correcting page proofs, but most of the work is done by the publisher of the journal or by the group or individual responsible for the publication. Chapter 16 describes the publishing process that begins with the acceptance of the paper through its publication. Publishers have different ways of handling the manuscript editing phase and forms of the manuscript that they return to the author for proofing. The publishing process is described in the chapter, but the author should recognize that it may differ across journals. Copyright also is presented in the chapter.

The scholarly publishing landscape has changed significantly over the last decade. All nurses and other health professionals need to keep abreast of changes in scholarly communication and select the best models for disseminating the results of their research and practice changes. Chapter 17 examines open-access publishing and varied models for this. The chapter also discusses predatory publishing and why nurse authors need to be aware of this issue. Strategies for avoiding the submission of a manuscript to a predatory journal are included in the chapter.

Many individuals have contributed to the preparation and writing of this book. The authors extend a special acknowledgment to Margaret Zuccarini, who recognized the need for this book in nursing. In addition to the book, as a resource for faculty, we have provided an *Instructor's Manual* that includes: a sample syllabus for a course in writing for publication in nursing; an online course with 17 modules (each module has a chapter summary, student learning activities, discussion questions, and online resources); and chapter-based PowerPoint presentations. **To obtain an electronic copy of these materials, faculty should contact Springer Publishing Company at textbook@springerpub.com.**

Marilyn H. Oermann
Judith C. Hays

PREPARING TO WRITE

GETTING STARTED

Writing for publication in nursing is essential to disseminate evidence, share initiatives and innovations with others, provide new information to keep nurses up to date, communicate the findings of research studies, and develop the science base of the profession. Writing manuscripts is hard work, but the process can be simplified by understanding how to develop a manuscript and submit it for publication.

This chapter introduces the steps the author follows in planning, writing, and publishing manuscripts in nursing. The focus of Chapter 1 is on early writing decisions, such as generating ideas, selecting a topic, and deciding on the type of article to be written. These are important decisions because they guide the author in selecting potential journals, which is addressed in Chapter 2.

REASONS TO WRITE

Writing for publication is an important skill for nurses to develop. By communicating initiatives and innovations in clinical practice, findings of research studies and evidence-based practice (EBP) projects, and new ideas, nurses direct the future of their practice and advance the development of the profession. As nursing attempts to build its evidence base, it is increasingly important for nurses to write about studies they are doing in their clinical practice: The findings of these studies provide the evidence for practice. Writing for publication cannot be considered the responsibility of only nurses in academic settings, for clinicians also have a major responsibility to describe the effectiveness of their nursing interventions and the innovations they have developed for patient care. Nurse educators, administrators, managers, and researchers have a similar responsibility: to share knowledge and ideas for the benefit of others.

There are five main reasons to write for publication: (a) to share ideas and expertise with other nurses; (b) to disseminate evidence and the findings of nursing research studies; (c) for promotion, tenure, and other personnel decisions; (d) for development of one's own knowledge and skills; and (e) for personal satisfaction.

Share Ideas and Expertise

Writing for publication provides a way of sharing ideas with other nurses. Through publications, nurses can describe best practices; innovations developed for patients, staff, and students; and new techniques they are using in clinical practice, teaching, management, and administration. Publications keep nurses abreast of new developments in nursing. Writing for publication also provides a forum for nurse leaders and staff nurses to share advances in clinical practice, leadership, teaching, and research (Derouin et al., 2015; Kooker, Latimer, & Mark, 2015; Tyndall, Scott, & Caswell, 2017).

Disseminate Evidence and Research Findings

For nurses involved in research studies and EBP projects, writing for publication is critical. Disseminating research findings and the outcomes of projects to evaluate the effectiveness of nursing interventions is essential to build the knowledge base of nursing, provide new evidence for practice, and develop studies that build on one another. Many clinicians are currently engaged in EBP projects. Some of these projects are to review and synthesize the available evidence to decide on best practices or if a change in practice is warranted. In other settings, nurses are studying the effects of nursing interventions, contributing to the evidence base of nursing. However, those contributions are not realized unless nurses disseminate the findings of their studies and projects. Dissemination needs to be wider than the nurse's own clinical agency, for example, presenting at conferences and publishing in professional journals. By publishing in journals, nurses can share their evidence and research findings with readers worldwide (Oermann, 2012).

Professions have theories to guide their practice, a body of specialized knowledge and competencies, a code of ethics and values, and a role in society. In practice disciplines such as nursing, an added responsibility is the use of research findings and other evidence to guide decisions about patient care. Research findings can only be applied to practice if they are published and made available for use by other clinicians and nursing professionals. All too often, nurses conduct important research without disseminating the findings of these studies to others.

Meet Promotion, Tenure, and Other Job Requirements

For nursing faculty in colleges and universities, writing for publication is required for promotion, tenure, and other personnel decisions. Not all articles carry the same weight in these decisions. Typically, databased papers, which report the findings of a research study, published in peer-reviewed journals are highly valued and more important in tenure and promotion decisions than other types of publications such as non-databased articles, chapters, and books.

Peer-reviewed journals, also called *refereed journals*, use peer reviewers to critique a manuscript as a basis for the acceptance decision. Peer reviewers are experts, external to the journal staff, who provide an independent, critical assessment of the quality of the manuscript, including the scientific process (International Committee of Medical Journal Editors, 2016). Although the responsibilities of peer reviewers differ with each journal, in general, they critique the manuscript, identify areas for revision, and give expert opinions on the quality of the paper. With some journals, the peer reviewers also suggest to the editor if the manuscript should be accepted, revised and resubmitted, or rejected. The peer-review process is discussed in Chapter 15 of this book. Publishing an article in a peer-reviewed journal is important in tenure and promotion decisions because it indicates that the quality of the paper was assessed by experts based on standards. Most nursing and healthcare journals are peer reviewed, although the process and standards vary for their reviews of papers.

The importance given to writing chapters and books varies across institutions. Most chapters are not peer reviewed and thus do not carry the same weight in tenure and promotion decisions as does an article in a peer-reviewed journal. Completion of a book requires a significant amount of time; prior to the tenure decision, that time might be better spent writing papers for journals. Because the standards for tenure and promotion vary widely across schools of nursing, faculty should be well informed about this process in their own institutions.

While nurses in clinical settings are not faced with tenure and promotion decisions, writing for publication is often a requirement for job mobility in that setting and career advancement. Whether or not the article is databased or published in a peer-reviewed journal is less important than writing for journals read by nurses who need this new information and perspective to guide their practice.

Expand Personal Knowledge and Skills

Another reason to write for publication is the learning gained in the process of preparing the manuscript. Rarely is the nurse able to write a manuscript without completing a thorough review of the literature. This literature review and the thinking that is done in developing the manuscript contribute to the knowledge base and understanding of the author.

Writing skills are useful in many settings as nurses fulfill both professional and personal roles. Writing about a topic facilitates understanding the subject. A good writer—that is, a well-practiced writer—brings a valuable skill to endeavors that range far beyond writing for publication.

Gain Personal Satisfaction

Writing also gives the nurse a sense of personal satisfaction in sharing expertise with other nurses and contributing to the development of the profession. Most journals do not pay authors for their manuscripts; however, writing for publication is personally fulfilling. It is a way of sharing stories and experiences in patient care, teaching, leadership, and other areas.

BARRIERS TO WRITING

Writing is time consuming, and authors may be frustrated as to their progress in preparing the manuscript. Developing a publishable paper requires practice, and the more writing the author does, the easier it will be to complete the manuscript. Similar to the development of clinical skills, writing improves with practice. Some of the barriers to writing are a lack of understanding of this process, writer's block, lack of time, and fear of rejection.

Lack of Understanding of How to Write for Publication

Many faculty members have had limited experience in writing for publication and are unsure of the process, but need to publish in their academic settings. Similarly, clinicians may be reluctant to assume the role of author because they too are unsure of the process of manuscript development and have not been prepared for this role in their educational programs (Derouin et al., 2015; Shirey, 2013; von Isenburg, Lee, & Oermann, 2017).

Before beginning any manuscript, the author needs to first understand the writing and publishing processes. Often, students believe that the A+ paper they completed as a requirement in one of their nursing courses is publishable; this may or may not be true. Papers prepared for a course may be at too low a level for readers of a journal who have specialized knowledge and more advanced understanding of the topic. Or, the course paper may not be in an appropriate writing style for the journal to which it is submitted: The paper may be too theoretical or the literature review may be too long. Or, the paper may not contain material that is original or represent an added value to readers. An understanding of how to write for publication and for a particular journal, and that journal's readership, helps the author avoid situations such as these.

Writer's Block

Some authors experience writer's block that keeps them from writing. This may occur from anxiety about the project, uncertainty as how to proceed, and past unsuccessful experiences with writing. It is important for authors to be clear about the topic and intent of their writing project—recording these on paper before beginning, discussing them with colleagues, and "presenting" ideas to others often help to avoid writer's block. Brainstorming, identifying alternate ways of approaching the topic, and diagramming or outlining ideas are strategies that can be used to overcome writer's block. Another strategy is to draw a concept map of the topics in the manuscript and how they relate to each other, providing a visual representation of the ideas and encouraging thinking about how best to proceed.

If these techniques are not effective, authors can review the literature, prepare the references, and engage in other activities that do not require the same degree of creativity as does writing. Often a short break from writing and use of some of the strategies identified earlier will resolve writer's block, but if not, authors should seek a mentor who can guide them through this process and completion of the paper.

Lack of Time

The extensive time required for preparing a manuscript is another barrier to writing. Time is needed for preliminary work such as developing the idea and reviewing the literature, for preparing the draft and rewriting it until suitable for submission, and for subsequent revisions suggested by the editor and reviewers. Lack of time, as a barrier to writing for publication, is a problem encountered by nursing faculty, staff nurses, and clinicians across healthcare fields (Tyndall et al., 2017; von Isenburg et al., 2017).

Fear of Rejection

One other barrier to writing is fear of rejection. In submitting manuscripts, authors open themselves to criticism and possible rejection; for some nurses, this is a barrier to writing for publication. Having a manuscript rejected is part of the writing process and may not be related to the quality of the writing. The manuscript may be rejected because a similar one has already been accepted, or the information in the manuscript is not new enough for publication in that particular journal. Rejections for reasons such as these do not mean that the ideas are questionable or poorly presented. Even if the manuscript is rejected because of criticisms of the research design, ideas in the manuscript, or format, the author can use this feedback as a way of learning more about the writing process, for developing writing skills further, and for revising the manuscript for submission elsewhere.

PERSONAL STRATEGIES

Writing manuscripts requires setting dates for completion and personal strategies to keep on target, meet deadlines, and use wisely the limited time available. A manuscript can be doomed to failure if the author does not manage the time allotted for writing and completing other aspects of preparing the manuscript for submission to a journal.

Set Due Dates

First, a due date should be set for completion of the manuscript, whether it is a journal article, chapter in a book, research proposal, or another writing project. The due date for completing the final copy should be realistic considering the writer's work and personal responsibilities and should not be altered; modifying the due date for completion of a manuscript often becomes a pattern, and the manuscript is never finished or takes too long to complete.

Second, after setting the due date for completion of the final manuscript, the author can divide the content areas into manageable parts and identify dates for completing each of these. In this way, smaller content areas are viewed as separate writing assignments with individual due dates. If the author is working from an outline, which will be discussed in a later chapter, dates can be assigned to different sections of the outline. Third, in addition to dividing the manuscript into sections, each with its own due date, the author can assign dates to complete other activities related to the manuscript, for example, preparing the references and registering at the journal's website. It is important not to waiver from these due dates because, with busy schedules, delays are difficult to make up later.

Even with firm dates, some writers have difficulty getting started and others have difficulty finishing. Viewing the manuscript in terms of smaller writing assignments and completing a few sections of the content often provide sufficient momentum and reinforcement to continue writing until the manuscript is completed.

Identify Prime Time for Writing

Authors should identify their prime time for writing, when they are most productive and creative; this time needs to be protected for writing activities. The author should avoid interruptions and distractions during the time allotted for writing. Checking emails and answering the phone, even if they take limited time, affect concentration and distract from thinking about the topic and how best to present it to readers. Similar to other skills, writing takes practice and a small amount of time allocated for writing is better than filling time with other activities. For some people, a large block of time is most effective, but for others, smaller segments of time are easier to allow for in a busy work schedule. For example, authors might set aside 1 to 2 hours a day for writing, plus the weekend, or 3 to 4 hours a few days of the week. In addition to removing distractions, the author should have a comfortable chair, good computer screen, and writing resources at hand.

STEPS IN WRITING FOR PUBLICATION

Every article written for publication begins with a planning phase; progresses to writing a draft, revising it, and submitting the final copy to the journal; and concludes with its publication. These phases, which provide a framework for the organization of the book, are discussed in more detail in later chapters.

Planning Phase

Prior to writing the manuscript, the author proceeds through a series of steps. These steps are important to assist the author in selecting a topic that is publishable, choosing an appropriate journal with readers who are interested in the topic, and gearing the content and format to the journal. The *manuscript* or *paper* is the unpublished document submitted to a journal for review. Once that paper is published, it is referred to as an *article*.

Identify Purpose of Manuscript

The first step in the planning phase is to identify the topic and purpose of the manuscript. In some cases, the purpose is to present research findings, describe an EBP project, or explain how practice changes were made based on a review of the evidence. The intent of other manuscripts may be to present new nursing interventions and approaches to managing patient problems, describe nursing interventions for patients with particular health problems, analyze trends and issues in practice, and present new directions in nursing education or management.

For some manuscripts, identifying the purpose is easy because the author has a specific goal in mind at the outset, such as presenting the findings of a project done in the clinical setting. Other times, though, generating the idea for the manuscript or deciding how to develop it is more involved. Every manuscript needs a primary message that is communicated to readers; this message directs how the manuscript is then developed and guides the selection of a journal for submission.

Before proceeding, the author should be able to answer these questions: What is the purpose of writing the manuscript? Why is this information important for readers? What difference will it make in clinical practice, teaching, administration, and research? The author should be able to answer these questions clearly and succinctly.

Once the purpose of the manuscript is clearly thought out, the author should record it somewhere—for example, as a document saved in the computer—and keep it in view during the writing phase. This helps to stay on target as the writing proceeds. Often novice writers have enthusiasm about a topic but conceptualize ideas that are too global. A useful strategy in the early planning phase is to write the purpose of the manuscript in one sentence to confirm that it is clear and focused.

Decide on Importance of Topic

After deciding on the purpose of the manuscript, the author needs to ask if the ideas to be presented are worth writing about. Will the paper present important information that readers need? The goal in this step in the writing process is to avoid preparing a manuscript that has a limited chance of being accepted for publication. Exhibit 1.1 presents questions the author can ask to evaluate if the manuscript is worth writing and if the content is important enough to warrant publication. The author should answer these questions before spending any more time on the manuscript.

EXHIBIT 1.1

Assessing Importance of Content of Manuscript

- Does the manuscript present new ideas?
- Is the topic already in the literature? If so, how does the planned manuscript differ from the existing literature?
- If the content is not new and articles have already been published on similar content, what is different about the manuscript to make it worthy of publication? What new perspective is offered?
- If the manuscript is published, how important is the message? Will it make a difference in patient care? Will it change nursing practice, education, administration, management, or research?
- Who is the audience, and will readers be interested in the topic?
- Is this a manuscript a journal would be interested in publishing?

Search for Related Articles

In generating ideas for a manuscript, the author should keep in mind that journals are interested in publishing new ideas and communicating information to readers that they may not already know. If the topic or idea is not new, then the question is whether it presents a unique perspective or a different way of looking at a well-known topic.

To determine this, the author should do a literature review on the topic and related content areas. The literature search may reveal that the topic is indeed new to the nursing literature, or at least to the readers for whom the manuscript is intended. An article may have been published for the general nursing audience, but the intended manuscript focuses instead on how the content would be used by nurses in a specialty area. Or, the articles are research oriented and the intended topic is related to clinical practice or professional issues. If there have been articles published on the same topic, they may have been in journals other than those targeted for the manuscript being planned, or the focus at present will add to what is already known about the topic.

The goal in searching the literature at this point is to scan articles to determine if others have been published on the same topic. Authors should not spend much time with the search in case the decision is made not to write about that topic because it has already been addressed in the literature. If the author finds, though, that the manuscript will present new information, this beginning literature search may be used later as the manuscript is developed. For this reason, the author should record complete information about the articles and other publications reviewed for ease in returning to them at a later time.

The next steps in the process of writing for publication are to identify the audience to whom the manuscript will be directed and to select a journal that might be interested in publishing it. These steps are discussed in Chapter 2. The goal is to match the purpose and type of manuscript with an appropriate journal and readers who would be interested in it.

Identify Type of Article to Be Written

The purpose of the manuscript indicates the type of article to be written. While there are many ways of categorizing articles in the nursing and healthcare literature, one way is research; review and EBP, including systematic reviews, integrative literature reviews, critical appraisals of research studies with implications for practice, and reports on EBP projects; clinical practice; and other forms of writing such as case reports and editorials. These types of manuscripts differ in their goals, format, and writing style, and frequently reach different audiences. Often, manuscripts are rejected because they do not match the type of articles that the journal publishes. Identifying the type of manuscript, therefore, helps the author make a decision about possible journals for submission. Nurses also prepare manuscripts and other documents for patients and nonprofessional audiences. These require careful writing to avoid using technical terms and to be at a level that readers without any healthcare background can understand. Nurses also prepare chapters and books.

Research Articles

Research (databased) articles present the findings of quantitative and qualitative studies. Quantitative research papers typically follow the IMRAD format: Introduction, Methods, Results, and Discussion, or an adaptation of this, depending on the journal and type of research (Jirge, 2017). In addition to the general IMRAD structure, reporting guidelines have been developed for writing manuscripts on specific types of studies (Oermann, 2017; Oermann et al., 2018). For example, the Consolidated Standards of Reporting Trials (CONSORT) provide guidelines for reporting randomized controlled trials. The format for presenting qualitative research depends on the type of study and purpose of the research report. Authors can look for guidelines to use at the Enhancing the Quality of Transparency of Health Research (EQUATOR) website (www.equator-network.org). This website is a portal of hundreds of guidelines for preparing manuscripts on different types of research studies (EQUATOR Network, 2017). Some of these guidelines are described in Appendix C.

With some manuscripts, the intent is to present the original research study with less of a focus on its clinical implications. For example, *Nursing Research* reports quantitative and qualitative studies, the latest research techniques, and methodological strategies. Although articles in that journal may present clinical research studies, the focus is more on the research itself rather than translating the findings for use by clinicians. Many clinical journals also publish research articles in their area of practice, and these generally emphasize the clinical implications of the research findings and are written for clinicians as readers. Journals in other areas of nursing, such as nursing education and administration, often publish databased papers but expect authors to emphasize the implications of those studies for teaching, administration, and other areas of practice.

Review and EBP Articles

Many nurses engage in projects to critically appraise evidence to answer questions about their practice and to evaluate the effectiveness of using those new approaches in patient care. In an integrative literature review, the author completes a comprehensive review of the literature on a topic, critiques the research, and then draws conclusions about the findings. The review of the literature is guided by a research question or problem to be solved, and the author may generate recommendations for practice based on the review. In EBP, nurses identify a clinical question or problem for which more information is needed, search for evidence to answer that question, critically appraise studies and assess the quality of the evidence, and make decisions about the use of the evidence for practice. Outcomes of these reviews are potential manuscripts for publication in nursing and other journals. In clinical settings, nurses use evidence to change practice and evaluate the effectiveness of those new approaches. The findings of those projects also can be prepared as manuscripts.

Clinical Articles

Another type of manuscript addresses topics in clinical practice. Clinical articles may be written for nurses across specialties or for nurses practicing in a particular clinical area. The goals of the *American Journal of Nursing* (AJN) are to disseminate evidence-based, peer-reviewed clinical information and original research, discuss relevant and controversial professional issues, and promote nursing perspectives to the healthcare community and public (AJN, 2018). In contrast, articles in journals such as *Cancer Nursing* are more focused on specific patient populations and health problems.

The format for writing clinical articles differs with the journal but usually includes a description of the patient problems and nursing interventions, with an emphasis on the clinical implications of whatever topic is presented. Some journals have different departments or columns, such as clinical updates, ethical cases, and drug news, each of which has a certain format for its articles. The information about the types of articles published in a journal and specifications for preparing them are included the author guidelines at the journal's website.

Other Types of Articles

Nurses write many other types of papers for publication. For example, case reports provide new information on nursing practice or care of patients with particular health problems through the presentation of a case. These manuscripts often begin with why the case was selected and its importance to nursing practice and continue with a description of the case and related care by nurses and other disciplines. Manuscripts also report quality improvement studies and projects done in the clinical setting. Articles may describe innovations, new practices, and issues in teaching, administration, and management. Other papers may focus on policy, ethics, legal aspects, historical studies, theory development or testing, issues affecting nurses in an area of clinical practice, and editorials. Nurses may respond to an article in a letter to the editor and complete book reviews for publication in a journal, both of which provide valuable experiences for a novice author.

Writing Phase

The writing phase involves preparing the first and subsequent drafts of the manuscript, completing the final revision, and submitting the manuscript to the journal. The steps in the writing phase include the following:

- Develop a formal or an informal outline to guide writing
- Write the first draft, focusing on presenting the content rather than on grammar, spelling, punctuation, and writing style
- Revise the first and later drafts, continuing to focus on the content of the manuscript
- Then revise the manuscript for grammar, spelling, punctuation, and writing style
- Prepare tables, figures, and the references, paying close attention to the journal's format for references
- Prepare the final version of the manuscript, accompanying materials required by the journal, and the submission or cover letter
- Submit the manuscript to the journal

Publishing Phase

The final phase in writing for publication occurs after the manuscript is submitted to the journal. The manuscript is critiqued by peer reviewers who have expertise in the topic or methodology and can assess its quality. Peer reviewers provide feedback to authors on needed revisions to strengthen the manuscript and to the editor on the suitability of the manuscript for publication in the journal. It is through this process that the best papers are accepted for publication, ensuring quality of the information and meeting ethical standards.

Editors of nursing journals are nurses who have expertise in the content area of the journal. The final decision on acceptance of a manuscript is made by the editor, considering the peer reviews, the editor's own assessment of the quality and suitability of the paper for the journal, and other factors such as how many similar papers have been published or are in the queue to be published and upcoming themes planned for the journal. Different editorial decisions are possible, ranging from acceptance of the manuscript without revision or pending revision; a request that the manuscript be revised and resubmitted, in which case the paper will be peer reviewed again; to rejection.

If the manuscript is rejected, the author should revise the paper using feedback from the peer-review process and submit it to another journal. With the wealth of nursing and other healthcare journals available, if authors are willing to revise their papers, it is likely they will find a journal interested in their manuscript. Writing for publication requires perseverance and a willingness to use feedback and guidance from others to craft a paper that is appropriate for a particular journal and audience.

The publishing phase also includes responsibilities of the author once the manuscript is accepted for publication. At this point, the author answers queries from the journal or production editor, reads carefully and corrects the page proofs, and returns promptly all materials to the publisher.

SUMMARY

Writing for publication is an important skill for nurses to develop. By disseminating new initiatives and innovations in clinical practice, research findings, and other ideas about nursing, nurses direct the future of their practice and advance the development of the profession. There are barriers to writing, but the nurse can overcome these by setting due dates for completion of writing projects, meeting these deadlines, and using wisely the available time for writing.

Every article written for publication begins with a planning phase; progresses to writing a draft, revising it, and submitting the final copy to the journal; and concludes with its publication. The manuscript or paper is the unpublished document submitted to a journal for review; once published, it is referred to as an article. The first step in the planning phase is to identify the topic and purpose of the manuscript. After deciding on the purpose of the manuscript, the author needs to assess if the ideas to be presented are worth writing about. Will the paper present important information that readers need? To determine this, the author should do a literature review on the topic and related content areas. The literature search may reveal that the topic is indeed new to the nursing literature or at least to the readers for whom the manuscript is intended.

The next steps in the process of writing for publication are to identify the audience to whom the manuscript will be directed and select a journal that might be interested in publishing it. While there are many ways of categorizing articles in the nursing and healthcare literature, one way to categorize is as research articles, review papers that disseminate the outcomes of a synthesis of individual studies and articles addressing EBP, clinical practice articles, and other types of articles, such as reports on quality improvement studies, case reports, and editorials.

The writing phase involves preparing the first and subsequent drafts of the manuscript, completing the final revision, and submitting the manuscript to the journal. The final phase in writing for publication occurs after the manuscript is submitted to the journal. The manuscript is critiqued by peer reviewers, who have expertise in the topic or methodology, and can assess its quality. Peer reviewers provide feedback to authors on needed revisions to strengthen the manuscript and to the editor on the suitability of the manuscript for publication in the journal. As the manuscript proceeds through the production process, the author answers queries about the paper and reads carefully the page proofs.

Writing for publication is hard work, but the satisfaction gained from completing a manuscript and making a lasting contribution to the literature outweighs the effort and time. Writing is a skill that can be developed with practice. When one manuscript is completed, the author should begin planning the next one.

REFERENCES

American Journal of Nursing. (2018). *About the journal.* Retrieved from https://journals.lww .com/ajnonline/Pages/aboutthejournal.aspx

Derouin, A. L., Hueckel, R. M., Turner, K. M., Hawks, S. J., Leonardelli, A. K., & Oermann, M. H. (2015). Use of workshops to develop nurses' and nursing students' writing skills. *Journal of Continuing Education in Nursing, 46,* 364–369. doi:10.3928/00220124-20150721-03

EQUATOR Network. (2017). Reporting guidelines for main study types. Retrieved from http:// www.equator-network.org

International Committee of Medical Journal Editors. (2016). Recommendations for the conduct, reporting, editing, and publication of scholarly work in medical journals. Retrieved from http://www.icmje.org/recommendations

Jirge, P. R. (2017). Preparing and publishing a scientific manuscript. *Journal of Human Reproductive Sciences, 10*(1), 3–9. doi:10.4103/jhrs.JHRS_36_17

Kooker, B. M., Latimer, R., & Mark, D. D. (2015). Successfully coaching nursing staff to publish outcomes. *Journal of Nursing Administration, 45,* 636–641. doi:10.1097/nna.0000000000000277

Oermann, M. H. (2012). Building evidence for practice: Not without dissemination. *MCN, American Journal of Maternal/Child Nursing, 37,* 77. doi:10.1097/NMC.0b013e318245dd7a

Oermann, M. H. (2017). Reporting guidelines: Tools for preparing your manuscript. *Nurse Author & Editor, 27*(4), 2. Retrieved from http://www.naepub.com/reporting -research/2017-24-4-2

Oermann, M. H., Nicoll, L. H., Chinn, P. L., Conklin, J. L., McCarty, M., & Amarasekara, S. (2018). Quality of author guidelines in nursing journals. *Journal of Nursing Scholarship.* Advance online publication. doi:10.1111/jnu.12383

Shirey, M. R. (2013). Building scholarly writing capacity in the doctor of nursing practice program. *Journal of Professional Nursing, 29,* 137–147. doi:10.1016/j.profnurs.2012.04.019

Tyndall, D. E., Scott, E. S., & Caswell, N. I. (2017). Factors facilitating publication by clinical nurses in a Magnet® hospital. *Journal of Nursing Administration, 47,* 522–526. doi:10.1097/ nna.0000000000000525

von Isenburg, M., Lee, L. S., & Oermann, M. H. (2017). Writing Together to Get AHEAD: An interprofessional boot camp to support scholarly writing in the health professions. *Journal of the Medical Library Association, 105,* 167–172. doi:10.5195/jmla.2017.222

SELECTING A JOURNAL

The first step in writing for publication is to identify the topic or focus of the manuscript. The next steps are to identify the intended audience for the manuscript and a journal that might be interested in publishing it. This chapter discusses how to evaluate possible journals, select an appropriate one, and write a query email to gauge the interest of the journals' editors.

WHO IS THE AUDIENCE?

The author needs to be clear as to the intended readers of the manuscript. Identifying the audience is an important early step because the manuscript needs to be written for readers who are interested in the content and written at a level appropriate for them. A manuscript written for a general nursing audience but then submitted to a specialty journal read predominantly by advanced practice nurses will probably be rejected, and the author will lose valuable time. One of the next steps in the process is to identify a journal that publishes manuscripts on that topic for the same audience. Otherwise, the manuscript will be inappropriate for the journal to which it is submitted.

The author can begin by asking who will likely read the manuscript and need the content in it. Most articles are read by people who need answers to questions about their practice, teaching, management, or research, or about other aspects of their work. Authors should consider whether the targeted readers are nurses in general practice or in a specialized area of nursing practice; whether they are staff nurses, advanced practice nurses, faculty, managers, or in other roles; whose needs would be met by reading the manuscript; and who would benefit from the content in the manuscript. Exhibit 2.1 provides questions to help the author characterize the audience of the manuscript.

The audience also may be consumers. Many health journals to which nurses contribute are written for the public. Writing for patients and consumers has implications for the depth and complexity of the content, technical words used in the writing, presentation style, and length of the manuscript. Chapter 9 discusses writing for patients and nonprofessional audiences.

EXHIBIT 2.1

Identifying the Audience of a Manuscript

- For whom will the article be written?
- Is the manuscript geared to a specialized audience, or is the content intended for nurses in general?
- If specialized, what is the reader's area of clinical nursing practice (e.g., pediatrics)?
- What is the primary role of the reader, such as staff nurse, advanced practice nurse, educator, manager, and others, that would influence how the manuscript is written?
- What is the work setting (e.g., hospital) of the reader?
- What are the needs of the reader that the manuscript will meet?
- Who will benefit from reading the article?
- How will the information improve readers' practice, teaching, management, or research, or other aspects of their work?
- What should the intended reader already know about the content area, and how will the manuscript build on this understanding?
- What is the educational level of the audience?

Once the author has identified the intended readers of the manuscript, this information should be used in selecting journals. During the writing process, the author keeps the intended audience in mind when deciding on the content and how it is presented to the readers, types of examples to use, and the writing style.

WHAT ARE THE PURPOSES OF THE PAPER?

Closely related to the audience of the manuscript is its purpose. Because science is a social enterprise and develops within a larger society, it depends upon clear communication among its practitioners and consumers (Penrose & Katz, 2010). The purpose of scientific communication varies widely. Original research, including its critical evaluation and replication, is the backbone of medical and scientific communication (American Medical Association [AMA], 2007). The purpose of such communication is to advance our understanding of healthcare by specifying research questions or hypotheses to be addressed using rigorous protocols. But there are many other reasons to communicate the work of nurses and other scientists and practitioners.

Some authors review, analyze, and summarize evidence concerning a population at risk, a health problem, a theory or model, an historical event, or a treatment regimen and then recommend next steps in research or practice. Other authors describe new approaches to nursing care of patients and populations, new initiatives to improve care in their settings, and quality improvement studies in a writing style that may be more informal than research articles but is nevertheless highly informative to readers. Some authors represent panels of experts that prepare consensus statements or practice guidelines based on available evidence on a healthcare topic of importance (AMA, 2007). Opinion pieces, such as editorials and letters to the editor, marshal the most persuasive evidence available to promote a specific point of view. Before authors can select an appropriate journal, they need to be clear about the intended purpose of the article and readers.

STRATEGIES FOR IDENTIFYING APPROPRIATE JOURNALS

Selecting a journal is an early and critical step in writing for publication. The number of nursing and healthcare journals is so large that the choice can feel overwhelming. Journals differ widely in their topics, the types of articles published, and readership. Selecting an appropriate journal is important because the author's goal is to submit the manuscript to a journal whose readers have a need for current information in that subject area and will look for the type of manuscript planned, for example, a research report. The choice of journals for manuscript submission, therefore, should be carefully made; otherwise, it is unlikely that the manuscript will be accepted.

If a paper is submitted to an inappropriate journal, three actions may occur. First, the editor may return the manuscript to the author, having decided not to send it to experts for peer review due to its lack of suitability regarding the topic or type. Second, the paper may be reviewed by peer experts but then rejected because reviewers reported a lack of fit with the journal's mission and readers. In this case, the reviewers' comments may not be helpful because they lacked expertise in the topic. With these first two possibilities, valuable time is lost. Third, the manuscript may be accepted and subsequently published but in a journal never read by the intended readers who most need the information provided in the article.

Match With Topic

The primary consideration in selecting a journal is whether the journal publishes articles in the subject area of the proposed manuscript. Is the topic appropriate for the journal? Although the author may be familiar with the most prominent journals in a particular area of nursing, it is likely that other journals also publish articles on the topic or in related content areas. The author should review all possible journals in nursing and other healthcare fields that might be interested in the manuscript and should keep a list of at least five relevant journals with related materials such as author guidelines. If an editor is not interested in reviewing the proposed manuscript, or the manuscript is rejected, then the author has other possible journals to consider for submission.

Match With Type of Article

The second consideration in choosing a journal is whether it publishes the type of article being planned. Different types of articles are identified in Chapters 5 through 9: research reports, reviews, quality improvement reports, clinical practice articles, case reports, and articles focused on policy, history, education, methods, and ethics. Not all journals publish the type of manuscript being considered. For example, some clinical journals may not publish research reports, especially those with extensive statistical analyses, and it is unlikely that a scientific journal such as *Nursing Research* would publish a quality improvement study. The formal writing style of research reports may not be appropriate for journals geared to clinicians, and a reader-friendly style of writing often found in clinical journals would not be used for manuscripts submitted to scientific journals. Similarly, if the intended manuscript will provide an extensive review of the literature in a particular area of nursing practice, then the author needs to identify a journal that publishes comprehensive reviews.

The review of journals may also suggest alternative strategies for publishing on a topic. For instance, a nurse reporting on an initiative to reduce noise in the ICU might prepare the manuscript for a journal that publishes quality improvement studies or for a clinical journal read by critical care nurses.

Match With Intended Audience

Is the audience that the author wants to reach the same audience that will read the target journal? Every journal uses a style of presentation that meets the needs of its targeted readers. The search for appropriate journals for a manuscript should include a review of the readership of that journal. The audience may be highly specialized and narrow in focus, or the journal may be geared to a more general readership. The primary audience for the *Journal of Infusion Nursing*, for instance, is nurses who deliver infusion therapy, a specialized area of nursing practice, in comparison with the *American Journal of Nursing*, for which the primary audience is nurses in general.

The author can develop an understanding of a journal's target audience in several ways. First, find the journal's mission or aims and scope. These describe the type of readers the journal serves. For example, *Nurse Educator* publishes articles for faculty in schools of nursing and nurse educators in other settings (*Nurse Educator*, 2018). *Advanced Emergency Nursing Journal* is intended for "advanced practice clinicians, clinical nurse specialists, nurse practitioners, healthcare professionals, and clinical and academic educators in emergency nursing" (*Advanced Emergency Nursing Journal*, 2018, para. 1). Second, review articles in multiple issues of the journal to gain an understanding of the range of issues and problems relevant to its readers in specific roles and the format and writing style appropriate for those readers. Finally, the author can use personal experience as a guide; the journals read most often by the author can be a good starting point when developing a list of journals that may be targets for the planned submission.

In the same way that reviewing journals inform what types of manuscripts are most appropriate, reviewing journals can suggest different audiences and expand the possible journals for submission. For example, the author may have planned to develop a manuscript for critical care nurses but realized after review of journals that nurses working in noncritical care settings are facing challenges of a similar nature and would benefit as much or more from the information in the planned manuscript.

INTERNET RESOURCES FOR IDENTIFYING JOURNALS

To choose the "right" journal for the manuscript, the author needs to review available journals in nursing and other healthcare fields. There are a number of different ways to identify possible journals: using the Directory of Nursing Journals, other websites to search for potential journals, and bibliographic databases, such as PubMed and the Cumulative Index to Nursing and Allied Health Literature (CINAHL), which index journals. Authors should also check resources available at their school's library website.

Directory of Nursing Journals

One of the best places to start when searching for possible journals for a manuscript is the Directory of Nursing Journals at the International Academy of Nursing Editors website (nursingeditors.com/journals-directory). There are approximately 250 journals in the directory. This directory is a key resource because all of the journals in it have been evaluated based on the Committee on Publication Ethics (COPE) Principles of Transparency and Best Practice in Scholarly Publishing (COPE, 2014). By using the directory, authors also avoid selecting a journal with questionable publishing practices, often referred to as *predatory journals*, which are discussed in Chapter 17. The journals in the directory include a link to the journal website, where the author can review the mission of the journal and target audience, review articles in the current and past issues, and obtain the author guidelines, which are the instructions for preparing the manuscript for submission to the journal. The journals in the directory also include the journal editor's email address for authors to send a query about the editor's interest in reviewing the manuscript.

Other Websites to Search for Journals

Another website to use for searching for possible journals for a manuscript is the Journal/Author Name Estimator (JANE) at jane.biosemantics.org (The Biosemantics Group, 2017). The JANE website has a large textbox where the author can input a projected title, abstract, or keywords and click Find Journals. The JANE algorithm uses an open-source search engine to identify the 50 (out of millions of) papers published over the past 10 years in PubMed that are most similar to the information added to the textbox. The author can also specify languages and types of manuscripts. The search engine then ranks related journals deemed appropriate to the proposed title, abstract, or keywords. Journal suggestions for the most closely related journals are ranked by confidence level of the search engine's algorithm and include the journal's article influence score based on 5 years of citation data. For example, the title "Pressure Ulcer Prevention in Long Term Nursing Care Facilities," further limited to English language, journal article, and randomized controlled trial, yielded 35 suggested journals. The *Journal of Clinical Nursing, Journal of Nursing Care Quality, Advances in Skin & Wound Care,* and *Journal of Wound Ostomy & Continence Nursing* were the top four journals listed that publish articles on this topic. Not all types of articles are included in a search in JANE; for example, editorials, history articles, and practice guidelines are excluded. To protect users' intellectual work, inputted data are not stored.

JANE uses data from PubMed, which provides access to the MEDLINE database. MEDLINE is the U.S. National Library of Medicine (NLM) bibliographic database, with more than 24 million references to journal articles in the life sciences (NLM, 2017). Journals included in MEDLINE are based on the recommendations of a review committee to ensure their relevance and quality. PubMed, in addition to providing access to the MEDLINE database, also includes citations to articles in some additional life science journals, online books and chapters, and other types of publications. Because JANE uses data from PubMed, which contains these other types of references and might also have articles from predatory journals, JANE tags journals that are indexed in the MEDLINE database and also indicates open-access journals in the Directory of Open Access Journals (The Biosemantics Group, 2017). When using JANE for a search, authors should use journals tagged as indexed in MEDLINE.

Publishing company websites provide lists of their journals with access to some current and past issues, information about the journal, and the author guidelines. For example, authors could search for journals published by Elsevier at its website (www.elsevier.com/catalog?producttype=journals) by selecting journals and nursing as the subject area. Nursing journals published by Wolters Kluwer can be searched at the Lippincott NursingCenter website (www.nursingcenter.com/articles-publications/all-journals). Nursing journals published by Wiley can be found at this website (onlinelibrary.wiley.com/browse/publications?type=journal&activeLetter=). Authors can add Nursing for the search and select Journals as the Publication Type. Disadvantages of this method, however, are that it restricts the search for journals to these main publishers, does not include any review for journal quality, and is time consuming.

Search for Journals in Bibliographic Databases

Another strategy for identifying possible journals is to search in one of the bibliographic databases such as PubMed and CINAHL to locate journals that publish papers in the topical area. By reviewing abstracts of some of the articles in the journals being considered, the author can learn more about the focus of the journal and types of papers published in it.

PubMed

PubMed provides access to MEDLINE, which is the NLM bibliographic database with more than 24 million references to journal articles in the life sciences (NLM, 2017). Authors can search for journals at the PubMed website (www .ncbi.nlm.nih.gov/pubmed) via the link Journals in NCBI Databases (on the right side of the page). That link allows authors to enter a topic in the search bar and obtain a list of the journals in the PubMed database on that topic. Journals on the list that are in MEDLINE are designated, and only those should be considered. The PubMed database is freely accessible on the Internet and does not require a subscription to search in it.

CINAHL

CINAHL provides searchable databases of nursing and allied health literature published from 1937 to the present (EBSCO Industries, 2018). Authors who have access to a medical, academic, government, corporate, or public library that subscribes to one of the EBSCO*host* databases can search CINAHL for journals that publish articles about the topic of their manuscript by doing a subject search. Databases are also searchable to retrieve material specific to clinical specialties. These databases can be set to retrieve articles according to "special interest," such as advanced practice nursing, critical care, emergency care, and hospice/palliative care, which the author can use to identify possible target journals. Although CINAHL is available by subscription (with access typically through a library), authors can find a complete list of journals available in full text online in both Excel and Hypertext Markup Language (HTML) formats at www.ebsco.com/products/research-databases/cinahl-plus-with-full-text.

Scopus

Scopus is a large database of peer-reviewed literature that includes journals, books, and conference proceedings. It indexes literature from more than 5,000 publishers and includes nearly 23,000 journals as well as books (Elsevier, 2018). Scopus can be used to identify journals for submission of a manuscript, and it provides other information about research impact, such as citation counts of individual articles and a researcher's index (citation impact of an author). Although Scopus requires a subscription to access the full range of the database, authors can search for possible journals on the Internet. For example, entering nursing in "Search for a source" at the website (www.scopus.com/sources.uri?zone=TopNavBar&origin=searchbasic) will generate a list of more than 300 nursing journals in the database.

Web of Science

Web of Science is another database that can be used to search for journals. This database requires a subscription to access and is often available through academic libraries. The Web of Science Core Collection covers more than 20,000 high-impact journals (Clarivate Analytics, 2018). Nursing journals are indexed in the InCites Journal Citation Reports in the Science Citation Index Expanded and Social Sciences Citation Index in the Core Collection. Authors can select Nursing as a category in each of these indexes to obtain a list of the journals and their Journal Impact Factor (based on the number of citations to the journal within the Web of Science database) (Oermann & Shaw-Kokot, 2013a, 2013b). As of January 2018, there were 116 nursing journals in the Science Citation Index Expanded and 114 nursing journals in the Social Science Citation Index. One of the issues with the Web of Science database is the small number of included nursing journals (Oermann & Shaw-Kokot, 2013a, 2013b).

OBTAINING AUTHOR GUIDELINES

After identifying possible journals, the author should read carefully each journal's information for authors page, also referred to as author guidelines. The information for authors usually describes the following:

- Topics the journal is interested in publishing
- Types of articles published (e.g., research, clinical practice, case studies, commentaries, theory, others)
- Manuscript preparation, including the title page, abstract, text, references, figures and tables, photographs, permission to reprint
- Length of manuscript allowed (in pages or word count) and for different types of manuscripts in the journal (original research, departments, sections, case reports, and others)
- Reporting guidelines to use for specific types of manuscripts, such as the Consolidated Standards of Reporting Trials (CONSORT) for reports of randomized controlled trials, in addition to the journal instructions
- Disclosure of conflicts of interest, authorship criteria, copyright transfer, and other ethical requirements
- Editorial process, peer review, and related information
- Other guidelines for writing the manuscript and submitting it (Nambiar, Tilak, & Cerejo, 2014; Oermann et al., 2018)

The information for authors is found on the journal website or via a link to download it. This information also might be included in an issue of the journal. A study of author guidelines of nursing journals indicated that most were comprehensive and informative. However, few journals required use of reporting guidelines such as CONSORT even though they improve the completeness of manuscripts on different types of studies (Oermann et al., 2018).

This is consistent with an earlier study of 15 leading nursing journals: only half of those journals promoted use of the CONSORT (Jull & Aye, 2015).

After reviewing the author guidelines and narrowing the list of possible journals, the author should read a few articles in each journal to get a better perspective on the types of papers published, their format and length, the writing style, and other characteristics. It is helpful to keep an electronic file of author guidelines or to bookmark journal websites for use with later writing projects.

OBTAINING OTHER RELEVANT INFORMATION ABOUT THE JOURNAL

In selecting a journal, some other considerations enter into the decision, such as the length of time for peer review and the journal's acceptance rate. Most of this information is not included on the journal's website, and the author needs to email the journal office for it.

Frequency of Publication, Response Time, and Acceptance Rates

The author should gather information about the frequency with which the journal is published, the average length of time for peer review and editorial decisions and between acceptance and publication, and what proportion of submitted articles are accepted. The time from acceptance to publication of a manuscript is usually shorter for journals that are published more often.

For journals that publish the acceptance date of the manuscript, the author can easily determine the length of time between acceptance and publication. Keep in mind that many journals, whether monthly, bimonthly, or quarterly, have backlogs; the projected time between acceptance and publication may be a factor in the author's consideration of journals. It is sometimes worthwhile to ask colleagues about their experiences with the response time of journals, and some editors will estimate for prospective authors the probable wait-time for publication of accepted manuscripts. The length of time from submission through publication also depends on how promptly reviewers respond with comments and authors resubmit their revised manuscripts. Many journals now publish papers ahead of print (epub ahead of print), and some publish the final submitted manuscript as a Word document (prior to copyediting) at their website. These forms of publication speed access to the content.

Editors and publishers routinely calculate the acceptance and rejection rates of their journals. This information is not published on websites. However, editors may respond to individual queries about this statistic.

Other Measures of Quality, Impact Factors, and CiteScores

There is no gold-standard system for ranking the quality of nursing journals. The author may make an informed judgment as to the quality and prestige of the journals by identifying the ones that present new and important information for readers and whose articles are clearly written.

Another way of assessing the quality of the journal is by reviewing the number of times articles in a journal are cited in other journals. The journal impact factor and CiteScore are two journal metrics based on citation rates. The impact factor is the number of citations to articles published in a specific journal in a 2-year period, divided by the total number of articles published in that journal over the same 2-year period (Minnick, 2017). Impact factors are based on citations to journals indexed in Web of Science. The InCites Journal Citation Reports provide citation data and impact factors of 116 nursing journals in the Science Citation Index Expanded and 114 in the Social Sciences Citation Index as of January 2018 (Clarivate Analytics, 2018). Many journals appropriate for a manuscript, however, may not be indexed in Web of Science and thus may not have an impact factor (Oermann & Shaw-Kokot, 2013b). In addition, the impact factors are low for many nursing journals because they are not well cited in other journals in the database. The lack of citations is no indication of quality or impact. Articles in journals with a low or no impact factor may be highly significant, and may be used by clinicians, teachers, and managers to improve their practice.

Another journal metric similar to the impact factor is CiteScore, which is based on journals indexed in the Scopus database versus Web of Science. CiteScore is the average number of citations to a journal over a 3-year time period compared to the 2 years used for determining impact factors (Oermann & Conklin, 2017). CiteScore counts all of the documents in the journal (editorials, letters to the editor, news items, conference papers, and others) as having the potential to be cited (Zijlstra & McCullough, 2016). This is important because the CiteScore, similar to impact factor, is the ratio of citations to the total number of documents that could be cited. CiteScore is freely available in Scopus and is easy to access. Authors can go to the Sources page in Scopus (www.scopus.com/sources) and enter the name of the journal under Search, or can access this metric at journalmetrics.scopus.com. CiteScore is a relatively new journal metric, introduced in December 2016. How widely it will be used is not yet known.

CONTACTING EDITORS: EMAIL QUERIES

Journal editors are committed to mentoring and coaching new authors (Kearney & Freda, 2006) and are approachable. Knowing that an editor is interested in the topic can be an important motivating factor for submitting first to that journal. On the other hand, the editor may not be interested in reviewing the manuscript because the journal does not publish that topic or type of manuscript, the journal has recently published too many articles on related topics, or a similar one has already been accepted. Therefore, a query can be emailed to the editors of the prospective journals asking about their interest in reviewing the manuscript. The author does not need to send a query email prior to submitting a manuscript, but doing so often saves time in the long run.

Queries may be sent to more than one editor simultaneously. The manuscript, however, can only be submitted to only one journal at a time. If several editors have been queried regarding their interest in a manuscript, professional courtesy suggests that those editors whose journals were not selected for the submission should be notified by the author of the decision not to submit to that journal.

EXHIBIT 2.2

Sample Query Email

Dr. Ann Brown
Editor, *Nursing Journal*
1234 Main Street
Anytown, Anystate 56789
abrown@herjournalemail.com

Dear Dr. Brown

I am interested in submitting a manuscript to the *Nursing Journal*. The manuscript describes an evaluation we conducted of an online teaching program for patients with heart failure and their caregivers. We assessed the effectiveness of this teaching program at three points in time, at discharge and at 3 and 6 months after discharge.

Are you interested in reviewing this manuscript? Thank you for your consideration.

Sincerely,
Mary Smith
Mary Smith, DNP, FNP-BC, AACC
Nurse Practitioner

A query email should be no longer than a few sentences to one paragraph. It should indicate the type of manuscript; for example, description of a clinical practice innovation, research report, case review, and so forth, and should explain in a few sentences what the manuscript is about. In the email, the author should include the anticipated completion date and contact information. The abstract for the manuscript may be included, if available. Penrose and Katz (2010) cautioned authors to avoid trying to "sell" the editor on the topic, but rather to present their material with an awareness of its limits. A sample query email appears in Exhibit 2.2.

The query should be emailed to the editor or managing editor of the journal. This information is available in the author guidelines and also at the journal website. Editors' email addresses are also available in the Directory of Nursing Journals at the International Academy of Nursing Editors website (nursingeditors.com/journals-directory).

MAKING THE DECISION

Exhibit 2.3 provides a checklist to help the author decide on the "right" journal. In making this decision, the author considers the appropriateness of the journal for the topic, type of manuscript, and intended audience; the quality of the journal; and other information about the publication that the author

EXHIBIT 2.3

Identifying the "Right" Journal

- Does the journal publish articles in the general subject area of the manuscript?
- Is the topic of the manuscript consistent with the goals and mission of the journal?
- Has the topic of the manuscript been published already in the journal? If so, will the manuscript be different enough to warrant publication?
- Does the journal publish the type of manuscript proposed (e.g., research, clinical practice, issue, theoretical, review articles, case reports, and others)?
- Who are the readers of the journal, and are they the same as the intended audience of the manuscript?
- What is the quality of the journal, and are important articles published in it?
- How frequently is the journal published (e.g., monthly, bimonthly, or quarterly)?
- What is the projected time for the manuscript review? Between acceptance and publication?
- Does the journal publish ahead of print?
- Is the journal peer reviewed?
- What databases (e.g., MEDLINE, Cumulative Index to Nursing and Allied Health Literature [CINAHL], Web of Science, others) is the journal indexed in?
- Does the journal charge a fee for publishing the article (open-access journals)?
- Is the journal editor interested in reviewing the manuscript?

has collected. Open-access journals, discussed in Chapter 17, charge a fee to publish, which would be another consideration in selecting a journal. The journals identified for submission, though, may not be the ones with the most important papers nor the ones cited more frequently by other authors. The journals chosen for the manuscript should be the ones read by nurses or others who are interested in the topic and need the information. Thus, with many manuscripts, the decision as to which journals are appropriate rests heavily on who reads the journal, who "cares about" the content in the manuscript, and who will use it for improved practice.

One other consideration is the risk of rejection. Highly ranked journals receive more manuscripts for review than do lower tier journals and have higher rates of rejection. With rejections, the author loses the time it took for the manuscript to be processed and reviewed. Authors may inquire of the journal editor about rejection rates, although this information may not be available. Novice authors should seek advice from experienced authors in the same field about target journals that provide a higher probability of acceptance and whose editors understand their role to include the mentoring of new authors.

Prioritizing Journals for Submission

From the review of journals, the author should select about five journals for submission of the manuscript and should prioritize them. If the editor of the journal of first choice is not interested in reviewing the manuscript, or it is rejected, then the author can send the manuscript to the next one on the list without having to review the journals again.

The author also can prepare a secondary list of journals that publish related topics or may be appropriate if the manuscript is adapted for their audience. This list is valuable if the primary journals are not interested in reviewing the manuscript, the author decides not to submit it to one of them, or the manuscript is rejected. Often, the manuscript can be adapted to another journal without much effort. For instance, if the manuscript is on nursing interventions for dyspnea, and the primary journals are not interested in reviewing it, the author might reframe the discussion around caring for the dyspneic patient in the home. Then, the choice of journals extends to those that focus on home care. For rejected manuscripts, the author might refer to this secondary list of publications for ideas on how to rewrite the manuscript to fit the different aims and scope of those journals. For example, a research report that has been rejected because of a small sample size may be rewritten as a clinical project or case study with greater emphasis placed on the implications of the study.

SUMMARY

The first step in writing for publication is to identify the topic or focus of the manuscript. From that point, the author decides on the intended readers. The manuscript needs to be written for defined readers and then submitted to a journal that publishes articles on that topic for the same audience.

Considerations in selecting a journal include whether the journal publishes articles in the subject area of the proposed manuscript; whether it publishes the type of article being planned, for example, research reports, reviews, quality improvement studies, clinical practice articles, case reports, and others; whether the readers of the journal are the same as the intended audience of the manuscript; the quality of the journal; and how frequently it is published. Open-access journals charge a fee to publish, which would be another consideration. There are a number of different ways to identify possible journals. These include using the Directory of Nursing Journals, using a website such as JANE, and searching in bibliographic databases.

The author should select about five possible journals for submission of the manuscript and prioritize them. A query email can be sent to the editors of the prospective journals asking about their interest in reviewing the manuscript. While many queries can be sent, the manuscript can only be submitted to one journal at a time. If the paper is rejected, or the author withdraws the submission, the manuscript can then be submitted to the next journal on the list. Other decisions made prior to writing the manuscript are discussed in Chapter 3.

REFERENCES

Advanced Emergency Nursing Journal. (2018). About the journal. Retrieved from http://journals
.lww.com/aenjournal/Pages/aboutthejournal.aspx

American Medical Association. (2007). *AMA manual of style: A guide for authors and editors* (10th
ed.). New York, NY: Oxford University Press.

The Biosemantics Group. (2017). Jane: Journal/author name estimator. Retrieved from http://jane
.biosemantics.org/faq.php

Clarivate Analytics. (2018). Web of science core collection. Retrieved from https://clarivate
.com/products/web-of-science/web-science-form/web-science-core-collection

Committee on Publication Ethics. (2014). *Principles of transparency and best practice in
scholarly publishing.* Retrieved from https://publicationethics.org/files/Principles_of_
Transparency_and_Best_Practice_in_Scholarly_Publishingv2.pdf

EBSCO Industries. (2018). CINAHL Plus with full text. Retrieved from https://www.ebscohost
.com/biomedical-libraries/cinahl-plus-with-full-text

Elsevier. (2018). *Scopus.* Retrieved from https://www.elsevier.com/solutions/scopus/content

Jull, A., & Aye, P. S. (2015). Endorsement of the CONSORT guidelines, trial registration, and
the quality of reporting randomised controlled trials in leading nursing journals: A cross-
sectional analysis. *International Journal of Nursing Studies, 52,* 1071–1079. doi:10.1016/
j.ijnurstu.2014.11.008

Kearney, M. H., & Freda, M. C. (2006). "Voice of the profession": Nurse editors as leaders.
Nursing Outlook, 54, 263–267. doi:10.1016/j.outlook.2006.04.002

Minnick, J. (2017). The many flavors of the journal impact factor. *Clarivate Analytics.* Retrieved
from http://stateofinnovation.com/the-many-flavors-of-the-journal-impact-factor

Nambiar, R., Tilak, P., & Cerejo, C. (2014). Quality of author guidelines of journals in the biomedical and physical sciences. *Learned Publishing, 27,* 201–206. doi:10.1087/20140306

Nurse Educator. (2018). About the journal. Retrieved from http://journals.lww.com/
nurseeducatoronline/Pages/aboutthejournal.aspx

Oermann, M. H., & Conklin, J. L. (2017). CiteScore and nursing journals. *Nurse Author & Editor,*
27(2), 3. Retrieved from http://naepub.com/publishing/2017-27-2-3

Oermann, M. H., Nicoll, L. H., Chinn, P. L., Conklin, J. L., McCarty, M., & Amarasekara, S. (2018).
Quality of author guidelines in nursing journals. *Journal of Nursing Scholarship.* Advance
online publication. doi:10.1111/jnu.12383

Oermann, M. H., & Shaw-Kokot, J. (2013a). Addressing the impact factors of nursing education
journals. *Journal of Nursing Education, 52*(9), 483–484. doi:10.3928/01484834-20130822-10

Oermann, M. H., & Shaw-Kokot, J. (2013b). Impact factors of nursing journals: What
nurses need to know. *Journal of Continuing Education in Nursing, 44*(7), 293–299.
doi:10.3928/00220124-20130501-14

Penrose, A. M., & Katz, S. B. (2010). *Writing in the sciences: Exploring conventions of scientific discourse* (3rd ed.). New York, NY: Pearson Longman.

U.S. National Library of Medicine. (2017). *Fact Sheet MEDLINE®.* Retrieved from https://www
.nlm.nih.gov/pubs/factsheets/medline.html

Zijlstra, H., & McCullough, R. (2016). CiteScore: A new metric to help you track journal performance and make decisions. Retrieved from https://www.elsevier.com/editors-update/
story/journal-metrics/citescore-a-new-metric-to-help-you-choose-the-right-journal

3

AUTHORSHIP AND PREPARING TO WRITE

Decisions about the focus of the manuscript, audience, and journal are important early in the writing process. Other decisions pertain to authorship; if these are not made before beginning the writing project, they may create problems and conflict among the authors later on. This chapter addresses authorship and author responsibilities in preparing to write.

AUTHORSHIP

The word "author" comes from the Latin word meaning "to produce." Authorship implies production, creation, and origination of new material. In the field of scientific writing, each individual designated as an author on a manuscript or other type of paper should have contributed something substantial to it. Authorship confers professional and personal rewards but involves considerable responsibility (American Medical Association [AMA], 2007). Authors bear responsibility for the truthfulness and trustworthiness of their work, in turn for which fairness dictates that they receive public credit.

Recommendations for the Conduct, Reporting, Editing, and Publication of Scholarly Work in Medical Journals

Who should receive credit as an author of a published manuscript? The *Recommendations for the Conduct, Reporting, Editing, and Publication of Scholarly Work in Medical Journals* specify that authorship credit should be given only when the author made substantial contributions to:

1. The conception or design of the work; or the acquisition, analysis, or interpretation of data for the work
2. Drafting the work or revising it critically for important intellectual content
3. Final approval of the version to be published
4. Agreement to be accountable for all aspects of the work in ensuring that questions related to the accuracy or integrity of any part of the work are appropriately investigated and resolved (International Committee of Medical Journal Editors [ICMJE], 2017)

Although many journals subscribe to these four Recommendations, some journals require only a subset of them (Hayter et al., 2013). As well, some journals require signature(s) certifying compliance with one or more of the Recommendations.

These criteria, where applied, have important implications for authors. First, each author listed in the byline must have participated in designing the project or acquiring, analyzing, or interpreting the data. Their participation may have involved identifying the questions for the study and designing it, identifying the need for a clinical project and planning its development, or critiquing and synthesizing the literature. Individuals who make important contributions to the analysis and interpretation of the data—even though they may not have been involved in the conception and design of the study— qualify for authorship if they meet the other criteria (ICMJE, 2017).

Next, authors must participate in writing the paper, critiquing it as a basis for subsequent revisions, or substantively revising the paper. Given that journals may require disclosure of evidence in support of authorship (Marušić et al., 2014), authors should be able to document their participation in a group writing activity such as through logs, data entry sheets, records of meetings held, and drafts of manuscripts. This recordkeeping may also be important after the paper is published to meet the final criterion for authorship if there arise questions about its content or methods at any point postpublication.

All coauthors must take responsibility for the content of the manuscript submitted for publication. Regardless of the number of drafts that circulate among groups of authors, all authors of a manuscript need to approve the final version, not only by signing the copyright transfer form, but also by approving the content.

Scientific publication requires the assistance of many individuals who do not meet the criteria for authorship. Editors have distinguished between authorship on the one hand and contributorship or coinvestigation on the other hand (Hayter et al., 2013). Contributors and coinvestigators include those who made suggestions for research questions; acquired funding for the study; recruited subjects or collected the data; provided statistical or technical writing support, editorial assistance, or review; contributed scientific expertise; or provided general supervision for the group such as a department chair or dean (AMA, 2007; American Psychological Association [APA], 2010; ICMJE, 2017). For clinical projects involving patients, physicians, and nurses who care for patients enrolled in a study do not qualify for authorship unless the previous four criteria are met. We discuss at the end of this chapter alternatives available to authors for acknowledging the important contributions of persons who do not meet the four criteria for authorship.

In addition to these four criteria included in the *Recommendations for the Conduct, Reporting, Editing, and Publication of Scholarly Work in Medical Journals*, there are additional responsibilities required of all authors. These include preparing the manuscript for submission; maintenance of the integrity of the copyright; and compliance with ethical, legal, and policy requirements of the journal. The latter includes disclosure of any conflicts of interest or sponsorships that could be interpreted as having been influential over their work and confirmation that they had access to all available data relevant to their research questions (APA, 2010). Conflicts of interest and data access are discussed as potential abuses of authorship responsibility. Manuscript preparation and copyright requirements are discussed in Chapters 14 and 16.

Information for Authors

Policies related to authorship, if available for a journal, can be found in the sections describing information for authors or author guidelines, as discussed in Chapter 2. Unfortunately, the information provided to authors may be insufficient or ineffective (Kornhaber, McLean, & Baber, 2015). Ambiguous professional norms regarding authorship make it difficult for authors to act ethically and hinder authors from knowing that a particular action constitutes wrongdoing.

Journal editors are responsible for making the authors' responsibilities explicit and concrete; for being honest, fair, collegial, and open in their dealings with authors; and for codifying these values in their information for authors (Marušić et al., 2014). Where such policies are not made explicit, authors should clarify with the editor of the target journal what are the expectations and requirements of authorship or risk ethical breaches.

ABUSES OF AUTHORSHIP

Authorship establishes both credit and responsibility for work in nursing, other health fields, and science in general. Misuse of authorship undermines this recognition and responsibility. During the process of writing for publication, authors make many decisions that have important ethical and legal implications. The publication of good science has many stakeholders: patients and their families, the media, general readers, publishers, students, faculty, and peer reviewers. But it is ultimately the responsibility of authors and editors to disseminate scientific work in a manner that maintains scholarly integrity within a profession (ICMJE, 2017). We address two ethical issues that affect authors: unjustified authorship and conflicts of interest.

Guest Authors and Ghost Authors

Ethical issues related to authorship center around the question of who is entitled to be listed as the author of a scientific publication. There is a trend of increasing numbers of articles with multiple authors published in all scientific fields, including healthcare (Kornhaber et al., 2015). While multiple authorship can reflect the increasing complexity of a field, the listing of many author names on a short paper or project description suggests that some individuals listed may be undeserving of authorship credit. The criteria established by the ICMJE provide a framework for determining who should be included as an author of a manuscript and who does not deserve authorship, but authors may not be aware of the criteria or may disagree with their extent and rigor (Marušić et al., 2014). Nursing students and authors should be apprised of these standards for authorship qualifications, and awareness of them should be reinforced.

One type of inappropriate authorship is that of an honorary or guest author. Guest authors are often persons in authority over the actual author but who are listed as authors without having met all appropriate criteria. Guest authorship is a prevalent breach of publication ethics (Resnik, Tyler, Black, & Kissling, 2016).

Authorship cannot be conferred upon someone as a gift or seized by someone in a position of power; it is a status that can only be assumed voluntarily by an individual who accepts all the responsibilities inherent in it (AMA, 2007). It is intellectually dishonest to list as a courtesy the name of someone who does not meet all criteria for authorship. It is unlikely that such individuals would be willing or able to take public responsibility for the accuracy of a paper's content if it was challenged. Inclusion of those not meeting a high standard of contribution also dilutes the meaning of authorship (AMA, 2007).

Some journals have formalized their efforts to reduce the potential for guest authorship by requiring disclosure by authors of the nature of all contributions made by each. Authors must document their specific contributions to conception and design, acquisition of data, and so forth (AMA, 2007). One reliability study of such contribution checklists suggests, however, that the actual contributions by authors may differ substantially from what authors report on these disclosure forms (Marušić et al., 2014). As more journals explicitly adopt the *Recommendations* as criteria for publication and provide authors with instructional guidelines for determining authorship, the attitudes and behavior of authors will likely change.

A related ethical issue is that of "ghost" authorship. Ghost authors may have met all of the criteria for authorship but are not listed as such in the author byline (AMA, 2007). In some fields, it is a common practice for a medical writer to be hired to write the manuscript, but this "ghost author" does not receive authorship credit. Instead, the name of a prominent scientist in that field is attached before the manuscript is submitted. In such cases, neither the person whose name is listed as author nor the ghost writer qualifies for authorship credit, the former because he or she understands the science but is not accountable for the writing, and the latter because she or he can defend the writing but not the science. Ghost authors may be the actual writers, such as authors' editors and researchers at facilities who write the article but cite others as the authors. Kennedy, Barnsteiner, and Daly (2014) reported nearly 28% of 10 leading nursing journals included articles written by ghost authors. Companies that offer to pay ghost writers to write articles that nurse scientists would then submit as the actual author are promoting unethical behavior.

Ghost authorship may be appropriate in some circumstances. Ghost authors may be freelance writers who are bound by contract not to receive authorship credit, corporate or governmental agency public relations officers, or authors' editors hired to draft or substantially revise a manuscript.

Although they do not qualify as authors, ghost writers should be identified to journal editors and their contributions explained to readers in an acknowledgment.

Conflicts of Interest

To facilitate readers' determination of the accuracy and value of published works, authors must disclose any financial or other competing interest that might cast doubt upon their impartiality. Relevant disclosures of potential conflicts include receipt of salaries, consulting fees, personal stock or research grants in products or services relevant to one's publication, or participation in a speakers' bureau for a product relevant to the study (APA, 2010). Does the author or his or her institution or business stand to gain financially from the mention of a commercial product in a publication? If so, questions may arise about whether this financial interest has affected the study results (APA, 2010). If the writer holds stock in a company whose products are promoted in the publication, the writer has an obligation to disclose this association to the editor, who then has a duty to inform readers. Similarly, if a researcher received grant support for a study, he or she should report the source of the funding in any published research report so that readers may determine if the content of the research report relates to the potential vested interest of the funding agency. Other examples of relevant disclosure include copyright holdings or receipts of royalties on an assessment tool used in the study (APA, 2010).

Authors disclose potential conflicts of interest in a variety of ways depending on the journal. Authors may add a statement in the acknowledgment sections, describe the circumstances in the cover letter to the editor, or include the information on the disclosure form, if one is provided by the journal.

WRITING IN A GROUP

Nurses often coauthor scientific manuscripts in a team setting (Ness, Duffy, McCallum, & Price, 2014), which can substantially improve publication productivity and dissemination of scientific findings (Kramer & Libhaber, 2016). Writing in a group can also produce frustrations and stumbling blocks that are avoidable with preplanning. Ground rules (Marušić et al., 2014) and a timeline (Clark, 2014) articulated in advance may help the group to proceed efficiently and effectively. The group involved in writing the manuscript should meet with all members present to discuss these areas: (a) who meets the criteria for authorship and whose contributions should be acknowledged in other ways, (b) the types of manuscripts that might be prepared, (c) the roles and responsibilities of each group member and tentative order of names on each planned manuscript, and (d) the time frame for completion of the manuscript(s). As in any group effort, the more coauthors involved in planning and writing the manuscript, the more difficult it is to coordinate the writing efforts and keep track of the group's progress. Small working groups focused on an individual writing project may be more manageable. One person in each group working on a manuscript should coordinate the work, track progress, and keep the group on schedule.

Responsibilities and Roles of Group Members

An early responsibility of the group is to review the criteria for authorship and decide who intends to meet them (Clark, 2014). Other contributors would then be recognized in the acknowledgment section of the manuscript. Discussions of the group and decisions reached should be recorded by one of the group members and kept securely in case questions and issues arise later.

The next responsibility of the group is to determine how many and what types of manuscripts will be prepared, including the audiences to be reached and potential journals. If the project involves research, the authors need to decide how the study findings will be disseminated and whether multiple papers may result and for which types of audiences and journals. If multiple manuscripts may emerge from the work completed by the group, this should be decided in the beginning so the roles and responsibilities associated with preparing the manuscripts may be distributed appropriately among the group.

The first priority for dissemination of the work is professional journals, but manuscripts also may be prepared for consumer audiences and other nonprofessional groups. The group might also discuss presentations to be made at conferences, including oral presentations and posters, so that these activities are reflected when the work is divided among the group.

Once the decisions are made about the types and number of manuscripts, the third function of the group is to determine the roles and specific responsibilities of group members for writing the manuscript (APA, 2010; ICMJE, 2017). Research teams may adopt a number of different strategies to complete the writing process. One member may write a first draft and then circulate it to other members for review and refinement. With some teams there is a natural distribution of labor related to content expertise, which may lend itself to dividing the writing among group members. For example, one member may write the description of the conceptual basis of the study and another the methodology of the study. Some teams write the manuscript "from the inside out," that is, first assigning the task of tabling all of the data to one member, followed by other members drafting the results, methods, introduction, and discussion, sequentially. Writing groups should divide the work according to the skills, habits, and preferences of its individual members (Marušić et al., 2014).

Documentation of the process and actions of the group are essential (Marušić et al., 2014). A procedure should be established for dating the drafts of the paper and, when writing as a group, labeling sections written and revised by different authors. This is important to keep track of contributions and know who to contact if there is a question about the substantive content or why a particular revision was made. Some word-processing programs have an option to automatically include the date with each draft. Another feature that is helpful with group writing is line numbering, in which each line of the manuscript is given a number automatically. This makes it easier to revise the manuscript and respond to comments about its content. The annotations feature of word-processing software helps coauthors communicate comments about specific parts of the manuscript.

Depending on the decisions made by members of the writing group, individual members will be assigned specific roles. These include the roles of first author, corresponding author, coauthors, and acknowledged contributors to the manuscript. These roles may shift as the writing project progresses, and with this shift may come a change in the order of author names. But discussion of assigned roles early in the process is important for accountability and productivity in the writing group.

First Author

Typically, the first or lead author contributes the most to the project and manuscript (APA, 2010). The first author is often the person who initiated and developed the clinical project, or in the case of research is the primary investigator, and is responsible for moving the group toward completion of a manuscript to describe its work (Fontanarosa, Bauchner, & Flanagin, 2017). The assignment of first and subsequent authors should reflect relative contributions to the manuscript rather than organizational status (APA, 2010).

The first author has more responsibilities associated with writing the paper than do the other authors and may be the most experienced in writing for publication. The first author coordinates preparation of the manuscript and is ultimately responsible for the integrity and documentation of its development. While the group should determine the roles and responsibilities of each author, some common activities completed by the first author are presented in Exhibit 3.1.

Corresponding Author

The corresponding author communicates with the editor, beginning with the query letter, and is designated as such on the title page of the manuscript or in the cover letter. Although the first author usually serves as the corresponding author, the group may decide that another person should assume this role.

The corresponding author is the contact between the authors and the editor, discussing revisions to be made, working with the editor to assure that these are adequately made, and returning the revisions and related materials on time. The corresponding author also receives notification of page proof availability and is responsible for their review and answering all queries in the time frame requested. The contact between the corresponding author and editor helps to establish the credibility of the group and its dependability. Positive working relationships between authors and editors are important in terms of

EXHIBIT 3.1

Responsibilities of First Author

- Leads the discussion about authorship; the manuscripts to be prepared, their content, and how to organize each one; the order of author names; who will assume responsibility for different parts of the manuscript and for multiple papers if more than one will be prepared; and the time frame.
- Obtains author guidelines and assures that they are met.
- Arranges for word processing of manuscript.
- Completes own writing assignment.
- Edits drafts and suggests revisions to coauthors.
- Maintains copies of all drafts, with dates, and notes about revisions.
- Edits a final version of the manuscript for a consistent writing style throughout.
- Reads and corrects the final typed manuscript.
- Facilitates approval of the final manuscript by coauthors; has each author date and initial the final copy, indicating their approval of it, and files these.
- Keeps copies of references used in preparing the manuscript and for background work.
- Sets up group meetings and keeps records of the discussions.
- Assures that coauthors adhere to the time frame and takes the actions established by the group when coauthors do not.
- Obtains permissions if needed.
- Makes sure that the correct number of copies of the manuscript and other required materials are submitted with it.
- May assume responsibilities of corresponding author.
- Coordinates subsequent revisions of the manuscript following peer review.
- Coordinates signing of the copyright agreement by coauthors.
- Reviews page proofs (the typeset manuscript pages that are reviewed for errors before publication) and returns them promptly to the publisher.

future publications. Once the paper is published, the corresponding author communicates with readers by distributing reprints of the article and answering questions.

Coauthors

Coauthorship of articles has become the norm, especially given the increasing specialization of healthcare, multidisciplinary collaborations, and multisite research projects (AMA, 2007; Resnik et al., 2016). There is no absolute limit imposed on the number of coauthors permitted on scientific manuscripts (AMA, 2007; APA, 2010), and the number of coauthors listed has grown over time (Fontanarosa et al., 2017). Coauthors assume responsibility not only for their sections of the manuscript but also for the intellectual content of the paper as a whole. Remember that each author should be able to defend the manuscript publicly.

Writing groups should review the order of author names early and often in order to avoid conflict and problems later on (Clark, 2014). The following principles should be considered by writing groups for determining the ordering of authors.

- No contributor should be considered unless the individual has met the four criteria for authorship discussed previously or otherwise complied with the journal's policies.
- Any contributor who meets criterion #1 should be afforded the opportunity to meet criteria #2 through #4.
- Authors should be listed according to level of contribution, from most to least.
- Decisions about the order should be discussed early in the project and reviewed regularly as the project progresses and the manuscript emerges.
- Decisions about the order are the prerogative of the authors, not the journal editor.
- Authors should be provided space to explain the order of authorship if deemed necessary.
- Editors may require disclosure of author contributions.
- Changes made to the author order following submission should be approved by all authors and communicated to the editor. This includes changes related to an author's death or incapacitation (AMA, 2007; ICMJE, 2017).

With the growing number of authors listed with publications, it is more and more difficult to determine the contributions of each person to the project based on the order of author names. If disclosure of the contributions made to the research and to the manuscript were more widespread, the contributors could accept credit and responsibility with more transparency. An example of a contributor list using this system is found in Exhibit 3.2.

EXHIBIT 3.2

Example of Presentation of Contributions

ARTICLE CITATION

Oermann, M. H., Kardong-Edgren, S. E., Odom-Maryon, T., & Roberts, C. J. (2014). Effects of practice on competency in single-rescuer cardiopulmonary resuscitation. *MEDSURG Nursing, 23*(1), 22–28.

NAMES ON BYLINE

Marilyn H. Oermann, Suzan E. Kardong-Edgren, Tamara Odom-Maryon, Caleb J. Roberts

CONTRIBUTOR LIST

Study design: MHO, SEKE; data collection: SEKE, TOM, CJR; data analysis: TOM, CJR; and manuscript preparation: MHO, SEKE, TOM, CJR. John J. Doe conducted the literature search for the study. (Note that he is not listed in the article citation.)

Group Authors

Group or collaborative authorship is growing (Fontanarosa et al., 2017) and may occur when a research project involves multiple academic centers or when organizations or working groups produce a publishable manuscript. In these cases, the manuscript may legitimately be considered as having been authored by the group rather than by individual authors. Authorship of a group-generated document should be determined based on two considerations: appropriate credit for individual contributors and user-friendly indexing of citations for online search and retrieval. When a group authors a manuscript, authorship may legitimately be assigned in several ways (AMA, 2007; ICMJE, 2017).

One or more authors who meet the standard criteria described previously may take the responsibility for writing the paper on behalf of or for the specified group and be listed as authors in the byline; participants who did not meet all of the criteria are listed in the acknowledgments.

The group name may appear in the byline as the sole collaborative author group, with all contributing members of the group listed in the acknowledgments or other space in the article.

Authorship may be attributed to the group as a whole, without identification of group members. In this case, every member of the group must meet criteria for authorship, and one member should be identified as the corresponding author for the group.

Acknowledged Contributors

Acknowledgments are generally used to recognize people who contributed to the research, project, or preparation of the manuscript but do not qualify for authorship. In the acknowledgment section of a manuscript, the author can give credit to people who assisted with the work, such as individuals who:

- Critically reviewed the research proposal, design, or methods
- Gave advice on the project
- Collected the data
- Analyzed the data
- Provided statistical support
- Provided technical support
- Assisted in writing and preparing the manuscript
- Critically reviewed the manuscript

Acknowledgments also should specify the financial and material support provided for the project (ICMJE, 2017). An example of an acknowledgment for grant support is: "Financial Disclosures: This project was supported by an educational/research award from the Nurse Practitioner Healthcare Foundation through a grant from Purdue Pharma LP, Stamford, Connecticut" (Staveski, Wu, Tesoro, Roth, & Cisco, 2017, p. 75).

Persons mentioned in the acknowledgment section of a manuscript must grant permission to include their names. The inclusion of names in the acknowledgment may suggest endorsement of the content of the manuscript, and for this reason acknowledged contributors should have the opportunity to read the manuscript and consent to be acknowledged.

The acknowledgment section may also contain statements that the authors had full access to datasets. Such disclosure is important under two conditions: when a study was funded by a commercial entity with financial interest in the outcome and when studies are based on data from public archives or repositories. In the latter case, a link to the dataset should be provided, along with any information about independent reliability checks of the analyses by noncompensated scientists (AMA, 2007).

The fourth responsibility of the writing group involves establishing a time frame for completion of each phase in the writing project and manuscript as a whole. The time frame should include the expectations of each group member with accompanying due dates and when the group will meet. The discussion of the time frame should also include the actions to be taken if coauthors do not complete their responsibilities by the due date. This is an important area of discussion because if the due dates are not established and adhered to, the writing project may never get completed. The actions to be taken when coauthors do not complete their responsibilities on time might include being dropped entirely from the writing group and listed as a contributor in the acknowledgments or involve a change in responsibilities and reordering of author names. The group should specify its decisions at this point in the discussions, not when required because of noncompliance.

Students Writing With Faculty

Writing groups that include both faculty members and students require special considerations. The relative contributions of each person, professor and student, often are perplexing when the student earns academic credit for his or her work on a project and the professor is being compensated for teaching the student.

Manuscripts coauthored by faculty and students may demonstrate elements of either guest or ghost authorship or both. Unfortunately, under pressure to publish in order to meet criteria for tenure and promotion, some faculty members request or demand authorship credit on any manuscript related to student work guided by faculty. However, unless professors meet all the four criteria for authorship specified by the *Recommendations* (ICMJE, 2017), they should not be listed as authors (guest authorship). If a student and a faculty member jointly plan and carry out a project, and both contribute to drafting and revising the manuscript, both should be listed as authors. It is unethical for a professor to ask a student to draft a manuscript and not give the student authorship credit, or worse, to assign a paper as a course requirement and then submit the student's work for publication without listing the student as an author (ghost authorship).

The best approach is to negotiate clear expectations for the roles of student and professor with regard to course work and writing for publication. If the student is expected to complete a project for course credit, the teacher should evaluate the work for a grade first, and then discuss the work necessary to author a manuscript for publication. It is at that time that the relative contributions of each person to the manuscript can be negotiated and authorship credit can be assigned fairly. As a general rule, a student is listed as first author on any multiple-authored manuscript that is substantially based on the student's thesis or dissertation (APA, 2010).

SUMMARY

Each individual designated as an author on a manuscript or other type of paper should have contributed sufficiently to it. The *Recommendations for the Conduct, Reporting, Editing, and Publication of Scholarly Work in Medical Journals* specify that authorship credit should be given only when the author made substantial contributions to (a) the conception and design of the study, or to the analysis and interpretation of the data, (b) drafting the manuscript or revising it for important content, (c) the approval of the final version of the manuscript, and (d) agreement to be accountable for all aspects of the work in ensuring that questions related to the accuracy or integrity of any part of the work are appropriately investigated (ICMJE, 2017).

Acknowledgments are generally used to recognize people who contributed to the research, project, or preparation of the manuscript but do not qualify for authorship. People mentioned in the acknowledgment section of a manuscript must grant permission to include their names.

When writing with multiple authors, the first step is to decide on authorship and who qualifies. The second step is to determine the order of author names on each manuscript under development. Typically the first author contributes the most to the project and manuscript. The order of coauthors' names should be determined by their relative contributions to the work. Coauthors assume responsibility not only for their sections of the manuscript but for the intellectual content of the paper as a whole.

Authors complete other preparations before beginning to write. These preparations allow authors to focus on their writing once they begin.

REFERENCES

American Medical Association. (2007). *AMA manual of style: A guide for authors and editors* (10th ed.). New York, NY: Oxford University Press.

American Psychological Association. (2010). *Publication manual of the American Psychological Association* (6th ed.). Washington, DC: Author.

Clark, C. (2014). A formula for collaborative writing. *Journal of Nursing Education, 53*(3), 119–120. doi:10.3928/01484834-20140220-10

Fontanarosa, P., Bauchner, H., & Flanagin A. (2017). Authorship and team science. *Journal of the American Medical Association, 318*(24), 2433–2437. doi:10.1001/jama.2017.19341

Hayter, M., Noyes, J., Perry, L., Pickler, R., Roe, B., & Watson, R. (2013). Who writes, whose rights, and who's right? Issues in authorship. *Journal of Advanced Nursing, 69*(12), 2599–2601. doi:10.1111/jan.12265

International Committee of Medical Journal Editors. (2017). Recommendations for the conduct, reporting, editing, and publication of scholarly work in medical journals. Retrieved from http://www.icmje.org/urm_main.html

Kennedy, M. S., Barnsteiner, J., & Daly, J. (2014). Honorary and ghost authorship in nursing publications. *Journal of Nursing Scholarship, 46*(6), 416–422. doi:10.1111/jnu.12093

Kornhaber, R. A., McLean, L. M., & Baber, R. J. (2015). Ongoing ethical issues concerning authorship in biomedical journals: An integrative review. *International Journal of Nanomedicine, 10*, 4837–4846. doi:10.2147/IJN.S87585

Kramer, B., & Libhaber, E. (2016). Writing for publication: Institutional support provides an enabling environment. *BMC Medical Education, 16*, 115. doi:10.1186/s12909-016-0642-0

Marušić, A., Hren, D., Mansi, B., Lineberry, N., Bhattacharya. A., Garrity M., . . . Peña, T. (2014). Five-step authorship framework to improve transparency in disclosing contributors to industry-sponsored clinical trial publications. *BMC Medicine, 12*, 197. doi:10.1186/s12916-014-0197-z

Ness, V., Duffy, K., McCallum, J., & Price, L. (2014). Getting published: Reflections of a collaborative writing group. *Nurse Education Today, 34*(1), 1–5. doi:10.1016/j.nedt.2013.03.019

Resnik, D. B., Tyler, A. M., Black, J. R., & Kissling, G. (2016). Authorship policies of scientific journals. *Journal of Medical Ethics, 42*, 199–202. doi:10.1136/medethics-2015-103171

Staveski, S. L., Wu, M., Tesoro, T. M., Roth, S. J., & Cisco, M. J. (2017). Interprofessional team's perception of care delivery after implementation of a pediatric pain and sedation protocol. *Critical Care Nurse, 37*, 66–76. doi: 10.4037/ccn2017538

REVIEWING THE LITERATURE

In order to be an effective writer, authors must develop the skill of conducting a literature review. Often, prior to writing the manuscript, the author has already reviewed, critiqued, and synthesized the literature as a basis for a research study, an innovation, or a project to be described in the paper. Before commencing to write the paper, that literature review may need to be updated or, if the focus of the manuscript differs somewhat from the original project, another review of the literature may be needed. Sometimes, however, the author begins to consider a topic for a manuscript but has not yet searched the literature. Such a review enables the author to decide if the manuscript is worth writing in the first place and to gain an understanding of material that has already been published on the topic. Either way, the author cannot begin writing without completing a review of the literature.

This chapter prepares the author for conducting and writing a literature review for a manuscript. Although literature reviews for research studies, theses and dissertations, course work, evidence-based practice, and other purposes vary in the types of literature used, their comprehensiveness, and how they are summarized for the reader, the process of reviewing the literature is the same. The chapter describes bibliographic databases useful for literature reviews in nursing, selecting databases to use, developing search strategies, analyzing and synthesizing the literature, and writing the literature review for a manuscript and other types of papers. The goal of this chapter is to develop authors' skills in conducting literature reviews for writing papers in nursing. Chapter 6 discusses writing integrative and systematic review articles.

PURPOSES OF LITERATURE REVIEW

A literature review is a critique and synthesis of current knowledge about a topic for research or for use in clinical practice, teaching, administration, and other areas of nursing. There are three main purposes of reviewing the literature.

The first purpose is to describe what is already known about a topic. The literature review provides the background on a research topic, a question about clinical practice, a new project, or other decisions in nursing. It reveals existing knowledge about a topic and related areas. Based on the literature search, the author then decides whether or not to write the paper. The author may have an idea to share with readers, but finds from the review of the literature that the topic has already been adequately covered and another article is unnecessary. Alternatively, a review may confirm that the proposed paper will contribute new ideas or a different perspective on the topic. The review provides the background readings for the manuscript.

The second purpose is to identify exactly where the gaps are in knowledge and where questions still remain. Research studies and other types of projects should build on prior work and fill those gaps. When reviewing the literature to guide practice decisions, nurses can assess the available evidence and identify where further study is needed to build the evidence base on a problem or intervention.

The third purpose is to assist in determining how the proposed manuscript will contribute new knowledge to nursing. Hicks (2014) notes that a good literature review serves as a family tree for visualizing the genealogy of knowledge on a specific topic. How does the author's work contribute to the literature and answer existing questions? How does it reinforce what is already known? Answering questions such as these is important because it will help the author decide how to present the content to best meet the needs of particular readers.

TYPES OF LITERATURE REVIEWS

This chapter presents guidelines for conducting literature reviews when writing a manuscript, but these same principles apply when reviewing the literature for papers for courses; a thesis or dissertation; and grants, projects, and other initiatives in which the nurse may be involved.

Literature Reviews for Papers for Courses

When writing the literature review for a term paper and other papers for courses, the author begins with identifying a topic (or the one assigned by the teacher), locates research and other types of articles on that topic using bibliographic databases, critiques and synthesizes the literature, and then writes the review. The keys to this process are understanding the purpose of the paper and pacing oneself to have adequate time to complete the review and write the necessary number of drafts of the paper by the course deadline.

Literature Reviews for Theses and Dissertations

For a thesis, which is a master's-level research project, and a dissertation, which is a more extensive and original research study completed at the doctoral level, the same process is used for completing the literature review. The student begins with a topic, approved by the faculty advisor and committee, and then locates, critiques, and synthesizes prior research, identifying how the study contributes new knowledge to nursing or confirms what is already known about the topic.

The literature review for a thesis and dissertation is comprehensive, revealing prior studies on the problem and related areas, and provides the rationale for conducting the research. The student needs to be thorough in identifying the relevant literature, use preset criteria for analyzing studies, and synthesize findings to reveal what is known about the problem and what needs to be examined further. Students defend the research proposal and completed thesis and dissertation, under the scrutiny of the student's committee and other faculty, depending on the procedures established by the college or university. The literature review is a major part of this process, providing the background and rationale for conducting the study and demonstrating how the completed research adds new knowledge to nursing.

Literature Reviews for Grants, Projects, and Other Initiatives

Nurses review and critique the literature as background for developing grants, evidence-based practice and clinical projects, quality improvement studies, and other initiatives. The literature review provides the rationale for these, indicating how they fulfill important needs. Depending on their purposes, the types of literature reviewed may include original research reports, descriptive articles, anecdotal reports, monographs, books, and published case reports. The process of conducting and writing the literature review is similar to other types of papers.

Literature Reviews for Manuscripts

The literature review completed for a course assignment, a thesis or dissertation, and grants, projects, and other initiatives may lead to the preparation of a manuscript and serve as the basis for writing its introduction and literature review section, depending on the format of the manuscript. For other manuscripts, though, the author begins with an idea and then searches the literature to learn what has already been published on the topic and to develop the background for the paper. Regardless of the beginning point for the literature review, the same process is used for identifying, critiquing, and synthesizing the literature.

However, compared with these earlier papers, there are differences in how the literature is presented in a publishable manuscript. In a manuscript there are restrictions on the number of pages, and the author needs to limit the summary of the literature to allow adequate pages for other sections of the paper. As such, the literature reviews in most manuscripts are short and focused, providing the background of the topic and rationale for the research or project described in the manuscript.

Format to Use

Each journal has its own format for how the literature is reported. In many journals, the literature is integrated in the introduction. With this format, the introduction presents the topic of the paper, purpose of the research or project, and why the topic is important, using the literature to explain the background and rationale for the research or project. A single paragraph may first state succinctly what is the current best evidence on the topic and the need for the study, then it specifies what new information in the manuscript will meet that need. A second paragraph states the purpose of the study. Papers submitted to medical journals often follow this format, and the *AMA Manual of Style* suggests that the introduction should not exceed two or three paragraphs (American Medical Association [AMA], 2007).

In other journals there is a section devoted to the literature review. With these papers, the topic and its importance are discussed in the introduction, often using research and other types of articles as support. The literature is then presented in the next section of the paper. Because ways of presenting the literature review differ across journals, it is important for the authors to read the guidelines for the journal and examine a few sample articles published by it.

Extent of Literature and Style of Presentation

The extent of literature presented and writing style used also differ across journals. For research manuscripts, the literature review is extensive and includes an analysis of prior studies and synthesis of the findings. A comprehensive review of the literature is important to reveal the gaps in knowledge, which led to the study being presented.

What about other journals? The research paper may be submitted to a clinical journal that publishes reports of research. When writing for a journal that focuses more on clinical practice, the literature review will be less extensive. In many journals, the presentation of the literature emphasizes the practice implications of prior studies; the author needs this information prior to writing the literature review.

Identifying a list of target journals, their goals, and their writing styles is important. Particular to each journal is the expected extent and presentation of background literature. In some journals, a more formal and academic style of writing is used to present the literature, whereas in other journals an informal style is used. An example of each style is presented in Exhibit 4.1.

Current Literature Reported Accurately

Editors and reviewers critique the recency and accuracy of the literature review for each manuscript submitted to peer-reviewed journals in order to decide whether or not to publish it for their readers' information. The literature cited in the paper should present the current state of the research and evidence on the topic and should be accurate. For a research paper, the author may have

EXHIBIT 4.1

Writing Styles for Literature Reviews

FORMAL, ACADEMIC STYLE

Studies on patient views of the quality of their healthcare have focused mainly on patient satisfaction with hospital care and the care provided by nursing staff during that hospitalization (Doe et al., 2018; Johnson & Jones, 2017; McDonald, Doe, & Alexander, 2017; Smith, 2018). Patient satisfaction is influenced by the expectations of patients, their prior experiences with the healthcare setting, and their perceptions of quality care (Baker, 2016; Miller, Jones, Smith, & Brown, 2016).

INFORMAL STYLE

Many studies have been done in nursing on how satisfied patients are with their nursing care in hospitals and other settings (Johnson & Jones, 2017; Smith, 2018). We know from these studies that patients expect a certain level of nursing care, and these expectations influence their satisfaction with care. Nurses do not always know what aspects of nursing care are important to patients—we need to learn more about this from our patients (Miller, Jones, Smith, & Brown, 2016).

completed the literature review a year or more prior to beginning the manuscript; in these cases, the literature review should be updated to capture the most recent work on the topic. The latest work published on the topic should be cited.

Accuracy is essential in interpreting and synthesizing the literature as well as in citing the references. Errors in citing references in the text of papers and on the reference lists must be avoided. Errors obstruct readers from retrieving cited documents and undermine an accurate count of how often publications were cited, which invalidates measures of publication impact. Errors impede the location of references by others interested in building on the science base. Authors should take time in preparing the references to verify their accuracy before submitting the manuscript and again in the page proofs. Use of reference management software such as EndNote can help prevent many of these citation errors.

Of particular importance, authors should repeatedly check the availability of web references, not only prior to submission of the manuscript but also when revising the paper and checking the page proofs. Websites and addresses can change frequently.

TYPES OF LITERATURE FOR INCLUSION IN REVIEW

There are different ways of classifying the literature that might be reviewed for manuscripts in nursing. One way of categorizing the literature is by empirical, theoretical, descriptive, or anecdotal reports, as well as reviews. The literature also includes primary and secondary sources.

Empirical

The empirical literature includes reports of research published in journals as well as unpublished studies such as master's theses and doctoral dissertations. These are the original reports of the research study, including its aims, methods, results, discussion of the findings, and implications. In writing research papers, the author focuses predominantly on empirical literature. Because the author has reviewed this literature as a basis for developing the research proposal and conducting the study, frequently only newly published articles need to be examined prior to beginning the manuscript.

Theoretical

Theoretical literature describes concepts, models, and theories in nursing and related fields. Articles, books, and other documents describing theoretical perspectives are useful for developing a conceptual framework for a research study and presenting in a manuscript the concepts and theories that guided the study or project. For example, the literature review for a manuscript on loneliness among older adults may include theoretical articles on loneliness, social isolation, social support, and aging, among others.

Descriptive

Many articles in nursing journals do not describe research or theory but instead report on practices important to nurses in their professional roles. Articles on patient care, new clinical practices and initiatives, educational innovations, nursing management, trends in nursing, issues, and other topics are in this category of literature. These are important to provide the background information for a manuscript and allow the author to assess what others have written about the topic.

Anecdotal Reports

Anecdotal reports are articles that present personal experiences and views of individuals rather than a systematic evaluation or study of the topic. An article about the benefits of preceptors to new graduates, based on comments by the graduates, preceptors' evaluations, and observations by others in the clinical setting, is an example of an anecdotal report; the effects of using preceptors were not measured through research. Anecdotal reports may be interesting to read and present innovative ideas for consideration, but because they are not based on any type of study with controls or comparison groups, they should be used sparingly in a literature review. For some manuscripts, however, anecdotal reports are useful in presenting the need for study in an area and for getting readers interested in the paper.

Reviews

Some journals publish articles that are reviews of the literature. Traditional literature reviews summarize what is known about a particular topic. Integrative reviews critique the research and synthesize the findings, using a well-defined and rigorous approach, to answer specific clinical and other types of questions. Reviews are valuable to authors in writing for publication because they synthesize the current state of the literature, indicating what is already known and gaps in knowledge. Review articles, though, are secondary sources, and for many papers authors will need to access the original documents cited in the review article. Review articles are discussed in detail in Chapter 6.

Primary and Secondary Sources

Primary sources are original sources of information written by the person who developed the ideas. They are original because they are the first published accounts of the research study, theory, innovation, or idea. For research reports, the primary source is the paper written by the researcher who conducted the study. In primary sources, the reader finds detailed information about the research problem, methodology, results, and discussion, described by the researchers themselves.

In the theoretical literature, the primary source is the theorist who developed the model, theory, or framework. For other types of literature, the primary source is the originator of the innovation or idea.

In secondary sources, the information is summarized and reported by someone other than the originator. Summaries of research, literature reviews, descriptions of clinical projects, and discussions of models and theories reported in articles, books, and other references by an author other than the original are secondary sources. The problem with using secondary sources is that the author has interpreted and summarized the writings of someone else. With secondary sources on research, sometimes only limited information is provided about the methodology and findings, or the discussion may highlight only some of the important outcomes.

For secondary theoretical literature, the author may have misinterpreted the model, theory, or framework, or allowed his or her own views to influence the discussion. For other literature, authors of secondary sources may omit vital details that would influence use of the innovation or idea in practice and may be biased in the information reported and how it is presented in the paper. In searching the literature in preparation for writing manuscripts and other papers, only primary sources should be used unless those sources cannot be found.

Most literature reviews predominantly include articles published in peer-reviewed journals, which have been critiqued by experts as a basis for their acceptance. These articles can be accessed by searching bibliographic databases, such as MEDLINE (Medical Literature, Analysis, and Retrieval System Online) and CINAHL (Cumulative Index to Nursing and Allied Health Literature), which index thousands of journals. By searching these databases, the author can develop a comprehensive review of the literature. Searching the literature is discussed later in this chapter.

Some manuscripts also may include in the literature review chapters, books, websites, and other grey literature. *Grey literature* is described as the material produced by governments, academics, and business and industry interests in both print and electronic formats, but uncontrolled by commercial publishers, that is, where publishing is not the primary activity of the material's authors (Godin, Stapleton, Kirkpatrick, Hanning, & Leatherdale, 2015).

Grey literature is generally accessed by searching the web, because most of these documents are not indexed in the bibliographic databases used for a literature review. Information obtained from websites and other unpublished documents is typically not peer reviewed and may not be available for readers to access in later years. For most manuscripts and papers, authors should rely on journal articles as sources of information for their literature reviews, an exception being surveillance data located in government documents and tables provided to the public on websites ending in .gov. However, the Cochrane Collaboration, the Institute of Medicine, and the Agency for Healthcare Research and Quality (AHRQ) all recommend searches of grey literature to ensure the comprehensiveness of literature reviews (Hartling et al., 2017), and systematic strategies for searching gray literature are emerging (Godin et al., 2015). Recent research suggests that inclusion of grey literature has a limited, if any, impact on conclusions drawn from major review articles (Hartling et al., 2017).

DIFFERENCES IN LITERATURE REVIEWS FOR RESEARCH AND USE IN PRACTICE

Literature reviews for developing a research proposal and writing a research report differ from those conducted when the goal is to locate background information about patient care, an issue in practice, a project being considered, and other topics not related to planning or reporting research.

Review for Research Purposes

Literature reviews for research projects examine studies already completed in a topical area of scientific research. The literature focuses one's understanding of the problem, the gaps in knowledge, and the basis for conducting the study. One reviews primarily the empirical literature. A robust literature review for research projects provides readers with a valid summary of existing evidence and showcases the argument that supports the need for the current study. While the study is being conducted, the researcher continues to periodically review the literature to keep current with other relevant studies. When the findings of the study are ready for dissemination, a follow-up literature review may or may not be needed, depending on how consistently the literature was reviewed up to this point.

The literature review for a research report presents prior studies on the topic, not descriptions of practice or anecdotal reports. These other types of articles, as well as chapters and books, provide sources of information for the author to use in writing the introduction and discussion section of the paper. They contribute to establishing the background of the problem and making a case why the study was indicated.

The other type of literature typically reviewed for research proposals and manuscripts relates to theoretical literature, which describes the concepts and theories to guide the research. A review of theoretical articles and books provides the background for developing the conceptual framework for the research study and for understanding the research results. Theories often enable the researcher to organize the literature around the concepts that are embedded in the theory, thus linking together in an organized way pieces of information and evidence.

Quantitative Research

In quantitative studies, the literature review directs the development and implementation of the study. The literature is examined prior to beginning the study to identify the work already done on the topic and where further study is indicated. The background and significance of the study are developed from this review of the literature, and theoretical literature is used to construct the conceptual framework for the research. The methodology, including the design, sample, measurement, treatment, and data collection procedure, is based on previous research. The literature review is also used in analyzing the data and reporting the findings such that the current study builds on earlier ones. Thus, in quantitative studies, the literature review is used in each phase of the research. Relevant literature may be cited throughout the research paper except for the results section, where references to the literature are generally not included.

Qualitative Research

In qualitative manuscripts, the style and format of the paper and how the literature is presented depend on the purposes of the research, methods used, the emergent findings, and their applicability to nursing care. Literature reviews of qualitative research can "maximize the understanding of a wide range of healthcare issues that cannot be measured quantitatively, . . . increase our understandings of the culture of communities, explore how service users experience illness and the health system, and evaluate components and activities of health services such as health promotion and community development" (Munn, Porritt, Lockwood, Aromataris, & Pearson, 2014, p. 109). Summaries of qualitative research should weigh highly the dependability and credibility of studies that are cited (Munn et al., 2014).

Review for Use in Practice

Literature reviews are also done to gain an understanding of best practices and new approaches to patient care, teaching, management, and other areas, and to provide the background for developing and implementing projects that are not related to research studies. To answer questions about practice problems, the nurse begins with a search of the literature to determine how others have approached these same problems and to identify effective strategies. Varied types of literature may be examined, including descriptive articles, anecdotal reports, case reports, chapters, books, and empirical studies, among others.

Similar to research reports, if the author reviewed the literature prior to developing a project, an innovation, or another initiative, then the author may need to update and expand the literature review when ready to write the manuscript. One literature review as a basis for developing new standards of practice, for instance, may not be sufficient for writing later about those standards and how they were used and evaluated in the clinical setting.

BEGINNING THE SEARCH

The author begins the literature review by identifying the topic of the paper. Whether the review is for a course, a thesis or dissertation, a research study, a project, or an idea to be developed into a manuscript, the author starts with a general topic and then narrows it down to one that can be searched easily in a bibliographic database. For example, the author may plan to write a manuscript on a project to improve the satisfaction of patients with their care in the clinic. The topic "Patient Satisfaction" is too broad for reviewing the literature. Using the advanced search fields in the CINAHL Complete database, we found more than 10,000 publications in the past 10 years alone with that Exact Major Subject Heading. Narrowing the topic to include publications in the "English Language" regarding "All Adults" who were "Outpatients" in the subset of nursing journals yielded a far more manageable number of citations. Some types of studies may require the authors to review very large volumes of published papers in order to cover a topic comprehensively, and strategies are available for managing hundreds or thousands of citations in digital file systems (Havill et al., 2014).

The author then searches the literature. In earlier years, this was done by looking up references in the card catalogue and in the annual indexes of the periodical literature, which were only in print format. This information is now compiled in electronic databases, which can be accessed via the Internet or may be provided on a local area network or in the library. These databases are searched electronically, making them fast and easy to use. The author reviews each publication in the database, produces a record that describes its identifiers and content, and then indexes it. This process allows the author to search the database for specific content areas and retrieve what is found.

Bibliographic Databases for Nursing Literature

There are varied bibliographic databases for conducting literature searches in nursing. The two databases that are most useful are MEDLINE and CINAHL. When the paper extends beyond nursing practice, there are other bibliographic databases, such as PsycINFO for psychological literature or Education Resources Information Center (ERIC) for education literature that also can be searched. In addition, many authors will use the library catalog to locate books and other types of resources. Selecting which databases to search is discussed later in the chapter.

Electronic databases provide easy access to the nursing literature when the author is ready to complete a literature review or needs to update the review. With Internet access, some of the databases can be searched from home for no charge, such as MEDLINE, or by subscription.

MEDLINE

The National Library of Medicine (NLM) provides a wide variety of resources related to the biomedical and health sciences. The NLM's premier bibliographic database is MEDLINE, which contains more than 24 million journal citations from 1949 to the present (NLM, 2017a). The citations in MEDLINE are from more than 5,000 biomedical journals worldwide, including nursing journals. MEDLINE is searched through PubMed®, available at www.ncbi.nlm .nih.gov/pubmed.

Articles are indexed using Medical Subject Headings (MeSH), which is the NLM's system for indexing articles and cataloging books. MEDLINE can be searched using MeSH or by key concepts, author last name followed by initials, journal title, publication date, and any combination of these (PubMed Help, 2017; NLM, 2017b). A search produces a list of citations to journal articles, each with information about the article and an abstract, if available; there are often links to the full-text document. Some of those full-text articles might be free, whereas others might include a link to the website of the publisher or other full-text provider.

The NLM also maintains PubMed Central, a web-based repository of biomedical journal literature with free and unrestricted access to more than 4.5 million full-text articles (www.ncbi.nlm.nih.gov/pmc); it provides access to molecular biology and genomic information, offers extensive healthcare information resources for the public through MedlinePlus (medlineplus.gov), and maintains the ClinicalTrials.gov database (clinicaltrials.gov/ct2/home) to provide the public with information about all types of clinical research studies.

Links to the many resources of the NLM can be found at www.nlm.nih.gov. The Library's catalog of books, journals, and audiovisuals can be searched through LocatorPlus.

CINAHL

CINAHL is a comprehensive database of nursing and allied health literature. The first edition of CINAHL was published in 1961, indexing the literature from 1956 to 1960, from 16 journals. Currently CINAHL Complete indexes more than 400 journals in nursing (Elton B. Stephens Company [EBSCO], 2017). The database also includes access to books and book chapters, nursing dissertations, selected conference proceedings, standards of practice, educational software, and audiovisual media. In addition to full-text journals, other documents that are available as full text are legal cases, clinical innovations, critical pathways, drug records, research instruments, and clinical trials (EBSCO, 2017).

Material is indexed according to the CINAHL subject headings specifically designed for nursing and allied health literature. The structure is based on MeSH. The CINAHL database is available at medical libraries and libraries with health information, providing access for students and employees for no charge. With this access authors can search the database and often obtain full-text articles. Personal subscriptions to CINAHL are available through varied vendors for a fee.

Other Bibliographic Databases

For many manuscripts, the author will want to review the literature in areas other than nursing. It is worth the time prior to beginning the paper to conduct a thorough search of the literature using multiple databases, as appropriate. This provides the author with a broad view of what has already been published on the topic, not only the work done in nursing. Selecting other databases to review depends on the topic of the manuscript. A brief description of selected other databases is found in Table 4.1. This list is not exhaustive, but does provide examples from the wealth of databases that might be used for reviewing the literature.

Database Structure

Each publication in a bibliographic database has a single *record* with *fields* that contain specific information describing the publication. For instance, the record for a book would include the author's name, title of the book, edition, publisher, and date. There are also fields in the record to indicate the main subject or subjects covered in the book.

Each journal article in a bibliographic database is indexed similarly. It has a single record with specific information about that article: the author's

TABLE 4.1 SELECTED BIBLIOGRAPHIC DATABASES

Database	Subject Area
BIOSIS Citation Index	Research databases on life sciences information, including biodiversity, biotechnology, drug discovery, gene therapy, and other topics
CINAHL Complete	Nursing and allied health literature
Cochrane Library	High-quality, independent evidence for practice and healthcare decision making; includes evidence from Cochrane and other systematic reviews, clinical trials, and other evidence reports
ERIC	Abstracts of journal articles, books, research syntheses, conference papers, and technical reports in education (including research and practice), and other education-related materials administered by the U.S. Department of Education
Family and Society Studies Worldwide	Four databases that cover journals and other literature in the areas of family studies and related topics
Health Source: Nursing/Academic Edition	Nursing and other biomedical fields; includes 500+ scholarly full-text journals
MEDLINE/PubMed	Journal articles in life sciences with a concentration on biomedicine and health; includes nursing literature
PsycINFO	Covers psychology and related disciplines including medicine, psychiatry, nursing, education, pharmacology, and other areas
Scopus	Abstract and citation database which includes peer-reviewed titles from international publishers, open-access journals, conference proceedings, trade publications, and quality web sources
Social Work Abstracts	Social work and related journals on topics such as homelessness, AIDS, child and family welfare, aging, substance abuse, and others
Web of Science	Multiple databases with information from journals, books, book series, reports, conferences, and others; includes Science Citation Index Expanded (SCI Expanded), Social Sciences Citation Index (SSCI), Arts & Humanities Citation Index (A&HCI), and Conference Proceedings Citation Indexes, among others; covers medicine, nursing (although limited), sciences, social sciences, and humanities. A Core Collection, Journal Citation Reports, annually compiles SCI Expanded and SSCI to publish impact factors

name, title of the article, journal in which published, publication date and information, and terms or phrases that describe the content of the article. These terms or phrases are important in searching the literature, although sometimes the nurse may begin by searching for particular authors who have done similar work.

Terms for Indexing

MeSH, which stands for Medical Subject Headings, is the NLM's controlled vocabulary thesaurus. A *thesaurus* is a carefully constructed set of terms in a structure that permits searching at different levels of specificity (NLM, 2017b). The MeSH terms describe the content of an article; thus, authors can search using those same terms to locate articles on a topic about which they are writing. In addition to its use for indexing articles from the thousands of journals in the MEDLINE/PubMed database (NLM, 2017c), MeSH is also used for the NLM's database on books, documents, and audiovisual materials.

MeSH consists of a set of terms or subject headings that are arranged in both an alphabetical and a hierarchical structure (NLM, 2017b). It uses a tree structure whereby terms are grouped under broad headings, which then have more specific subject headings under them. For example, the heading "education" is at the most general level of the hierarchical structure; more narrow levels have specific headings such as "baccalaureate nursing education." Exhibit 4.2 provides an example of the MeSH subject headings and levels for the topic "baccalaureate nursing education."

An advantage of using CINAHL is that the subject headings follow MeSH structure but are specific to the terms used by nurses and allied health professionals, making it easy to search for articles on topics most relevant to nurses. For example, if the author is preparing a paper describing a nursing model, there is a major heading "nursing models, theoretical," with many different models and theories listed by both the author's last name and formal name of the model or theory. The search in MEDLINE would be less precise because the

EXHIBIT 4.2

Example of MeSH Subject Headings

Anthropology, Education, Sociology, and Social Phenomena Category
    Education
      Education, Professional
        Education, Nursing
          Education, Nursing, Associate
          Education, Nursing, Baccalaureate
          Education, Nursing, Continuing
          Education, Nursing, Diploma Programs
          Education, Nursing, Graduate
          Nursing Education Research

headings are more general, such as "nursing theory" and "models, nursing." Subject headings in CINAHL Complete are available by clicking the box for "Suggest Subject Terms" above the topic field.

As another example, if the author is writing a paper on a new staffing pattern for maternity nursing, there is a subject heading in CINAHL for obstetric nursing and other headings such as hospital units, alternative birth centers, nursing care, and primary nursing. There are many subheadings for obstetric nursing that might be searched depending on the focus of the paper, for example, administration, economics, manpower, organizations, and trends. Table 4.2 compares the major terms for an article indexed in MEDLINE and the same article in CINAHL.

Keywords

When articles are indexed in a database, an indexer decides what terms or phrases best represent the content in the article, using the MeSH terms or subject headings in CINAHL. This ensures that all articles on a particular subject are indexed in the same way, which is essential when searching for that information.

The indexed terms are often called *keywords* in the author guidelines for journals. Many times, the guidelines ask authors to submit a short list of keywords with the manuscript when it is submitted. These words are then used for indexing the paper, if accepted. To identify keywords for this purpose, the author should go to the thesaurus of the database in which the journal is indexed and select keywords that best describe the content. The indexes are usually listed in the journal on the masthead or table of contents page. If unsure of where the journal is indexed, then the author should use MeSH terms or CINAHL subject headings. A MeSH browser is available at www.nlm .nih.gov/mesh/MBrowser.html. Where authors have access to a proprietary

TABLE 4.2 COMPARISON OF SUBJECT INDEXING IN MEDLINE AND CINAHL FOR A PUBLISHED ARTICLE

MEDLINE MeSH Terms	CINAHL Major Subject Headings
Adolescent	Fatigue
Child	Sleep
Fatigue/etiology*	Cancer patients—In Infancy and Childhood
Female	Childhood neoplasms
Humans	
Male	
Neoplasms/complications*	
Sleep wake disorders/etiology*	

Note: *Major topic of article.

Source: Based on Nunes, M. D. R., Jacob, E., Adlard, K., Secola, R., & Nascimento, L.C. (2015). Fatigue and sleep experiences at home in children and adolescents with cancer. *Oncology Nursing Forum, 42,* 498–506. doi:10.1188/15.ONF.498-506

CINAHL database, subject headings can be searched from the header above the main search page.

SELECTING THE DATABASE

After choosing the topic and narrowing it down, the next step is to select the most appropriate database for the search. For most clinical topics in nursing, the author should use both CINAHL and MEDLINE and also may search the library catalog. Searches on nonclinical topics often will extend beyond these into other relevant databases such as those listed in Table 4.1. If unsure of the databases to use, the author should consult with a librarian or should review potential databases and types of articles indexed in them.

Identifying the databases to search is an important decision for the author because otherwise critical articles may be missed. Even though electronic resources are easy to access and convenient to use, a comprehensive search also may involve a review of books and other sources of information.

SEARCH STRATEGIES

Once the databases are selected, it is wise to become familiar with how they are organized. The author should read through some records of articles indexed in them to gain perspective on the fields and information provided. Many of the databases offer different views of each record. For instance, one view may include the citation and abstract only while another view adds the terms (e.g., MeSH terms or CINAHL subject headings) and other indexing information.

Before beginning the search, the author should:

- Become familiar with the database and the literature indexed in it
- Learn how the database is organized and how to use it for a search
- Review sample records and different views of each record
- Locate the thesaurus and look up the terms that might be used for the search
- Review search strategies and tips included with information about the database
- Learn how to broaden the search (e.g., by using *or*), narrow the search (e.g., by using *and*), exclude terms in a search (e.g., by using *not*), and other ways of making the search more precise
- Learn how to save searches while in progress and at their completion
- Determine how to order documents if available

Selecting Search Terms

After selecting an appropriate database, the author should do a quick search to determine how much literature has been published on the topic. A good way of beginning is to look up in the thesaurus of the database the terms to use.

This preliminary search allows the author to restate the terms if needed before beginning the actual search. The initial search may reveal that the terms chosen are too broad and need to be more specific to produce more manageable results. If the author is planning on writing a manuscript on using videos for teaching patients with asthma, searching all fields in PubMed by using "patient education" yields around 90,000 citations. The term "asthma" results in close to 170,000 citations.

The author needs to choose more specific terms from the thesaurus to best describe the topic and retrieve relevant articles, or modify the search using other techniques. At the other extreme, the terms initially selected for the search may be too specific, thereby excluding some of the relevant literature.

Combining Search Terms

Searches can be modified by choosing other terms to search; by manipulating the fields such as limiting publication dates, looking for selected authors, or restricting the search to certain journals; and by using the Boolean connectors *and*, *or*, and *not*. These connectors indicate how the computer should combine the search terms and treat them in relation to one another. *And* retrieves results that include all the search terms; *or* means that the results must contain at least one of the search terms; and *not* excludes citations with the selected term (National Library of Medicine, 2017a).

In the example of a search of the literature on using videos for teaching patients with asthma, by including *and* between "patient education" *and* "asthma," the list is reduced to several thousand references, but this is still too many to be manageable. Limiting the search to English language produces still fewer citations. Even restricting those to the past 5 years yields more than 500 citations. Depending on the purpose of the paper and literature review, the author might decide to review the citations for the most current year to identify relevant ones. This literature would provide background information on educating patients with asthma, though not necessarily by using videos as the instructional method.

The author may decide to add "video" to the search, which results in 40 citations. Some of the references, though, may not be relevant, and the author can exclude those quickly by reading the abstract of the article. A look in the MeSH database reveals a number of specific terms related to video, which the author could use to focus the search even further. By searching for video recording rather than video, the search yields five citations, which are too few for the complete search.

Modifying the search to "patient education" *and* "video recording" (using quotes) results in more than 400 citations. Limiting the publication date to the past 5 years, adults 19 years and older, and English language, though, produces a more manageable number of citations. Although these articles do not focus on using videos for teaching patients with asthma, they provide background information on how videos have been used for educating patients with other health problems and in varied settings. This literature would contribute to a better understanding of what is known about educating patients by video instruction and as such should be reviewed by the author.

This is a good example of how different terms might be combined to retrieve the best citations for the paper and a manageable number without omitting important publications. The same process is used when searching the CINAHL database. Similar to setting limits in PubMed, such as English language only or by publication date, in CINAHL the author refines the search by including limits such as publication date and age limit. Selecting different "filters" in CINAHL eliminates those documents from the search. The author should allow time to experiment with terms and phrases until the search produces the type of literature needed for preparing the paper.

Searching Relevant Databases

With the search strategy planned, the author is ready to begin the search in all relevant databases. The author should search each target database first to refine the search terms. When the author finds a relevant citation, some databases allow for searching related articles. This feature produces a list of citations to articles that are indexed with the same terms or similar ones.

Reviewing the Literature: How Far Back?

The literature should be reviewed starting with the most recent references and working backward. However, the author should also be alert to landmark or classic studies that might have been published earlier. Determining how far back to review the literature depends on the topic. Reviewing literature published in the past 5 years is usually sufficient for most papers. If there are limited publications in this time frame, then the author can continue to work backward, asking why there are few publications in recent years. It may be a problem with the search terms or may suggest trends in nursing that should be considered in the manuscript. Some areas of nursing practice such as technology are changing so rapidly that articles published even a few years earlier are outdated.

Reviewing Reference Lists

As the citations of articles are retrieved, the author may decide to extend the search using alternate terms or searching different databases. One other technique for ensuring a comprehensive list of relevant references is to review the reference lists of the most relevant articles, chapters, and books to identify other citations that might have been missed. Sometimes the classic references are found there. Co-citation with one or more key articles has proven to be an efficient strategy for identifying relevant research otherwise missed (Cecile,

Janssens, & Gwinn, 2015). The author may also find citations to journals not included in the databases used for the original search or may identify other subject headings that might extend the search.

What Is Enough?

A word of caution: There comes a point at which the author must decide to end the search and begin writing the manuscript. Otherwise the author may delay writing and use valuable time to locate a few more references not even needed for preparation of the paper. In a digital age, producing a comprehensive review of the literature can feel like being blasted by a wall of sound. Badke (2017) recommends a stepwise process to identify the ultimate body of relevant literature:

1. Identify the major players writing on the topic, its history of development, and list of authors supporting each point of view.
2. Use technology to scan those authors' citation counts and related articles.
3. Pay particular attention to articles that discuss key published research.
4. Privilege published review articles from annualreviews.org (e.g., Annual Review of Nursing Research) over those from the grey literature (e.g., Wikipedia).
5. Write the review as a narrative conversation among voices of a chorus, where each part is specified, and agreements, divisions, strengths, and weaknesses of the parts are noted.

Saving Searches

When searching the literature, it is important to save the results of each search for use in preparing the manuscript and to avoid reviewing a citation more than once. Electronic databases allow authors to save the results of searches and individual citations. Searches in PubMed can be "sent" temporarily to the Clipboard, emailed or saved permanently as a text file in My NCBI, or exported into a reference management program called My Bibliography or other citation management software programs. Citations from CINAHL searches can be saved by clicking the "add folder" icon at the right side of each citation, which automatically places them in a temporary session folder; folder contents can then be printed, emailed, saved permanently in My EBSCOhost, or exported to various bibliographic management software programs.

The following guidelines provide strategies for authors to manage the searches in addition to saving the results of each search.

- Keep a record of (a) each database searched, (b) terms used for the search, (c) years searched, (d) other limitations placed on the search (such as English language only), and (e) resulting citations. Mark the date the search was completed. This record should be kept for writing the current paper and for subsequent searches on the same topic.

- Save the search terms in an electronic file, including terms originally chosen and modified after reviewing the thesaurus of the database. Include any synonyms for the original terms.
- Record how search terms were combined with sample citations produced from each combination; this is helpful in later searches about the same topic
- Note the dates of any changes in search terms so there is a running record of the progression of the search.
- If related records were searched, make a note of how these were accessed and the resulting citations.
- Note citations identified from reference lists of articles, chapters, and books, including the original work.
- Record articles, chapters, books, and other materials that will *not* be used for the paper. If another search is done, this will help the author avoid rechecking the same publication.
- Save a copy of publications that will be used in preparing the paper; full-text documents may be accessed during the search. This enables the author to have the material on hand when beginning to write.
- Record *all* citation information, because reference styles differ across journals. This avoids having to recheck a reference when a manuscript is submitted to a journal different than originally planned and using a different style. The author should never rely on memory when it comes to citations.

MANAGING CITATIONS

Considering the large number of citations retrieved in a search, authors need efficient ways of managing and retrieving them for research, writing, and other projects (Hicks, 2014). Frequently, a literature search done for one purpose may be expanded for subsequent papers and projects. Along the same line, a review completed for one need (e.g., a lecture or presentation or grant proposal) provides the basis for manuscripts about that work that is written subsequently. It is important to have a system for keeping track of citations for the current project and for use in the future.

Developing a Personalized System

For limited searches of the literature, the author can copy and paste the bibliographic information and abstract into a word-processing document for use later in writing the manuscript, or can copy and paste the citation into the paper. However, this is not an efficient way to keep track of citations for a comprehensive literature review. Saving citation information in a reference management program is more efficient and promotes easy access to the citations at a later time.

Reference Management Software

Reference management software, also referred to as *citation* or *bibliographic management software,* allows authors to save citations found in a search and access them later. Such software can sort, retrieve, and reformat citations in the style required by the journal. Hicks (2014) recently reported the availability of 30 such products. Reference management software such as EndNote is a proprietary product and can be purchased by authors; some software packages, such as Zotero, are free, and the school or institution library may have free software for use by students and employees. These software programs allow authors to search online bibliographic databases, store thousands of records, organize citations, create reference lists, and collaborate with others. They also enable authors to format manuscripts, complete with in-text citations and references based on the journal's style. If the author decides later to submit the manuscript to another publication that uses a different reference style, the software can reformat the in-text citations and reference list, thus avoiding the need to retype them. Prior to purchasing reference management software, the author should choose a program that is versatile and easy to use, and should first try out any available demo versions. Reference management software can be unreliable and may not format references according to specific author guidelines. Therefore, authors should check their reference lists scrupulously to ensure accuracy and retrievability.

ANALYSIS OF THE LITERATURE

The author has searched the literature and is now ready to read and analyze the materials. In this phase of the literature review, the author organizes the publications into content areas, develops a format for recording comments, and then analyzes each publication.

Organizing Publications

Initially, the author should scan the materials to gain an overview of each publication and its content. This prereading enables the author to develop a perspective on the literature as a whole.

Then the author should group the articles and other materials by topics or content areas that fit together. While the publications are usually organized by topics, they also might be grouped chronologically or by research design and findings. The decision about how to organize them depends on the purpose of the paper and content area. Organizing them into some specified rubric of categories facilitates the literature review because then all the articles and other materials about one category are read at a time. This helps the author gain an understanding of the content and what has already been published about it, and assists in managing an extensive literature review. Reading the materials in categories also is valuable when writing the draft because the documents are grouped as they might be in the paper.

Literature searches related to an extensive research agenda from which numerous manuscripts will emerge require careful preplanning. Havill et al. (2014) described their strategy for managing a search that initially involved more than 67,000 citations. Their strategy included defining concepts; selecting databases, limits, and search terms; and managing retrieval, duplications, and review.

As the articles and other documents are grouped into topics, the author should attempt to identify more specific content areas, *subtopics*, which in turn will help to organize the literature within each topic. For instance, in a literature review on what nursing students learn about patient safety, the authors grouped the literature into three topics: (a) patient safety content in nursing curricula, (b) learning and teaching methods, and (c) outcomes of student learning, the last of which was then grouped into three subtopics: (a) improvement of patient safety competence, (b) sensitivity to their role, and (c) a supportive learning environment (Tella et al., 2014).

Hard copies of articles can be placed in file folders, or portable document formats (PDFs) of the articles can be saved in electronic folders labeled with specific content areas and accompanying notes stored with them. Notes can be added to the folders with important comments about the publications that are critical to the literature review or might be cited in the paper, to keep track of different research methods and subjects, to identify trends in findings of studies or the development of ideas, and to highlight other points.

A similar system should be set up for keeping track of website searches. This system should include documenting how the web search was conducted and recording information about the material accessed at the website, including the author's name, title of the document, name of the website and its URL, publication date, and date accessed. This information is needed for the reference list of the paper should the site be included in it.

Format for Recording Comments

Before reading the publications and other resources, the author should decide how comments about them will be recorded. This facilitates writing the manuscript and saves the author time later. When reading research articles, consistency in note-taking is important in examining patterns across studies and later in synthesizing findings. Care should be taken when recording quotations so that they are accurate and the page number is noted; this will avoid having to return to the reference at the writing stage.

Exhibits 4.3 through 4.6 provide sample formats for recording comments about different types of literature reviewed. Regardless of the format, the key is to develop a consistent method of documenting comments so they are useful later when writing the manuscript.

Guidelines for Analyzing Literature

For some papers, the author's intent in reviewing the literature is to learn what has already been published on the topic to decide whether to proceed with the manuscript. Once this is determined, then authors need to examine critically

EXHIBIT 4.3

Format for Notes About Non-Databased[1] Publications

Reference Information[2]

Articles:

Authors' last and first names,[3] middle initial(s) _____
Title of article _____
Journal name and publication date _____
Volume, issue, and page numbers _____
DOI _____

Books:

Chapter authors' last and first names, middle initial(s) _____
Title of chapter and page numbers _____
Book authors'/editors' last and first names, initial(s) _____
Title of book and subtitle, if any _____
Volume number and title if more than one volume; edition number (other than
   first edition) _____
Place of publication, name of publisher, date of publication _____

Electronic Materials:

Authors' last and first names,[3] middle initial(s) _____
Title of document _____
Name of website _____
URL _____
Date accessed _____

Notes

1. What is the main point of this publication?
2. What are the major content areas included in it?
3. What background information will it contribute to the paper?
4. How might the publication be used for writing the paper?
5. What are strengths of the publication? Weaknesses?
6. Other comments:

_____
_____
_____

[1]Publications that do not report an original research study.
[2]Record complete citation. If using reference management software or have copy of
document, record enough information to match notes with reference.
[3]Some reference formats require first name of lead author.

each publication before using it as a basis for their own research and writing. Not every document retrieved from a literature review may be used for preparing a manuscript. Some papers are not used because of poor quality; other times the content is not relevant to the purpose of the paper.

EXHIBIT 4.4

Format for Notes About Databased Publications: Quantitative Studies

Reference Information[1]

Authors' last and first names,[2] middle initial(s) _____
Title of article _____
Journal name and publication date _____
Volume, issue, and page numbers _____
DOI _____

Purpose/ Research Questions	Design	Sample (and size)	Instruments (Validity and reliability)	Findings	Comments

[1]Record complete citation. If using reference management software or have copy of document, record enough information to match notes with reference.
[2]Some reference formats require first name of lead author.

EXHIBIT 4.5

Format for Notes About Databased Publications: Qualitative Studies

Reference Information[1]

Authors' last and first names,[2] middle initial(s) _____
Title of article _____
Journal name and publication date _____
Volume, issue, and page numbers _____
DOI _____

Type of Qualitative Study	Purpose	Methods	Sample	Findings	Comments

[1]Record complete citation. If using reference management software or have copy of document, record enough information to match notes with reference.
[2]Some reference formats require first name of lead author.

EXHIBIT 4.6

Format for Summarizing Purpose, Methods, and Results of Databased Articles for Literature Review

Author(s)/ Year	Purpose/ Research Questions	Design	Sample (and size)	Instruments (Validity and reliability)	Findings	Comments

Note: Add column for treatment/intervention if relevant.

The questions in Exhibit 4.7 are useful for analyzing nursing literature. These are general questions to guide the critique of articles and other documents for deciding whether or not to include them in a literature review, assessing their strengths and weaknesses, and planning how they might be incorporated as background for a paper.

Research reports need to be critically appraised to determine the quality of study and its applicability to answer the research or clinical questions. Studies have strengths and flaws that should be recognized by the author. Problems may exist in how the study was conceptualized and its rationale. There may be issues with the design—its methods, how variables were measured, the instruments used, procedures, and data analysis. The study might have been well designed, but a small sample size limits generalizing the findings to other groups and settings. There may be problems with the statistical analysis or how themes were identified and labeled in qualitative studies. Exhibit 4.8 provides a guide for critiquing the research literature in nursing.

Synthesizing the Literature

From this critique of individual articles and other documents, the author develops a view of the literature as a whole, an understanding of what is known about the topic, and what still needs to be learned. Synthesis gives authors a sense of how studies and other types of projects relate to one another and a perspective of how their own topic relates to prior work. Synthesizing the research literature is critical because it allows the author to identify relationships among

EXHIBIT 4.7

Guide for Analyzing Nursing Literature

- What is the purpose of the article, or other type of document, and is it consistent with the author's goals for writing the paper?
- What topics and subtopics are addressed in the article, and are these similar to the content planned for the author's own paper?
- Does the introduction state the problem, issue, need, and so forth, and its significance? Can similarities be drawn between these and the author's own work to be discussed in the paper? If not, how will the article be used in the preparation of the paper?
- Is there a clear and coherent rationale for why the article was written? Why is it important?
- If the article describes nursing practice, a project, an innovation, and so forth, is it comprehensive, providing the reader with information essential to using the content in its own setting?
- If the article suggests a change in practice, is evidence provided for this change?
- Is the literature review in the article accurate and up to date? Are primary sources used?
- Does the literature support the discussion and establish the background?
- Does the article make it clear how it fills gaps in the literature? Is this accurate?
- Does the article make significant contributions to the nursing field? Why or why not? What is the relationship between these contributions and the author's goals for writing his or her own paper?
- What concepts, models, and theories are described in the article, and are they relevant to the author's paper? How can these be used to develop the paper?
- Are key terms defined similarly?
- Does the article provide solutions to the problem, issue, need, and so forth, identified in the introduction? Are these solutions applicable to the author's own work?
- If the article evaluated the effectiveness of an intervention, was the methodology sound? Was it described sufficiently to be replicated?
- What is unique about the problem, issue, need, intervention, subjects, setting, and resources described in the article? Are these relevant to the author's own situation? Why or why not?
- What are strengths and weaknesses of the article? How can they be used in preparing the author's own paper?

studies, gaps in the research, and where further study is needed before using the findings in practice.

In developing evidence-based practice, the synthesis of related research provides the evidence to support a change in practice or indicates if further study is needed. If the synthesis provides sufficient evidence to support a change in practice that is also feasible, then nurses have a basis for considering

EXHIBIT 4.8

Guide for Analyzing Research Literature in Nursing

Title

Does it describe the study? Is it informative?

Abstract

Does it emphasize the study's purpose, method, major findings, and conclusions?
Is this a quantitative or qualitative study?

Introduction

Does it state the problem and its significance to nursing?
Does the introduction provide the background and rationale for the study?
What is the purpose of the study, and is it clear?
If a conceptual framework is presented, does it relate to the purpose and describe the concepts underlying the study and their relationships?

Literature Review

Is the literature critically reviewed?
Are strengths and weaknesses of earlier studies presented?
Does the review support the rationale for conducting the study as reported in the article?
Is the literature review up to date?
Are important studies included in it?
Are primary sources used?

Research Questions or Hypotheses

Are the research questions or hypotheses clear, specific, and stated appropriately?
Are variables defined if appropriate?

Design

Is the design consistent with the problem?
What type of design is used?
What are strengths and weaknesses of the design?

Sample

Is the sampling procedure described?
What criteria were used to select the sample?
Is the sample size adequate?
Is the sample representative, and how will this affect generalizing the findings?

Instruments

Are the instruments and other measures described, and are they appropriate?
Are they valid and reliable?

(continued)

EXHIBIT 4.8

Guide for Analyzing Research Literature in Nursing (*continued*)

Data Collection Procedure

Is the procedure clearly described?
Are methods for collecting qualitative data appropriate for the type of study?

Findings

Are the findings interpreted correctly, including any statistical analyses?
Are the statistics appropriate for analyzing the data?
Are the findings presented clearly and in relation to the study questions or hypotheses?
Are the findings presented logically?
Are any tables and figures easy to read, and do they support the text?

Discussion

Are the conclusions based on the study results?
Is the discussion related to the literature, and does it include how the study builds on earlier research?
Are the limitations identified, and could they have been resolved?
Can the findings be generalized and if so, to what populations?
Are there implications for practice, teaching, administration, and others, and are they relevant?

Strengths and Weaknesses

Overall, what are the study's major strengths and weaknesses?

a change in practice. Chapter 6 expands on synthesizing literature for evidence-based practice manuscripts.

When the publications have been reviewed and analyzed, the author's task is to integrate them and present a summary in the manuscript. First, the author returns to the original purpose of completing the literature review. Was the goal to develop the background for a research study, answer questions about clinical practice, use evidence in practice, develop new projects, or make other decisions? Was the literature review conducted for a paper in a course, thesis, dissertation, grant, or project in which the nurse may be involved? Was the purpose of the literature review to decide whether to write the manuscript, and if so how it should be developed to fill gaps in the literature? The synthesis should meet the original goals for reviewing the literature.

Second, for each topic and subtopic, the author should identify similarities and common points of view in the publications. For research reports, the author should indicate when findings are consistent across studies and when they are different and then propose explanations for those differences. For instance, were the studies done at varied points in time? Were there differences in methodologies and subjects that might account for the discrepancies in findings? Were different instruments used, or were there variations in statistical analyses that might account for the lack of consistency in the results?

Third, the author should recognize gaps in the literature. If so, the author can make a case for how the paper fills these gaps and contributes new and critical knowledge to nursing.

WRITING THE LITERATURE REVIEW

The first step in writing the literature review is to consider the audience of the journal to which the manuscript will be submitted. If writing the literature review for a research journal, it should be comprehensive, each research study should be critiqued as described earlier, and research findings should be synthesized, noting where further study is indicated. To the extent that cited material is relevant to the author's current manuscript, the author should identify gaps in the evidence base, tests of theory, the need for replication, and how methods differ.

For nonresearch journals, the literature review will not have the same depth, nor will the readers expect this same level of critique. Rather, the literature review is used to present the topic and why it is important for readers. The literature may be integrated throughout the paper rather than discussed in a separate section. Once again, the importance of identifying possible journals prior to writing the paper is apparent when deciding on how to present the literature review.

Introductory Statement

The literature review should begin with an introductory statement about what literature will be presented and why it is important to the problem or purpose of the paper. This introductory statement should not be too broad.

In the example that follows, the first introductory statement to the literature review is too broad; it does not tell the reader what types of literature will be discussed. The methods for assessing critical thinking could be standardized tests, strategies used in classroom instruction, or methods for evaluating cognitive skills in clinical practice. The revised statement indicates more specifically that the literature reviewed is on methods for assessing the critical thinking of nursing students in clinical practice.

Too Broad

Critical thinking is an important competency for nursing students to develop. Varied methods can be used for assessing critical thinking.

Specific and Focused

Five methods used to assess nursing students' critical thinking skills within the context of clinical practice include: (a) observation of students in practice,

(b) higher level questions, (c) postclinical conferences, (d) case method, and (e) written assignments. The literature is reviewed on each of these methods.

Important Studies

In writing the literature review, the author should highlight important studies and describe why they are significant. Classic studies should be noted and some discussion provided as to how they contributed to development of the topic. These papers are frequently pivotal works and can be used in the review to show the progression of research in an area. Other than these classic works, however, the literature review should describe current publications, within the past 5 years.

Lack of Publications on Topic

At times the author may not locate any relevant literature about a topic. If few or no studies can be found, the authors should explain the dearth by indicating the databases that were searched, the years searched, and other limits applied in the search. Details on the search strategy provide support for the statement that no studies were found in the literature review.

Grouping Publications

In the synthesis of the literature, authors should group studies, identify similarities and differences across them, and describe how individual studies relate to one another, rather than simply listing and discussing each publication without showing their relation to each other. The following example by Nunes, Jacob, Adlard, Secola, and Nascimento (2015, p. 498) demonstrates this principle.

> Fatigue is often characterized by physical symptoms, including lack of energy, decreased physical ability, and feelings of tiredness. It may be experienced before the initiation of treatment (Goedendorp, Gielissen, Verhagen, Peters, & Bleijenberg, 2008), during cancer treatment (Hinds, Hockenberry, Gattuso, et al., 2007; Perdikaris et al., 2009; Purcell et al., 2010), in disease-free survivors (Andrykowski, Donovan, Laronga, & Jacobsen, 2010; Bower et al., 2006), and at the end of life (Murphy, Alexander, & Stone, 2006; Teunissen et al., 2007; Ullrich et al., 2010).

There are nine different articles cited in this paragraph of the literature review, but rather than discussing each one separately, they are integrated in the review.

When findings are inconsistent, however, the author should report studies separately so the discrepancies are clear to readers. For instance, in the first example that follows it is not clear which studies had a low return rate of 25% and which had the higher rate of return (65%) after sending reminder postcards.

Original

Previous studies have shown a return rate of surveys ranging from 25% to 65% after clinic staff sent postcards reminding patients to send back their surveys (Adams, 2008; Gabow, 2009; Smith & Jones, 2014).

Revised

Previous studies have shown that sending reminder postcards from clinic staff to patients results in survey return rates ranging from 25% (Adams, 2008; Smith & Jones, 2014) to 65% (Gabow, 2009).

Presentation of Search Strategy

The author can indicate the search terms and how they were combined in the text of the paper or can prepare a table to display this. Exhibit 4.9 illustrates how to describe the search terms in the text versus presenting them in a table.

Some types of studies require a standardized search presentation format, which assists readers to evaluate findings across published studies. One such standard is the Preferred Reporting Items for Systematic Reviews and Meta-Analyses (PRISMA), which specifies the minimum set of items that should be reported when publishing outcomes of randomized trials and evaluations of interventions. The format shows succinctly the number of articles that were searched, discarded, and presented. Chapter 6 discusses PRISMA in greater detail.

EXHIBIT 4.9

Example of Search Strategy Described in Text and Presented in Table

Text

A combination of keywords and controlled vocabulary were used for three separate concepts: students, evaluations, and health professions education. Synonyms and word variations were included; for example, the student concept was searched with the Boolean operator "or" for student, students, learner, and learners. The concept for evaluations included the related terms feedback, surveys, and assessment. The specific health professions searched included medicine, nursing, dentistry, and pharmacy. The search was limited to the English language and publication dates of 2010 to 2016. Editorials, letters, case reports, and comments were not included.

Table

Set #	
1	"Students"[Mesh] OR student[tiab] OR students[tiab] OR learner[tiab] OR learners[tiab]

(continued)

EXHIBIT 4.9

Example of Search Strategy Described in Text and Presented in Table (*continued*)

Set #	
2	(("Curriculum"[Mesh:NoExp] OR "Teaching"[Mesh:NoExp]) AND (evaluation[tiab] OR evaluations[tiab])) OR "course evaluation"[tiab] OR "course evaluations" [tiab] OR "teacher evaluation"[tiab] OR "teacher evaluations"[tiab] OR "student evaluation"[tiab] OR "student evaluations"[tiab] OR "student survey"[tiab] OR "student surveys"[tiab] OR "course assessment"[tiab] OR "course assessments"[tiab] OR "student feedback"[tiab] OR "effective teaching"[tiab] OR "teaching effectiveness"[tiab] OR "course survey"[tiab] OR "course surveys"[tiab]
3	"Schools, Medical"[Mesh] OR "Schools, Nursing"[Mesh] OR "Schools, Dental"[Mesh] OR "Schools, Pharmacy"[Mesh] OR "medical school"[tiab] OR "medical schools"[tiab] OR "nursing school"[tiab] OR "nursing schools"[tiab] OR "dental school"[tiab] OR "dental schools"[tiab] OR "pharmacy school"[tiab] OR "pharmacy schools"[tiab] OR "Education, Dental"[Mesh] OR "dental education"[tiab] OR "Education, Medical"[Mesh] OR "medical education"[tiab] OR "Education, Nursing"[Mesh] OR "nursing education"[tiab] OR "Education, Pharmacy"[Mesh:NoExp] OR "pharmacy education"[tiab]
4	#1 AND #2 AND #3
5	#6 NOT (Editorial[pt] OR Letter[pt] OR Case Reports[pt] OR Comment[pt])
6	#7 Filters: English, 2010-
	Key: [Mesh]: Medical Subject Headings; [Mesh:NoExp]: Mesh heading; does not include narrower terms in tree; [tiab]: Title/Abstract fields; [pt]: Publication Type

Note: Search Strategy for PubMed

Accuracy of References

Meticulous citations are crucial for building the scientific base of a field of knowledge. The citations in a manuscript reflect the quality and thoroughness of the author's work and allow others to retrieve documents cited in the paper, as well as to assess the value of the author's work (Hicks, 2014). Errors in authors' names, article title, journal name, page numbers, and publication date may inhibit the retrieval of the publication and violate the rights of the original authors. Finally, careful referencing protects the author from plagiarizing previous work, which violates professional publishing standards (American Psychological Association [APA], 2010). It is important to be accurate with citations in the literature review, where many publications are often cited, and on the reference list. Each reference should be checked carefully for errors.

Reference management software does not guarantee accuracy of citations. There may be errors because of data entry mistakes made by the author, limitations of the software, or discrepancies between the software and author guidelines of a journal (Hicks, 2014).

PERMISSIONS

Copyright is a form of legal protection for authors, which prevents others from copying their original work. The copyright is held initially by the manuscript's author or coauthors, but the copyright typically transfers to the publisher either at the time the manuscript is submitted or when it is accepted. Publishers usually require assignment of the copyright to them, so they in turn may publish the article and distribute it in different forms. When authors are reviewing the literature and deciding to include previously published text, tables, figures, or other illustrations in their manuscripts, they need permission from the copyright holder, for example, the publisher of the journal or book, to adapt or reproduce the copyrighted materials. Copyright is described in more detail in Chapter 16.

Permission should be obtained for quotes that extend for a few paragraphs. The length of the quoted material should not diminish the "value of the original work" (AMA, 2007, p. 198). Entire tables, figures, and illustrations may not be reproduced without permission. This includes use of a table, figure, or other type of graphic in a paper prepared for a course. Using one or two sentences from a table is acceptable if the original source is referenced, but reprinting the entire table is not acceptable without copyright permission.

The request for this permission should be done early in the writing process to avoid delays in the submission and publication of the manuscript. Although permission to reprint is required before the article is published, some journal editors may request letters indicating permission has been received when the manuscript is submitted for review.

For journal articles, which are usually copyrighted by the publisher of the journal, the author requests permission from the publisher to reproduce any major selection of text, table, figure, or other illustration in the manuscript. Information on how to obtain this permission is included in the masthead of the journal, which lists the editor, staff, and other journal details, or on the information for authors page. This information is also found at the journal's website, and many journals have links to the Copyright Clearance Center to facilitate obtaining permission to adapt and reprint materials. For a book, the copyright holder is specified on the page following the title page. When the authors of the original works hold the copyright, they would grant permission to reprint their material and would be contacted directly.

The Copyright Clearance Center (www.copyright.com) manages the rights for many copyrighted works, for publishers, and for authors. At the website authors can purchase permission to adapt, reproduce, and distribute published materials, and post them to a website (Copyright Clearance Center, 2017).

EXHIBIT 4.10

Sample Permission Credit Lines

Journal

From Turmell, J.W., Coke, L., Catinella, R., Hosford, T., and Majeski, A. (2017). Alarm fatigue: Use of an evidence-based alarm management strategy (p. 51). *Journal of Nursing Care Quality, 32,* 47-54. Copyright 2017 by Wolters Kluwer Health. Reprinted with permission.

Book

From Bonnel, W., & Smith K. V. (2014). *Proposal writing for nursing capstones and clinical projects* (p. 29). New York, NY: Springer Publishing. Copyright 2014 by Springer Publishing. Adapted with permission.

As part of the permission to adapt and use copyrighted materials, copyright holders will often specify how the credit line should be written and also may require certain conditions when granting permission to use the material. Examples of credit lines are in Exhibit 4.10. In all situations, authors need to include a credit line with copyrighted materials and the copyright notice if applicable (AMA, 2007).

Permissions Letter

In most instances, requests for permission to reprint from journals can be done online. An electronic form is available from the publisher, through a service such as Rightslink that is linked with the article at the website of the journal from which the author is requesting permission, or at the Copyright Clearance Center using the Purchase Permissions feature. Requests for permission to reprint portions of a book, chapter, or website require a written request from the publisher. An example of a letter requesting permission to reprint copyrighted nonperiodical materials is in Exhibit 4.11. Authors should check at the publisher's website for a form to submit when requesting permission to reprint copyrighted nonperiodical materials. In the request, whether done electronically or by hard copy, the author should include the complete citation of the original work; a description of the material to be reprinted, such as the exact portion of the text, table, figure, or other illustration, including the page number(s) where it can be found; publication in which the material will be used; and how the original work would be adapted, if at all. For books, the publisher typically provides a permission form for the author to use for requesting permissions to reprint.

Authors will likely incur a fee, which may be significant, when requesting copyright permission. When seeking permission to reprint materials they have written, however, the fee may be waived. Another possibility is that permission to reprint may not be granted.

EXHIBIT 4.11

Sample Letter Requesting Permission to Reproduce Copyrighted Nonperiodical Materials

Permissions Department
Publisher
Mailing or Email Address

Dear Permissions Department:

I am requesting permission to include the figure Components of a Typical Graph in a manuscript I am writing for submission to *The Nurse Practitioner* or a similar scholarly journal. The figure was in: Lang, T. A. (2010). *How to write, publish, & present in the health sciences: A guide for clinicians and laboratory researchers.* Philadelphia, PA: American College of Physicians, p. 90.

Thank you for your consideration of this request.

Sincerely,
[author's name, credentials,
email and complete mailing address,
fax number, and other contact information]

Photographs

Patients, nurses, and other people shown in photographs need to provide written permission for reproduction of the photograph in the manuscript. In the letter asking their permission, the author should include the title of the manuscript, possible journal in which it might be published, and when the photograph was taken. The subject in the photograph must sign a release form that the author, in turn, submits with the manuscript.

PLAGIARISM

When the literature review is completed and authors begin writing the paper, they must be cautious to give proper credit to their sources. The exact words of another source should be placed in quotation marks. *Paraphrasing* refers to summarizing content, rearranging the order of words, or changing some words from source material (APA, 2010). Many writers, especially students, believe that plagiarism refers only to failure to indicate and cite properly a verbatim quotation. However, any time authors present the ideas of another as their own, without giving proper credit to their source, plagiarism has occurred.

Plagiarism can be considered a crime of theft of intellectual property. It is not a victimless crime; plagiarism can harm the author of the original source material, the scientific community, and the plagiarizer.

Authors can avoid plagiarism through adequate and appropriate documentation, but at times, this is not easy to do. All authors absorb and use the ideas of others, and a writer may forget the original source of an idea or even that there was an original source. However, unless authors specifically acknowledge the sources of ideas, they claim credit for them (AMA, 2007). Strategies to help avoid plagiarism are careful note-taking, recordkeeping, and documentation of data and sources (AMA, 2007, p. 158). Authors should not cut and paste from an original source, a website, or an electronic document. Over the extended time during which manuscripts are prepared, it may be difficult to remember that the text was from another source and not one's own ideas.

Can an author plagiarize unintentionally? In some cases, it is unclear whether the author lacked knowledge about proper documentation of sources or whether intentional plagiarism occurred, especially with students. Skillful paraphrasing without plagiarizing requires the writer to understand and synthesize the ideas and information from the original sources. Reading the materials, thinking about them before writing, and taking notes can all help authors to develop their own ideas about a topic. Exhibit 4.12 presents seven of Roig's (2015, pp. 6–9, 12) guidelines for preventing plagiarism when writing for publication.

EXHIBIT 4.12

Guidelines for Preventing Plagiarism When Writing for Publication

1. "An ethical writer ALWAYS acknowledges the contributions of others to his/her work.
2. "Any verbatim text taken from another source must be enclosed in quotation marks and be accompanied by a citation to indicate its origin.
3. "When we summarize others' work, we use our own words to condense and convey others' contributions in a shorter version of the original.
4. "When paraphrasing others' work, not only must we use our own words, but we must also use our own syntactical structure.
5. "Whether we are paraphrasing or summarizing we must always identify the source of our information.
6. "When paraphrasing and/or summarizing others' work we must ensure that we are reproducing the exact meaning of the other author's ideas or facts and that we are doing so using our own words and sentence structure.
7. "In order to be able to make the types of substantial modifications to the original text that result in a proper paraphrase, one must have a thorough command of the language and a good understanding of the ideas and terminology being used."

Source: From Roig, M. (2015). *Avoiding plagiarism, self-plagiarism, and other questionable writing practices: A guide to ethical writing.* Retrieved from https://ori.hhs.gov/avoiding-plagiarism-self-plagiarism-and-other-questionable-writing-practices-guide-ethical-writing. Reprinted by permission.

Copying one's own previously published material without proper citation of the source is also an example of plagiarism. Remember that once a publisher holds a copyright for published material, that material cannot be reused without permission. Even short verbatim quotes from an author's previously published content should be referenced back to the original source, and the author should seek permission from the copyright holder to reproduce lengthier portions.

SUMMARY

A literature review is a critique and summary of current knowledge about a topic, for research and for use in clinical practice, teaching, administration, and other areas of nursing. Literature reviews are conducted when writing a paper for a course, a thesis, a dissertation, grants, projects in which the nurse may be involved, and manuscripts.

There are three main purposes of reviewing the literature. The first purpose is to describe what is already known about a topic. The literature review provides the background needed for developing a research study, answering questions about clinical practice, developing new projects and initiatives, and making other decisions. It reveals existing knowledge about a topic and related areas. The second purpose is to identify gaps in knowledge and where questions still remain. The third purpose is to determine how the proposed study, project, innovation, or paper will contribute new knowledge to nursing.

The author first identifies the topic of the paper and then searches the literature.

There are varied bibliographic databases for conducting literature searches in nursing. The two databases that are most useful for nurse authors are MEDLINE and CINAHL.

Each article in a bibliographic database is indexed similarly. It has a single record with specific information about that article. The record has fields that include information such as the author's name, title of the article, journal in which published, publication date and information, and terms or phrases that describe the content of the article. MeSH is used for MEDLINE indexing and other databases produced by the NLM. CINAHL has its own controlled vocabulary thesaurus based on MeSH but with additional terms for nursing and allied health literature.

After choosing the topic and narrowing it down, the next step is to select the most appropriate database for the search. The author does a preliminary search to evaluate the effectiveness of the search terms. Searches can be modified by choosing other terms to search; by manipulating the fields such as limiting publication dates; and by using the Boolean connectors *and*, *or*, and *not*. These connectors indicate how the search terms should be combined and used in relation to one another.

The literature should be reviewed starting with the most recent references and working backward. Reviewing literature published in the past 5 years is usually sufficient for most papers. Reference lists of articles, chapters, and books also can be examined to identify citations that might have been missed.

The author should keep a record of (a) each database searched, (b) terms used for the search, (c) years searched, (d) limitations placed on the search, and (e) resulting citations. Considering the large number of references retrieved in a search, authors need efficient ways of managing these references and retrieving them for research, writing, and other projects, such as with reference management software.

Authors need to examine critically each publication before using it as a basis for their own research and writing, and for decisions about clinical practice. Not every document retrieved from a literature review may be used for preparing a manuscript. Some papers are not used because of poor quality; other times the content is not relevant to the purpose of the paper. When multiple studies exist in an area, authors should synthesize the literature, noting similarities and consistent findings across studies. The critical appraisal of research studies and synthesis of findings are essential for evidence-based practice.

In writing the literature review, authors should identify explicitly how their paper closes a gap in the literature and extends earlier work. They should emphasize how their research replicates an important study and contributes new knowledge to nursing.

When authors are reviewing the literature and deciding on previously published text, tables, figures, and other illustrations to include in their papers, they need permission from the copyright holder, for example, the publisher of the journal or book, to adapt or reproduce the copyrighted material in their manuscript. This is true even for the author's own article, chapter, or book because the copyright was transferred to and is then held by the publisher. Patients, nurses, and other people shown in photographs need to provide written permission for reproduction of the photograph in the manuscript. A general principle is that, whenever identifying information about patients, other individuals, and institutions is provided in a manuscript, they or their representatives should review the manuscript and give written consent.

Plagiarism is presenting the ideas of another as one's own, without giving proper credit to the source. Many writers, especially students, believe that plagiarism refers only to failure to indicate and cite properly a verbatim quotation, but plagiarism also can involve paraphrasing without citing the source of the ideas. Careful note taking and documenting sources, and using multiple sources of information, are strategies to avoid plagiarism.

REFERENCES

American Medical Association. (2007). *AMA manual of style: A guide for authors and editors* (10th ed.). New York, NY: Oxford Press.

American Psychological Association. (2010). *Publication manual of the American Psychological Association* (6th ed.). Washington, DC: Author.

Badke, W. (2017). The literature review in a digital age. *Online Searcher*, 41(3), 57–59. Retrieved from http://www.infotoday.com/OnlineSearcher/Issue/7096-May-June-2017.shtml

Cecile, A., Janssens, J. W., & Gwinn, M. (2015). Novel citation-based search method for scientific literature: Application to meta-analyses. *BMC Medical Research Methodology*, 15, 1–11. doi:10.1186/s12874-015-0077-z

Copyright Clearance Center. (2017). Get permissions. Retrieved from http://www.copyright.com/content/cc3/en/toolbar/getPermission.html

Elton B. Stephens Company. (2017). CINAHL® Complete. Retrieved from https://www.ebscohost.com/nursing/products/cinahl-databases/cinahl-complete

Godin, K., Stapleton, J., Kirkpatrick, S. I., Hanning, R. M., & Leatherdale, S. T. (2015). Applying systematic review search methods to the grey literature: A case study examining guidelines for school-based breakfast programs in Canada. *Systematic Reviews*, 4, 138. doi:10.1186/s13643-015-0125-0

Havill, N. L., Leeman, J., Shaw-Kokot, J., Knafl, K., Crandell, J., & Sandelowski, M. (2014). Managing large-volume literature searches in research synthesis studies. *Nursing Outlook*, 62(2), 112–118. doi:10.1016/j.outlook.2013.11.002

Hartling, L., Featherstone, R., Nuspl, M., Shave, K., Dryden, D. M., & Vandermeer, B. (2017). Grey literature in systematic reviews: A cross-sectional study of the contribution of non-English reports, unpublished studies and dissertations to the results of meta-analyses in child-relevant reviews. *BMC Medical Research Methodology*, 17, 64. doi:10.1186/s12874-017-0347-z

Hicks, R. (2014). I write, therefore, I cite: Why and how tools can help the author. *Journal of the American Association of Nurse Practitioners*, 26, 177–178. doi:10.1002/2327-6924.12115

Munn, Z., Porritt, K., Lockwood, C., Aromataris, E., & Pearson A. (2014). Establishing confidence in the output of qualitative research synthesis: The ConQual approach. *BMC Medical Research Methodology*, 14, 1–11. doi:10.1186/1471-2288-14-108

National Library of Medicine. (2017a). Fact sheet MEDLINE®. Retrieved from http://www.nlm.nih.gov/pubs/factsheets/jsel.html

National Library of Medicine. (2017b). Fact sheet Medical Subject Headings (MeSH®). Retrieved from http://www.nlm.nih.gov/pubs/factsheets/mesh.html

National Library of Medicine. (2017c). NLM databases & electronic resources. Retrieved from http://wwwcf2.nlm.nih.gov/nlm_eresources/eresources/search_database.cfm

Nunes, M. D. R., Jacob, E., Adlard, K., Secola, R., & Nascimento, L. C. (2015). Fatigue and sleep experiences at home in children and adolescents with cancer. *Oncology Nursing Forum*, 42, 498–506. doi:10.1188/15.ONF.498-506

PubMed Help. (2017). Bethesda (MD): National Center for Biotechnology Information (US); 2005. Retrieved from https://www.ncbi.nlm.nih.gov/books/NBK3830

Roig, M. (2015). Avoiding plagiarism, self-plagiarism, and other questionable writing practices: A guide to ethical writing. Retrieved from https://ori.hhs.gov/avoiding-plagiarism-self-plagiarism-and-other-questionable-writing-practices-guide-ethical-writing

Tella, S., Liukka, M., Jamookeeah, D., Smith, N. J., Partanen, P., & Turunen, H. (2014). What do nursing students learn about patient safety? An integrative literature review. *Journal of Nursing Education*, 53(1), 7–13. doi:10.3928/01484834-20131209-04

WRITING RESEARCH, EVIDENCE-BASED PRACTICE, QUALITY IMPROVEMENT, AND CLINICAL PRACTICE ARTICLES

WRITING RESEARCH ARTICLES

Research papers present the findings of quantitative and qualitative research based on original data. The chapter begins with a discussion of how to report research using the conventional format of an introduction and literature review; a methods section, including design and sample, measurements, and analytic strategy; a results section; and a discussion. This basic structure of research articles is known as IMRAD, that is, Introduction, Methods, Results, and Discussion. The chapter concludes by describing both pitfalls to avoid when reporting research findings and strategies to adopt when revising academic papers as research manuscripts.

Research articles may be written for journals that publish mainly research articles, or they may be prepared for clinical journals that report research in that practice specialty. Many journals publish research articles as well as other types. When developing research papers for clinical journals, the IMRAD format may or may not be explicitly required, but can serve as a formal or informal framework for the author to use in deciding how to organize the content.

This chapter does not explain the research process or different types of research that might be reported in the literature. Instead, it offers general principles for writing research manuscripts. As formatting requirements of each journal differ, the author will need to adapt these general principles for the type of journal to which the manuscript is submitted.

RESEARCH DISSEMINATION

Research projects are not complete until the findings are communicated to others. All too often nurses conduct important research studies but fail to disseminate the results of their work. Some nurses are not prepared for their role as authors and are unsure how to proceed; others may believe that their work does not warrant publication. However, findings based on rigorous research should be communicated to others, regardless of whether the findings were anticipated or not. Findings that do not support the hypothesis may be as important as ones that do, for other researchers and clinicians need this information as they plan studies and make decisions about clinical practice.

There are many reasons for disseminating the results of research in the literature. First, nursing research is of little value if the findings are not made available
for use by clinicians and others who need the research results for their work.
Nurses who conduct research are responsible for reporting the results in journals
that are read by nurses who can then use the information in their practice, teaching, management, and other roles. Effective patient care and service delivery
depend on the dissemination of findings from rigorous research (Hicks, 2014).

Second, by publishing the findings of research, nurses advance the body of
knowledge of nursing and contribute to the scientific basis of nursing practice.
Research is essential for professional practice because it generates the knowledge that defines that practice.

Third, communicating the findings of research promotes the critique
and replication of studies (American Medical Association [AMA], 2007).
Researchers can build studies on one another, extending and refining what is
known about the topic and enabling nurses to test the findings in other groups
and settings. By reading research reports, nurses can generate new questions
that lead to further studies.

Fourth, nurses need research data to establish evidence for their clinical
decisions and interventions. Evidence-based practice (EBP) involves the use
of the best evidence available for making decisions about patient care (Tweed,
D'Lima, Schneider, & Zimbro, 2016). This evidence includes clinically relevant
research combined with individual clinical expertise. Summarizing research
for EBP recommendations is described in Chapter 6.

Fifth, disseminating the findings of research is essential for research utili-
zation, that is, the process by which knowledge from research is incorporated
into clinical practice (Benton, 2014). Although there are varied research utiliza-
tion and EBP models, they all involve the critique of research findings and subsequent use of those findings in practice. Improving the quality of care requires
a commitment to provide nursing care that is based on sound research. Writing
a manuscript on a review of research findings, such as a systematic review
paper, and use of research for EBP are discussed in Chapter 6.

Sixth, dissemination of findings from studies supported by federal funding is the law. As of March 9, 2009, researchers supported by the National
Institutes of Health must submit an electronic copy of their final peer-reviewed
manuscripts to the National Library of Medicine's PubMed Central, so that
their work is available to the public within 12 months of publication, consistent
with copyright law (U.S. Department of Health and Human Services, 2017b).
Compliance is a condition of the award of funding. Copyright law regarding
scientific publications is discussed in Chapter 16.

RESEARCH REPORTS

Writing about research is similar to making a reasoned argument. The author's
goal is to demonstrate to readers that the study was important to do and follows logically from previous research, the methods were appropriate for

examining the problem, the findings are valid, and the implications for practice are consistent with the data. The research report summarizes the study and its purpose, methods, and findings. This report is the document that presents key aspects of the study for readers. Research reports vary in length, ranging from publishable manuscripts that are about 15 to 20 pages to master's theses and doctoral dissertations that are significantly longer and may range from 50 to 200 pages, depending on the study.

Writing Research Papers for Research Journals

The format for the research report follows the same format as the research process. It begins with an introduction and the purpose of the study, proceeds through a description of its methods and results, and concludes with a discussion of the findings. Research journals require the author to explain each component of the research study in sufficient detail for others to understand the problem, methods, and findings, and to replicate the study, if desired.

For example, Ngangana, Davis, Burns, McGee, and Montgomery (2016) used a systems model to study the perception of stressors among adult siblings who were sharing parental caregiving in the community. Their article was organized using the traditional format of a research report: introduction, method, results (called The Study and Findings, respectively, by this journal), and discussion. In the introduction, the researchers presented background material on the epidemiologic importance of this topic and gaps in the evidence base; in the method section, they described the study's aims, design, data collection, ethical considerations, and analytic strategy; and in the results, they presented a description of the sample and tests of relationships in the study data, using statistical analyses, followed by a discussion of the lessons learned from the results of their study. The article described in detail each component of the original research study.

WRITING RESEARCH PAPERS FOR SPECIALTY JOURNALS

The author may decide to prepare the research report for a journal that publishes research in a clinical specialty, for nurse educators, or nurses practicing in specialty roles in management, law, or other fields. In research reports in specialty journals, authors should be guided by the aims and scope of the journal and its guidelines for authors. In specialty journals, the literature review may be similarly or less extensive than for a research journal, and there may be similar or less discussion on the research methods themselves, as readers of specialty journals may not be interested in elaborate discussions of the statistical analyses used in the study nor have the background to understand this discussion. Most specialty journals focus on how the research findings might guide practice or work in specific nursing roles. For example, *Oncology Nursing Forum* requires headings for "implications for nursing" and "knowledge translation" in all abstracts and text. Such manuscripts should emphasize the practical implications of the study. As discussed in Chapters 1 and 2, the author needs to gear the paper to the journal and its stated audience.

In *Pediatric Nursing*, for example, Benjamin, Hendrix, and Woody (2016) described a vibration therapy intervention by nurses for children receiving immunizations. In a brief introduction, the authors reviewed the epidemiology of and barriers to vaccinations and gaps in the evaluation of clinically and cost-effective therapies to overcome such barriers. The literature review focused on five currently used therapies and concluded with a statement of the purpose of the study: "to determine whether vibration therapy without cold analgesia reduces pain among children aged 2 months to 7 years undergoing routine vaccination at an urban clinic, compared to children receiving standard vaccination treatment" (pp. 125–126). The methods section then described in detail the study design, subject, vibration instrument, vaccinations, and outcome measures. These were followed by a results section that focused on statistical differences between the groups, as well as inter-rater reliability scores. The discussion reflected on gate-control theory as a possible explanation of the findings, before reviewing limitations and recommendations for further research. Although the research format is apparent in the article, the emphasis was placed on assisting readers to understand precisely what was entailed in the intervention, how it was received by participants, and how problems encountered might be addressed in future trials.

Research projects that assess students or educational initiatives are subject to the same formatting guidelines as studies of patients, families, and communities. If the author is targeting an education journal that is research oriented, then a full description of background literature, research methodology, and implications for future research should be provided in IMRAD format. If, on the other hand, the target audience is primarily nurse educators who will be interested in the implications of the research findings for curriculum development, student support, or other applications, then the author should focus the manuscript on these elements.

Writing Randomized Controlled Trial Papers

Authors of randomized controlled trials (RCTs) are subject to stringent rules for publishing their studies. The rules were designed for reports of simple two-group parallel-arm studies. The rationale for these rules is that RCTs, which represent the most rigorous testing of interventions prior to widespread implementation in human populations, must be described with complete transparency in order to avoid biased, unreliable, or irrelevant interpretation of the results.

To this end, an international body of scientists and editors developed the **Consolidated Standards of Reporting Trials** (CONSORT) statement (Moher et al., 2010). The CONSORT statement includes a checklist of elements to include in the title, abstract, introduction, methods, results, and discussions sections of the manuscript. For example, the title should identify the study as a randomized trial, and the manuscript should include a flow diagram that presents how many participants passed through the RCT in each of four stages: enrollment, allocation, follow-up, and analysis. The template for the CONSORT flow diagram, shown in Figure 13.2, allows readers to judge whether the analysis was performed based on intention-to-treat. Newman et al. (2015) used a CONSORT flow diagram to show readers how many admissions to a neonatal intensive care unit ($n = 377$) were eligible for a study of extremely low-birth-weight neonates ($n = 78$) to be randomized to one of three continuous positive airway pressure interventions. The intent of the CONSORT checklist and diagram is to improve reporting of RCTs in the scientific literature, but the checklist and diagram may be more broadly useful for authors of all intervention studies when choosing elements to present to readers. Studies of nursing journals demonstrate the need for more widespread use of CONSORT in nursing journals (Jull & Aye, 2015; Oermann et al., 2018).

Writing About Other Types of Research Projects

Research published in the scientific literature does not have to involve complex studies with large samples. There are many studies by nurses on a smaller scale that are important for others to know about. These include studies of small patient groups or communities to which the nurse has ready access, including single case studies. The knowledge gained from research questions or program evaluations done by nurses of interventions and new initiatives for patient populations, for instance, may be important for advancing nursing practice and answering questions about one's own clinical practice. Reports of clinical studies conducted in one setting may guide replication research by nurses in another setting, which expands general understanding about care of patients across settings. Researchers can use findings from these smaller studies to design larger ones that develop general nursing knowledge.

An example of a research report of a pilot study was published by Kapu, Wheeler, and Lee (2014). They tested the impact of adding an acute care nurse practitioner (ACNP) to medical and surgical rapid response teams at Vanderbilt Hospital to avoid delays in implementing prescription management protocols for patients whose condition had deteriorated suddenly. The article included a brief case study of an 80-year-old patient whose care was dramatically improved by the availability of an ACNP in this role. Although ACNPs were added to only two units in one hospital over 1 year, this limited study made an important contribution to practice by building on previous work reported nationally and at Vanderbilt in response to Joint Commission mandates.

There are other situations in which the author initiated a research study but because of problems in implementation was not able to carry it out as planned. In developing a manuscript about the study, the author might develop a manuscript on the difficulties encountered in conducting this type of study and possible solutions. Articles that describe research methods are described in Chapter 8.

ELEMENTS OF A RESEARCH REPORT

Title

Every research paper needs a title. The title should be carefully worded to capture the objective of the study, as it is used for indexing and searches. Research shows that references to published papers correlate positively with the length of their titles and the use of colons (Hudson, 2016).

The intent of the title is to inform readers exactly what information will be presented in the paper and its relevance to the content discipline (Jirge, 2017). Titles should be specific (AMA, 2007), using keywords that represent the content of the article. Titles are compiled in reference works; therefore, authors should select keywords for the title based on the words that their target audience will find the most informative. Authors should avoid overly general titles that omit key elements of the population that was studied.

Titles should be "fully explanatory while standing alone" (American Psychological Association [APA], 2010, p. 23). The title should be easily shortened for a running head. One title may be written, or it may be developed with a subtitle that provides supplementary information about the paper. Subtitles should not be used to provide additional information for overly general titles but rather to add valuable information. For example:

Avoid: Nurse Practitioners: A Pilot Study of Their Impact on Medical and Surgical Rapid Response Teams in an Acute Care Setting
Better: Addition of Acute Care Nurse Practitioners to Medical and Surgical Rapid Response Teams: A Pilot Study (Kapu et al., 2014, p. 51)

Subtitles should be reserved for supplementary information that helps the reader retrieve needed information. Subtitles may contain information about the study's methodology, for example, "A Systematic Review" or "A Comparative Study." Subtitles should be avoided where key elements can be arranged simply and with style (APA, 2010).

Titles should be concise. APA (2010) recommends titles should be no more than 12 words and should avoid unnecessary phrases such as "A Study of" and "An Investigation of." By reading the title, the information conveyed in the article should be apparent to any interested reader.

Abstract

Abstracts are just as important as titles in directing readers to articles they will find important. The abstract provides a summary of the research. It describes the study purpose and background, methods used for the research, key findings, and conclusions. "A well-prepared abstract can be the most important single paragraph in an article" (APA, 2010, p. 26). A densely constructed abstract rich in keywords can convince the interested reader to read the entire article.

Abstracts should be accurate, nonevaluative, coherent and readable, and concise (APA, 2010). The abstract should specify the purpose of the study and report the content of the article's text without expanding upon it. Good abstracts use simple sentences and the active voice. Effective abstracts employ keywords that interested readers would logically employ as search terms in online searches. Abstracts should feature the most important results and the key conclusions. Quantitative and qualitative results reported in the abstract should not differ from the numbers or concepts in the manuscript's tables and graphics. The abstract should also not repeat the title of the article, cite references, or use abbreviations (AMA, 2007).

In some journals, structured abstracts are required. The journal's author guidelines will specify the information to be included in the abstract, including labels to be used for the headings. Structured abstracts may include one or more sentences under the following headings.

- Purpose: clinical importance and research question(s) or hypothesis
- Design: structure of study including year(s) and duration
- Setting: community or practice setting
- Subjects: selection criteria, number of subjects (by group, if appropriate), key sociodemographic data
- Intervention (if appropriate)
- Measures: independent and outcome variables
- Results: main outcomes, including effect sizes and confidence intervals and/or statistical significance
- Conclusions: discussion of the results "taking into account limitations, along with implications for clinical practice, and avoiding speculation and over-generalization" (AMA, 2007, p. 22)

Abstracts of an original research report are typically between 150 (APA, 2010) and 300 words (AMA, 2007), although journals often specify the length and format for abstracts. If the author guidelines do not specify a maximum length, the author should keep to a 250-word limit, as few journals would allow longer abstracts.

A second reason for limiting the length of the abstract has to do with the indexing of the article. If the abstract is too long, the complete abstract may not be included in some bibliographic databases. For example, the MEDLINE database abstracts published after the year 2000 are limited to 400 words or 10,000 characters (U.S. Department of Health and Human Services, 2017a).

Examples of abstracts for research reports are displayed in Exhibit 5.1. The first two examples are structured abstracts; although the third example is unstructured, it provides the same information about the study as the other two. More discussion about writing titles and abstracts for other types of articles is provided later in the book.

EXHIBIT 5.1

Sample Abstracts

STRUCTURED ABSTRACT: QUANTITATIVE STUDY

Cesarean Outcomes in US Birth Centers and Collaborating Hospitals: A Cohort Comparison

Abstract

Introduction: High rates of cesarean birth are a significant health care quality issue, and birth centers have shown potential to reduce rates of cesarean birth. Measuring this potential is complicated by lack of randomized trials and limited observational comparisons. Cesarean rates vary by provider type, setting, and clinical and nonclinical characteristics of women, but our understanding of these dynamics is incomplete.

Methods: We sought to isolate labor setting from other risk factors in order to assess the effect of birth centers on the odds of cesarean birth. We generated low-risk cohorts admitted in labor to hospitals (n = 2527) and birth centers (n = 8776) using secondary data obtained from the American Association of Birth Centers (AABC). All women received prenatal care in the birth center and midwifery care in labor, but some chose hospital admission for labor. Analysis was intent to treat according to site of admission in spontaneous labor. We used propensity score adjustment and multivariable logistic regression to control for cohort differences and measured effect sizes associated with setting.

Results: There was a 37% (adjusted odds ratio [OR], 0.63; 95% confidence interval [CI], 0.50–0.79) to 38% (adjusted OR, 0.62; 95% CI, 0.49–0.79) decreased odds of cesarean in the birth center cohort and a remarkably low overall cesarean rate of less than 5% in both cohorts.

Discussion: These findings suggest that low rates of cesarean in birth centers are not attributable to labor setting alone. The entire birth center care model, including prenatal preparation and relationship-based midwifery care, should be studied, promoted, and implemented by policy makers interested in achieving appropriate cesarean rates in the United States.[1]

STRUCTURED ABSTRACT: QUALITATIVE STUDY

Fatigue in hospital nurses—"Supernurse" culture is a barrier to addressing problems: A qualitative interview study

Abstract

Background: Fatigue in hospital nurses is associated with decreased nurse satisfaction, increased turnover and negative patient outcomes. Addressing fatigue in nurses has been identified as a priority by many organizations worldwide in an effort to promote both a culture of patient safety and a healthy nursing workforce.

Objectives: The overall aim of this study was to explore barriers and facilitators within the hospital nurse work system to nurse coping and fatigue. The purpose

(continued)

EXHIBIT 5.1

Sample Abstracts (*continued*)

of this paper is to describe emergent themes that offer new insight describing the relationships among nurse perceptions of fatigue, nursing professional culture, and implications for the nursing workforce.

Design: A qualitative exploratory study was used to explore nurse identified sources, barriers to addressing, and consequences of fatigue. Participants and setting: Twenty-two nurses working in intensive care and medical-surgical units within a large academic medical center in the United States participated in the interviews.

Method: Interviews with the participants followed a semi-structured interview guide that included questions eliciting participants' views on nurse fatigue levels, consequences of fatigue, and barriers to addressing fatigue. The interview transcripts were analyzed using directed content analysis guided by the Systems Engineering Initiative for Patient Safety (SEIPS) model. Additional themes that did not directly align with the SEIPS model were also identified.

Results: All nurses in the current study experienced fatigue; yet they had varying perspectives on the importance of addressing fatigue in relation to other health systems challenges. A new construct related to nursing professional culture was identified and defined as "Supernurse." Identified subthemes of Supernurse include: extraordinary powers used for good; cloak of invulnerability; no sidekick; Kryptonite, and an alterego. These values, beliefs, and behaviors define the specific aspects of nursing professional culture that can act as barriers to fatigue risk management programs and achieving safety culture in hospital organizations. Nurse fatigue and attributes of nurse professional culture also have implications for nurse satisfaction and retention.

Conclusions: Findings from this study further support the role of nursing professional culture as an important barrier to effectively addressing fatigue in nursing work systems. Future work is needed to identify and evaluate innovative culture change models and strategies to target these barriers.[2]

UNSTRUCTURED ABSTRACT: QUANTITATIVE STUDY

Effects of Vibration Therapy in Pediatric Immunizations

Abstract

A randomized clinical trial of 100 children (52 boys, 48 girls) ages 2 months to 7 years was conducted to evaluate the effect of vibration therapy without cold analgesia on pain. A convenience sample was recruited at two sites: a publicly funded, free immunization clinic and a private group pediatric practice. Participants were randomly assigned to receive vibration therapy via a specialized vibrating device or standard care. All children regardless of intervention group were allowed to be distracted and soothed by the parent. Pain was evaluated using the FLACC score, which two nurses assessed at three points in time: prior to, during, and after the injection(s). Data were analyzed using a two-independent samples-paired t-test.

(continued)

EXHIBIT 5.1

Sample Abstracts (*continued*)

Results show that vibration therapy had no effect on pain scores in the younger age groups studied (2 months ≤ 1 year, > 1 years ≤ 4 years). In the oldest age group (> 4 to 7 years of age), a heightened pain reading was found in the period from preinjection to post-injection periods (p = 0.045). These results indicate that the addition of vibration therapy (without cold analgesia) to standard soothing techniques is no more effective in reducing immunization pain than standard soothing techniques alone, and thus, is not indicated for use with immunization pain. Recommendations include further evaluation of interventions.[3]

---

[1]From Thornton, P., McFarlin, B. L., Park, C., Rankin, K., Schorn, M., Finnegan, L., & Stapleton, S. (2017). Cesarean outcomes in U.S. birth centers and collaborating hospitals: A cohort comparison. *Journal of Midwifery & Women's Health, 72,* 40–48. doi:10.1111/ jmwh.12553. Reprinted with permission of John Wiley & Sons.

[2]From Steege, L. M., & Rainbow, J. G. (2017). Fatigue in hospital nurses—'Supernurse' culture is a barrier to addressing problems: A qualitative interview study. *International Journal of Nursing Studies, 67,* 20–28. doi:10.1016/j.ijnurstu.2016.11.014. Reprinted with permission of Elsevier.

[3]From Benjamin, A. L., Hendrix, T. J., & Woody, J. L. (2016). Effects of vibration therapy in pediatric immunizations. *Pediatric Nursing, 42,* 124–129. Reprinted with permission of Anthony J. Jannetti.

IMRAD Formatted Reports

The conventional format for writing research papers is the IMRAD format: Introduction, Methods, Results, and Discussion, or an adaptation of this depending on the journal and type of research (AMA, 2007; International Committee of Medical Journal Editors [ICMJE], 2017) (Figure 5.1). IMRAD provides a structure for organizing the paper and specifies in advance the headings for it.

Some authors choose to include a separate section in the paper for the literature review rather than incorporating it in the introduction, and additional subheadings might be included to highlight more specific components of the background literature, measurement scales, or discussion of hypotheses. Even when more specificity is added in the form of subheadings, the overall IMRAD format is helpful because it follows the process used for the research study and provides a clear structure for the manuscript. The IMRAD format is also useful in writing research reports for clinical journals even if the structure is not explicit in the paper.

The IMRAD format follows the research process and answers four important questions of interest to readers:

- Why was the study done?
- What was done?
- What did the researcher find?
- What does it mean?

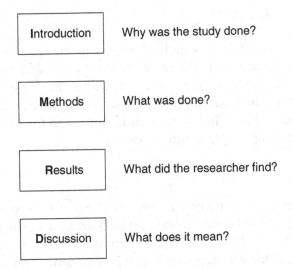

FIGURE 5.1 IMRAD format.

Why Was the Study Done?

The first question to be answered in the manuscript is why the study was done. A manuscript written for a research or specialty journal should begin with an explanation of the nature and extent of the problem and its importance to nursing, leading to the questions that need answers or hypotheses to be tested. Presenting *why* the study was undertaken and its importance is an effective strategy for gaining reader interest in the topic and convincing them to read the article. Answering why the study was done provides the basis for the introduction, which includes information about the background research on the problem, its significance for human health, and the logical next steps of research reflected in the research questions or hypotheses.

What Was Done?

Once the reader understands the problem, its importance, and the purpose of the study, the next question is what did the researcher do? How were the study questions answered or hypotheses tested? What procedures did the researcher use? This content reflects the methods section of the paper.

What Did the Researcher Find?

Once readers know the problem and how it was studied, the next question is what was learned? What were the findings of the study? In answering these questions, the author presents the data that were analyzed, observations, interview results, statistical findings, and so forth, in the results section of the paper. This part of the paper provides the evidence, based on the stated methodological procedures, that answers the research questions.

What Does It Mean?

In this last section of the research paper, the discussion, the researcher briefly summarizes the answers to the research questions, compares the new findings to previous findings from other related studies, and specifies the limitations and strengths of the current study. Finally, the authors answer the important question for readers, "What do these findings mean for clinical practice, teaching, clinical management, or future research?"

Introduction

The first section of the manuscript is the introduction, which is the author's opportunity to explain the nature and background of the study, its purpose, and its importance. The goals of the introductory section are to explain to the reader the need for the study and why it was done. This section of the manuscript provides a framework for reading the related literature; determining how the study builds on previous research on the topic; and understanding how the study leads logically to the purposes, questions, and/or hypotheses to be addressed. Introducing the problem statement early in the manuscript also clarifies why certain concepts and theories were used to guide the research.

In the beginning sentences, readers should learn about the problem that prompted the study and why the research is important to the readers and their constituencies. The author should begin the introduction with a discussion of the magnitude of the specific problem, using published data on its nature and scope. Who suffers from the problem? How extensive is the problem? What barriers prevent solving the problem? When written for a research journal, a good introduction clearly identifies research related to the health outcome and what is understood about its causes. When writing for a specialty journal, the author should be specific about how the study is linked to the nurse's own clinical, educational, or other specialty role or practice. These strategies not only set the stage for the remainder of the manuscript but also capture the reader's interest. After reading the introduction, the reader should be convinced that there is a genuine need for specific information and that the remainder of the manuscript will address that need in a focused way that will help the reader.

When the research project was originally planned, the author reviewed the literature and identified gaps in the research. In the introduction, the author should refer very briefly to these gaps in knowledge and how the current study addressed them. Exhibit 5.2 is an example of an effective introduction because it presents the current standard of care and practice for the patient population, the gap in the evidence base with respect to effectiveness and patient tolerance, and the benefit to neonatal patients were this gap to be filled. The brief summary in one paragraph prepares the reader for the more extensive background section to follow.

Some authors include too much discussion of the background of the study before they identify the specific problem under investigation. Instead, the statement of the problem should be clear to readers early in the introduction.

EXHIBIT 5.2

Sample Introduction

The use of nasal continuous positive airway pressure (CPAP) is the standard for care of preterm infants with respiratory distress syndrome (RDS) (Davis, Morley, & Owen, 2009; Verder, 2007; Verder, Bohlin, Kamper, Lindwall, & Jonsson, 2009). Various nasal interfaces are currently available to provide neonatal CPAP yet few studies have compared the effectiveness of these devices to determine efficacy, tolerance and measure differences in the incidence and/or the severity of nasal skin breakdown—a well described side effect of this useful treatment (Ramanathan, 2010; Rego & Martinez, 2002; Yong, Chen, & Boo, 2005).

From Newman et al. (2015). A comparative effectiveness study of continuous positive airway pressure-related skin breakdown when using different nasal interfaces in the extremely low birth weight neonate. *Applied Nursing Research, 18,* 36–41. doi:10.1016/j.apnr.2014.05.005. Reprinted with permission of Elsevier.

In Exhibit 5.2, the authors provide a succinct introduction to the problem and gap by the end of the first paragraph. They then expand on the dimensions of the problem and what is already known about it in subsequent paragraphs of the literature review.

Literature Review

The literature review describes what is already known about the topic and what needs to be studied, thereby justifying the current project. The literature review is critical to validate the need for the research. In the literature review, the author synthesizes related research, summarizes major findings from the studies, indicates when they are consistent, and suggests reasons for conflicting results. Gaps in knowledge and limitations of prior studies are emphasized to provide support for the current study. Continuity between previous research and the current study should be made explicit (APA, 2010). The author also may address methodological issues in the research, particularly when the design of the current study sought to resolve these. How to review the literature and write the literature review was presented in Chapter 4.

Typically, for research papers, only research studies are included in the literature review section. Exhibit 5.3 depicts a portion of a literature review that demonstrates how to organize studies for a research manuscript. Note that the review focuses primarily on the two studies with the best evidence (RCTs) and only briefly describes the extent of agreement among the findings in the larger body of literature relevant to the patient problem. The second paragraph summarizes background literature and rationale for the research method to be used in the current study. Descriptive articles, anecdotal reports, and other nonresearch papers may be used in the beginning of the manuscript to introduce the problem, but generally only research is incorporated in the literature review.

EXHIBIT 5.3

Sample Literature Review

Following an integrative review of 113 articles related to the use of nasal CPAP for preterm infants, only two randomized controlled trials (RCTs) included comparisons of nasal interfaces to determine the frequency of skin breakdown or nasal trauma (Rego & Martinez, 2002; Yong et al., 2005). Rego and Martinez evaluated the performance of two types of nasal prongs—Argyle™ and Hudson™—used to deliver nasal CPAP to preterm infants. Although both were found to be equally effective in the delivery of nasal CPAP, the Argyle™ prong was more difficult to maintain in the infant's nares and had a higher incidence of nasal hyperemia (first sign of skin breakdown) or erythma when compared to the Hudson™ prong. Yong et al. conducted an RCT to compare the incidence of nasal trauma associated with continuous nasal prongs or continuous nasal mask during nasal CPAP in neonates ≤1500 g. Although no significant differences were found in the incidence of nasal injury between the two interfaces (mask and prongs), there was a significant correlation between nasal trauma and length of therapy. Comparison studies examining prongs, mask or rotation of devices were not reported in the literature although this nursing care strategy was described to reduce pressure on nasal skin during the use of CPAP (McCoskey, 2008; Squires & Hyndman, 2009). Global recommendations in 46 of the 113 articles reviewed included frequent skin assessment, increased nursing care, and clinical expertise with clear agreement that nasal injury is a potential risk factor when using nasal interfaces during CPAP delivery in the preterm infant (Newnam et al., 2013).

Evidence based practice (EBP) supports clinical decision making based on scientific evidence with the clear aim of improving patient outcomes and reducing health care waste (Melnyk & Fineout-Overholt, 2011). Comparative effectiveness research (CER) has emerged as a research method to critically evaluate scientific evidence, identify major gaps in current evidence typically identified by systematic reviews, clinical guidelines developed by consensus review, and other methods to aggregate clinical research and then compare this information with current patient care practices (Tricoci, Allen, Kramer, Califf, & Smith, 2009). Researchers are discovering that information that emerges from real world settings is a valuable aspect of evidence and should be considered to determine best clinical practices. CER findings support clinical decisions based on results from alternative study designs including non-experimental research (Prosser, 2012). The framework for this research used principles of CER, including the direct comparison of clinical interventions (i.e., nasal CPAP) whose efficacy was previously supported by empiric evidence. . . EBP uses previous research findings to guide practice and does not compare practices through research methods.

Note: Selected parts of literature review.
Source: From Newnam, K. M., McGrath, J. M., Salyer, J., Estes, T., Jallo, N., & Bass, W. T. (2015). A comparative effectiveness study of continuous positive airway pressure-related skin breakdown when using different nasal interfaces in the extremely low birth weight neonate. Applied Nursing Research, 28, 36–41. doi:10.1016/j.apnr.2014.05.005. Reprinted with permission of Elsevier.

The intent of the literature review is to present the most relevant and recent studies that show why the current study is of critical importance to conduct. It is not an exhaustive review of the research, nor is the author attempting to give an historical perspective to the field of study. Avoid citing research that is tangential to the primary question of the study. At the same time, the review of the literature should not be so brief as to be intelligible only to specialists. The most recent and relevant published research should be featured, with exceptions for classic studies that defined the field. A literature review developed prior to the study should be updated with newer studies that may have emerged during the conduct of the study. Readers will gain a sense of the development of the research by reviewing the progression of studies.

The literature review may be incorporated into the introduction, as suggested by the IMRAD format, or presented as a separate section in the manuscript. This differs across nursing journals. The author should read selected articles from the target journal and follow guidelines for authors to gain a sense of how specific journals handle the literature review.

When writing research reports for clinical journals, the literature review is generally less extensive than for a research journal and is often incorporated into the introduction rather than presented as a separate section. Generally, readers of clinical journals are interested in whether the background literature and research methods are relevant for their patient populations. Some biomedical journals confine the entire introduction to two to three paragraphs (AMA, 2007).

Theoretical Framework

The literature review may contain the discussion of the conceptual or theoretical framework that guided the study, or the framework may be included in a separate section. The length and complexity of the description of the conceptual or theoretical framework vary across research reports. With some manuscripts, authors discuss the framework in detail, particularly when the hypotheses or interventions are organized around a theory's dimensions. In other research reports, often those prepared for clinical journals, the discussion of the framework may be limited or not even included in the manuscript. Whether to discuss the framework, and in how much depth, depends on the journal, goal of the paper, and objective of the research study. These discussions may or may not include a visual depiction of the framework.

Exhibit 5.4 provides three examples of theoretical frameworks incorporated into the introductions of research reports. In the first example, the study of fatigue among hospital nurses was guided by a systems model used previously to understand complex work situations. In the second example, a study aimed at improving pain relief strategies for young children receiving vaccinations was based on gate-control theory. In the third example, the authors defend the use of a systems model—also represented visually—in their study of stressors among adult siblings caring for a disabled parent.

Aim or Purpose

The last part of the introduction includes a statement of the approach that the current study will take to address the problem as described in the preceding paragraphs. This may be the closing paragraph of the introduction (APA, 2010). The author should include a statement of the (a) purposes of the study, (b) questions the research was designed to answer, and/or (c) hypotheses

EXHIBIT 5.4

Sample Theoretical Frameworks

EXAMPLE 1

The Systems Engineering Initiative for Patient Safety (SEIPS) model (Carayon et al., 2006b) was selected as the theoretical framework to account for the complexity of the work system and its relationship to nurse, patient, and organizational outcomes. The SEIPS model has been widely used to characterize the design of healthcare work systems and investigate the influence of the work system on processes, and employee and patient outcomes (Carayon et al., 2014; Holden et al., 2013). The model has also been used to identify barriers and facilitators to performance in nursing work systems (Gurses and Carayon, 2009; Gurses et al., 2009). SEIPS integrates a work system model and balance theory to define five components of the work system structure: person (in this case the nurse), tools and technology, tasks, environment, and organization (Carayon et al., 2006b; Carayon and Smith, 2000).[1]

EXAMPLE 2

This article proposes to evaluate the effectiveness of vibration therapy alone, using the Buzzy® device, as a clinic tool for alleviating pain during routine vaccination. This type of therapy involves the pre-immunization application of vibration stimulus, often in combination with cold packs, at the injection site. As hypothesized by the gate-control theory, vibration therapy interferes with pain receptors at the site of injection leading to a reduced perception of pain (Melzack & Wall, 1965). If effective, this therapy could offer clinicians a simple, cost-effective method to help patients receiving injections.[2]

EXAMPLE 3

Even though other nursing models were considered to guide this study (King's Conceptual System and Roy's Adaptation Model), the Newman Systems Model (NSM) was chosen because its concepts are more congruent with research about stressors and the family as a client system (Fawcett & Gigliotti, 2001; Reed, 1993;). . . . Accordingly, four NSM concepts—client system, stressors, sociocultural variable and developmental variables—guided this study.

(continued)

EXHIBIT 5.4

Sample Theoretical Frameworks (*continued*)

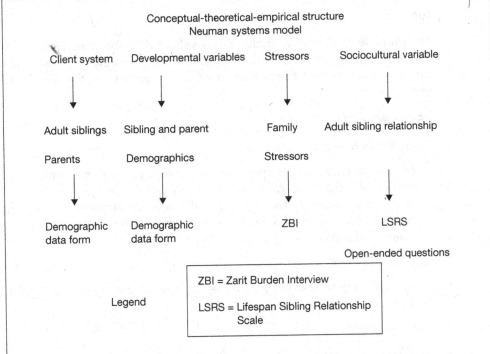

Conceptual-theoretical-empirical structure for the study of intra-family stressors among siblings sharing caregiving for parents (investigator developed).[3]

[1]From Steege, L. M., & Rainbow, J. G. (2017). Fatigue in hospital nurses—"Supernurse" culture is a barrier to addressing problems: A qualitative interview study. *International Journal of Nursing Studies, 67,* 20–28. doi:10.1016/j.ijnurstu.2016.11.014. Reprinted with permission of Elsevier.

[2]From Benjamin, A. L., Hendrix, T. J., & Woody, J. L. (2016). Effects of vibration therapy in pediatric immunizations. *Pediatric Nursing, 42,* 124–129. Reprinted with permission Anthony J. Jannetti Inc.

[3]From Ngangana, P. C., Davis, B. L., Burns, D. P., McGee Z. T., & Montgomery, A. J. (2016). Intra-family stressors among adult siblings sharing caregiving for parents. *Journal of Advanced Nursing, 72,* 3169–3181. doi:10.1111/jan.13065. Reprinted with permission of John Wiley & Sons, Inc.

that were tested. Exhibit 5.5 presents an example of these from a study on caregiving stress among adult children that included both quantitative and qualitative methods. A clear statement of the purpose of the research is essential to provide a rationale for the method chosen for the study and serves to link the background concepts with the specific procedures and variables discussed in the next section of the manuscript.

While the study's original (a priori) questions or hypotheses must be included in the introduction, subsidiary research questions may be presented in the results section of the manuscript. For instance, in a study comparing

EXHIBIT 5.5

Sample Aim, Research Questions, and Hypotheses

AIM

The purpose of this NSM-guided study was to describe perceptions of family stressors experienced by adult siblings who share caregiving responsibilities for their parents and the influence of the stressors on the adult siblings' relationships.

RESEARCH QUESTIONS

Quantitative Research Questions:

1. What is the extent of the overall burden of family stressors identified by adult siblings who share caregiving for their parents?
2. What is the relation between the overall burden of family stressors identified by adult siblings who share caregiving for their parents and the overall adult siblings' relationship?

Qualitative Research Question:

1. How would you describe your experience while sharing caregiving for your parent with your sibling?

HYPOTHESES

H1: The extent of the overall burden of family stressors identified by adult siblings who share caregiving for their parents will be high. This hypothesis was based on earlier reports that informal family caregivers usually experience high burden (Perrig-Chiello & Hutchison, 2010; Scharlach et al., 2006).

H2: The greater the burden of family stressors, the poorer the adult sibling relationship. This hypothesis was based on research by Checkovich and Stern (2002) and Tolkacheva et al. (2011), who found that negative encounters between family caregivers have effects on their relationship.

From Ngangana, P. C., Davis, B. L., Burns, D. P., McGee, Z. T., & Montgomery, A. J. (2016). Intra-family stressors among adult siblings sharing caregiving for parents. *Journal of Advanced Nursing, 72,* 3169–3181. doi:10.11.11/jan.13065. Reprinted with permission of John Wiley & Sons.

exercise interventions for older persons, the researcher might find evidence of gender differences in the use of interventions. These effects might be tested subsequently as interaction effects and reported in the results section as exploratory findings, but the effect would not be listed as a primary research question in the introduction. The main research questions should be presented in the introduction, keeping the report focused on the effectiveness of those treatments. Exploratory findings should be noted in the discussion section as being important lines of future research.

The introduction should not contain a statement about the research design unless the study was explicitly designed to refine a methodological limitation of previous studies. For example, the telephone coaching study expanded on data from a study described in two previous publications, the methods for which were briefly summarized in the literature review.

Methods

The next section of the manuscript explains the methods. How did the researcher carry out the study? What was done? In the methods section, information about the study design, subjects, measures, procedures, and data analysis is presented, in this order. Often, each subsection is labeled accordingly, making it easy for the reader to follow the methodology of the research.

The methods section needs to be detailed to demonstrate the degree to which the procedures are appropriate to the purpose of the study and the methods will yield reliable and valid results (APA, 2010). Enough detail should be provided such that researchers can replicate the study if desired and so that clinicians can evaluate the relevance of the findings for their patient population.

The methods section is written in the past tense since the study has been completed. Often the material from a research grant, thesis, or dissertation may be used in the manuscript if changed to the past tense, updated (where procedures changed from the original proposal), and shortened to comply with the page limits of the journal. Material written for research proposals and academic assignments may include an extensive rationale for each concept that will be measured, but this level of detail is usually unnecessary in a scientific manuscript, unless the focus of the study is on methodological issues or testing new measures.

If the research is an extension of an earlier study, the author can refer the reader to a previously published article for more detailed information about the methodology. For example:

> We identified a cohort of women within the data set who were admitted directly to hospitals for spontaneous labor and compared these to women admitted in labor to birth centers. . . . Data on both cohorts were collected simultaneously and prospectively, using the same validated instruments and procedures by midwives providing care. A detailed description of the data collection processes and instruments, including a validation study, has been previously published. (Thornton et al., 2017, p. 41)

Design

The first subsection is the study design. The design should follow logically from the background literature on the problem and be consistent with the purposes, questions, and/or hypotheses presented in the introduction. For designs that are well known, such as descriptive and experimental, no further information is needed other than indicating the design used for the research. Dates and period of study should be included (AMA, 2007). Sample statements of the design are found in Exhibit 5.6.

EXHIBIT 5.6

Sample Design Statements

QUANTITATIVE STUDY

This is a retrospective cohort study using secondary data from the Uniform Data Set of the American Association of Birth Centers (AABC). Data were collected prospectively at 79 US birth centers in 43 states between 2006 and 2011.[1]

INTERVENTION STUDY

A randomized clinical trial was conducted to evaluate the effect of vibration therapy on pain. Data collection included a convenience sample of subjects recruited at two clinical sites. Once informed consent and child assent (from children over 5 years) was granted, children were randomly assigned to one of two treatment groups: vibration versus typical treatment. Those assigned to the intervention group received vibration via the Buzzy vibrating device 10 seconds prior to receiving the injection. A sample of 100 children was recruited from a consecutive patient population attending clinics for routine immunizations. All children, aged 2 months to 7 years, were invited to participate in the study. Before inclusion, children were shown the device, allowed to hold it, and given the choice of whether or not they wanted to participate in the study. Exclusion criteria included the parent's inability to understand English. Random assignment to intervention (vibration therapy) ($n = 50$) or control ($n = 50$) group was determined by a computer-generated randomization list in clusters.[2]

QUALITATIVE STUDY

A semi-structured interview guide was created by the two authors based on prior research on fatigue in nursing and the SEIPS model of the work system. The guide included questions about personal experiences with fatigue, sources of fatigue, barriers and facilitators to fatigue and coping within the nursing work system, and nurse-identified consequences and potential solutions to fatigue. . . . Interview transcripts were analyzed for themes using directed content analysis as described by Hsieh and Shannon (2005). The authors utilized the SEIPS model to direct the coding of the transcripts (Carayon et al., 2006a).[3]

[1]From Thornton et al. (2017). Cesarean outcomes in U.S. birth centers and collaborating hospitals: A cohort comparison. *Journal of Midwifery & Women's Health, 72,* 40–48. doi:10.1111/jmwh.12553. Reprinted with permission of John Wiley & Sons, Inc.
[2]From Benjamin et al. (2016). Effects of vibration therapy in pediatric immunizations. *Pediatric Nursing, 42,* 124–129. Reprinted with permission of Anthony J. Jannetti Inc.
[3]From Steege, L. M., & Rainbow, J. (2017). Fatigue in hospital nurses—'Supernurse' culture is a barrier to addressing problems: A qualitative interview study. *International Journal of Nursing Studies, 67,* 20–28. doi:10.1016/j.ijnurstu.2016.11.014. Reprinted with permission of Elsevier.

For intervention studies, it should be clear to the reader how the study groups were determined and how the interventions differed across the groups. An example of this is seen in Exhibit 5.6.

For qualitative manuscripts, the method of the study, such as grounded theory, phenomenology, ethnography, and historical research, would be described. Exhibit 5.6 includes an example from an article on a qualitative study.

Setting and Subjects or Sample

The next subsection(s) concern who and where: the subjects who were studied and the setting in which the study took place. The description of the participants in the research is important for making comparisons across groups, generalizing the findings, and replicating the study (APA, 2010). Results can only be interpreted accurately when there is sufficient information provided about who was studied and their characteristics.

In writing the description of the subjects, the author can refer to the following list for information that may be included in this section, depending on the type of study.

- Source of subjects
- Number of subjects recruited, number who participated, and number in each study group if relevant
- How subjects were recruited
- Criteria for including and excluding participants
- How subjects were assigned within the study
- Randomization method if random assignment used
- Basis for decisions about sample size
- Procedures when subjects withdrew from study and actions taken, including how many and why
- Payments or other incentives provided to subjects

Demographic information about the subjects, such as age, gender, racial and ethnic background, and educational level, among others, is usually reported in the beginning of the results section of the manuscript, particularly when these are variables in the study. However, some authors elect to include information on the subjects in the methods section in order to focus the results section on the findings about the main concepts of their theoretical framework.

Likewise, the setting is an important dimension of a study, as the external environment may affect the participants and/or the researchers. Readers are assisted in interpreting the findings and in replicating the study if they understand the setting in which the research occurred.

An explanation should be included about human subjects requirements met for the research. This includes a statement about informed consent, review and approval of the research proposal by the institutional review board, and its review and approval by the institutions where the subjects were recruited. Frequently, one statement will suffice, such as "The study was approved by the institutional review boards of the university and participating hospitals prior to subject selection. Each subject signed an informed consent." For other studies, though, more information may be needed. This statement may be included in the description of the design, the subjects, or under a separate subheading, depending on the journal's guidelines for authors. Exhibit 5.7 presents the subsections on setting, participants, and ethical considerations from Ngangana et al.'s (2016) study of inter-sibling stressors during parental caregiving.

EXHIBIT 5.7

Sample of a Setting, Subjects, and Ethics Description

PARTICIPANTS

Purposive, self-selecting and snowball sampling were used to recruit respondents. Letters and flyers distributed to churches, adult senior day care centres, caregiver support groups, barbershops and beauty salons to recruit respondents. People interested in participating in the study contacted the researcher by e-mail or telephone. Only adult siblings who were sharing caregiving for their non-institutionalized parents experiencing a chronic illness and/or a disability were included in this study. A total of 84 participants were recruited for the study.

SETTING

The interview schedule was initially sent to 20 respondents, who were instructed to call the researcher if there were any concerns. After the 20 respondents returned the completed interview schedule without any calls about concerns or questions, the same interview schedule was distributed to other respondents as they were recruited.

The ZBI, LSRS, and the interview schedule were mailed to each respondent. Respondents answered the questions in writing and returned the forms to the researcher in a self-addressed stamped envelope.

ETHICAL CONSIDERATIONS

A university institutional review board approved the study. Consent forms were mailed to respondents along with the data collection forms. Respondents' confidentiality was maintained by separating the signed informed consent forms from the data collection forms when returned.

From Ngangana et al. (2016). Intra-family stressors among adult siblings sharing caregiving for parents. *Journal of Advanced Nursing, 72*, 3169–3181. doi:10.1111/jan.13065. Reprinted with permission of John Wiley & Sons.

Interventions

For intervention studies, the groups and treatments can be briefly described as part of the design or, if more explanation is needed, under a separate subheading. Interventions may also be highlighted in a figure and summarized in the body of the methods section. A visual aid with supplemental description may be helpful when reporting research for clinical journals because those readers may be particularly interested in the detailed descriptions of how a promising intervention was implemented to enhance patient care.

For example, Benjamin et al. described the vibration therapy in one paragraph.

> Those assigned to the intervention group received vibration via the Buzzy vibrating device 10 seconds prior to receiving the injection. The device was placed anatomically superior to the injection site, along the same skin dermatome. The nurse injected the immunization within approximately 0.5 centimeters from the device. The vibration device remained vibrating next to the skin while the injection was administered until after the needle was removed. If more than one injection was scheduled and two nurses were available for administration, then two vaccines were given simultaneously using two vibrating devices, one at each injection site. When one nurse was administering more than one injection in different locations (arm and leg, for example), then the vibration device was moved to each injection site prior to injection. If multiple injections were given sequentially, the most painful injection, such as MMR or Prevnar®, was always administered last, as recommended by the Centers for Disease Control and Prevention (CDC, 2012). The control group received the scheduled immunization injection without vibration. Both groups were allowed to be held, soothed, comforted, and distracted by both the nurse and parent, as would have been normally done. (Benjamin et al., 2016, p. 126)

Kessler and colleagues (2012) discuss optimal use of the "RE-AIM" model, that is, *Reach* and *Effectiveness* for individuals, their *Adoption* and *Implementation* in organizations and settings, and their *Maintenance* for both individuals and settings. APA (2010) offered these suggestions when writing a complete description of an intervention study. Authors should explain:

- All groups, including the screening criteria for each
- Content of interventions, including a summary of instructions to participants or, if they are unusual or represent a manipulation, verbatim in an appendix or a supplemental online section
- Procedures of manipulation or data acquisition, including equipment model, manufacturer, and settings, if any

- Persons who delivered the intervention, including their numbers, ratio to participants, professional training, and training in the intervention
- Setting, including quantity and duration of exposure, time frame of each intervention, and time between first and last intervention
- Incentives for participation

Procedures

For nonintervention studies, if the procedures used in carrying out the research were complex, a separate subsection on procedures may be included in addition to subsections on design and subjects. Therein, the author presents each step in detail. This section might include how surveys were distributed to subjects and returned to the investigator; how instruments and other measures were administered to subjects; the explanations given to participants; the qualifications of those who administered instruments or interventions; how groups were formed and interventions implemented; the setting, duration, and repetition of elements of the study; and other steps in collecting the data and carrying out the research. The principle for writing the procedures section is to describe what was done in enough detail for others to replicate it.

Measures

In the next subsection, the author describes the measures used for the study. This includes a discussion of the instruments, observations, and other measures for collecting the data. Widely used measures should be accompanied by a citation where the reader can find a description of the scale's content, validity, and reliability. For previously unpublished measures, full information about their validity and reliability should be provided. If the research involved the use of equipment, this should be indicated, including its manufacturer.

Exhibit 5.8 presents an abbreviated portion of the measures section from the study by Ngangana et al. (2016), who measured burden perceived by siblings caring for a noninstitutionalized parent. It is easy to see how the researchers measured each outcome for this study and how the instruments relate to the purposes of the research. Note the consistency between organization of the research questions (see Exhibit 5.5) and the order used to present the instruments (Exhibit 5.8). This type of organization is essential in a research report so readers can see the relationships among the components of the study.

Qualitative manuscripts would emphasize methods and sources of data collection, such as interviews and field notes, and how these data were recorded, transcribed, and then analyzed.

Data Analysis

The final subsection in methods deals with the procedures used for data analysis. In this section, the author describing a quantitative study lists the statistical methods, the alpha level considered acceptable, how variables were

EXHIBIT 5.8

Sample Description of a Measures Section

ZARIT BURDEN INTERVIEW

The Zarit Burden Interview (ZBI) is composed of 22 items that assess the degree to which caregivers perceive their responsibilities as having an adverse effect on their health, personal and social life, finances, and emotional well-being (Zarit et al. 1987). ZBI has been used to measure stressors associated with caregiving (Zarit et al. 1987). The total ZBI score consist of scoring for five domains— burden in relationship (six items), emotional well-being (seven items), social and family life (four items), finances (one item) and loss of control over one's life (four items)—were used to determine the amount of family stressor burden. The items are scored from 0 (never)–4 (nearly always), with higher scores indicating higher levels of burden. Total scores range from 0–88. Interpretation of the category of level of burden was based on the ZBI means as well as number of items endorsed and the mean score per item endorsed, as suggested by Zarit (personal communication, 13 July 2014). In addition, cut scores identified by Brodaty et al. (2014, p. 758) were considered; they maintained that "a score between 21–40 was used to determine mild-to-moderate burden in caregivers and a score of 41 or greater identified moderate to severe burden."

LIFESPAN SIBLING RELATIONSHIP SCALE:

The Lifespan Sibling Relationship Scale (LSRS) was used to measure attitudes towards the sibling relationship adulthood. The LSRS consists of 48 items divided into six sub-scales of eight items that measure sibling relationship in both childhood and adulthood. Child Affect (CA) and Adult Affect (AA) measure feelings of love, affection, pleasure, etc., about the sibling. Child Cognition (CC) and Adult Cognition measure cognitions or beliefs about the sibling and the sibling relationship (closeness and importance of the relationship). Child Behaviour (CB) and Adult Behaviour (AB) measure the degree of interactions through behaviours (phone call, visit and sharing secret) with and towards the sibling (Jeong et al., 2013; Riggio, 2000).

INTERVIEW SCHEDULE:

An investigator-developed interview schedule was used to ask adult siblings, How would you describe your experience while sharing caregiving for your parent with your sibling?

From Ngangana et al. (2016). Intra-family stressors among adult siblings sharing caregiving for parents. *Journal of Advanced Nursing, 72*, 3169–3181. doi:10.1111/jan.13065. Reprinted with permission of John Wiley & Sons.

modeled and analyzed, and computer programs used for the analysis. The goal of this section is to explain to readers how the data were analyzed. In qualitative reports, the author provides a detailed explanation of how the data were analyzed; what software program was used, if any, for organizing the analysis; coding strategies; how saturation was determined; and how the validity and reliability of the data were addressed.

Exhibit 5.9 provides examples of data analysis sections. In the first example, from a quantitative study, the statistical methods are listed for the reader; since these are common procedures, no further discussion is indicated. The second example is from a qualitative study.

EXHIBIT 5.9

Sample Statements of Data Analysis

QUANTITATIVE STUDY

Patient characteristics, including age, gender, and vaccination type (high vs. low pain), were first compared according to their intervention status (vibration vs. standard care) using a Chi-square test (see Table 1).

A series of two independent-samples paired t-test was performed to determine if the two methods (vibration therapy versus control) produce significantly different pain from immunization. The difference between pre-injection scores and injection scores for recipients of vibration therapy was compared to the same difference in control scores; similarly, the difference between pre-injection scores and post-injection scores was compared between vibration therapy and control, and finally, the difference between injection and postinjection scores was compared. Prior scores were subtracted from the later scores, so higher numbers indicate higher pain at later time points.

Differences between vibration therapy and standard care were assessed overall, as well as within age categories (ages 2 months to 1 year, ages 1 to 4 years, and 4 to 7 years), and type of injection received (high pain versus low pain).[1]

QUALITATIVE STUDY

Interview transcripts were analyzed for themes using directed content analysis as described by Hsieh and Shannon (2005). The authors utilized the SEIPS model to direct the coding of the transcripts (Carayon et al., 2006a). The two authors, a human factors engineer and a nurse, served as coders for the initial analysis and completed analysis on the cloud-based coding application Dedoose (SocioCultural Research Consultants, 2014). The two began by reading three transcripts for themes, and then developed an initial coding structure and book based on themes found in the transcripts and the components defined in the SEIPS Model. The authors then each independently coded all twenty-two interviews while meeting weekly to ensure that all coding matched throughout the entirety of each transcript.

After this initial analysis was completed, the second author went back through the coded excerpts and identified subthemes in the initial coding. The subthemes were presented back to the first author and discussed at multiple presentations

(continued)

EXHIBIT 5.9

Sample Statements of Data Analysis (*continued*)

to nursing and researcher audiences, including a broad population of nurses from the hospital where data were collected, to ensure validity of themes.[2]

[1]From Benjamin et al. (2016). Effects of vibration therapy in pediatric immunizations. *Pediatric Nursing, 42,* 124–129. Reprinted with permission of Anthony J. Jannetti Inc.
[2]From Steege, L. M., & Rainbow, J. (2017). Fatigue in hospital nurses—"Supernurse" culture is a barrier to addressing problems: A qualitative interview study. *International Journal of Nursing Studies, 67,* 20–28. doi:10.1016/j.ijnurstu.2016.11.014. Reprinted with permission of Elsevier.

Results

In the results section, the author presents the findings of the study. What was learned directly from the procedures just described? What new evidence was gathered? The findings should address the original purposes of the study and should answer each of the research questions or show results of hypothesis testing. This is the section in which the author presents the data and its analysis but without discussion of the findings. Authorial comments about their meaning, importance, implications, strengths, and weaknesses should be reserved for the subsequent section. The reader needs an understanding of the results before considering their relationship to previous research and their implications. An example of how to present the results from both quantitative and qualitative methods can be found in Exhibit 5.10.

The author is obligated to present all of the findings even (and especially!) when they run counter to what was anticipated, are counterintuitive, or do not support the hypotheses. In those cases, the author examines possible reasons for the findings in the discussion section.

Describe Subjects

For most research papers, though, the results section begins with a description of the study population, its demographic characteristics, the number of subjects who began the study, and the number who were excluded or were not included in the research because they withdrew, were lost in the follow-up, or for other reasons. If there were subgroups, the demographics characteristics of each group should be presented in the beginning of the results. With extensive demographic data, a table is helpful to summarize this information. When the results section begins with the report of the demographic data, the author should be careful not to replicate the information provided earlier in the methods section. If the demographic descriptors of the participants were presented in the methods section, the author should begin the results section with the findings related to the research questions.

EXHIBIT 5.10

Sample Results

QUALITATIVE DATA RESULTS:

Themes extracted from respondents' answers to the open-ended question indicate that the caregiving experience affected the lives of adult siblings in negative and positive ways. Three overall themes and related subthemes were identified: (1) Parental Care Rewards; (2) Parental Care Challenges; and (3) Sibling Help. Tables . . . display the thematic analysis results.

PARENT CARE REWARDS

Parent Care Rewards included six subthemes; all classified as beneficial stressors (Table . . .). The greatest number of respondents, 34 (43%), was for the subtheme, To Give Back—"Being able to give back to her what was done for me as a child." The least number of responses, five (6.3%), was for the subtheme, Sense of Being Appreciated by Parents—"The most rewarding part is that my parents appreciate me for every little thing I do for them and it makes me happy a lot." Of the 79 respondents, 16 (20.2%) provided data that were categorized as the subtheme, Historical Reflection—"She tells me stories that I had no knowledge about, i.e. family history, jokes." "Hearing stories from her childhood."

PARENT CARE CHALLENGES

Parent Care Challenges included nine subthemes (Table . . .). The majority of respondents, 23 (29%), reported responses that were associated with the Sense of Imbalance subtheme—"Not having enough time to commit to care 24 hours a day. Working full-time and caring for my own family is a challenge." Fourteen (17.7%) respondents reported responses that were consistent with the subtheme Loss of Self-Regulation of Personal Time—"Having my parent live with me. Everything I do their care must be factored in. I feel as if I no longer have my own life, I cannot do What I want, How I want, When I want". . . .

SIBLING HELP

Sibling Help included eight subthemes (Table 7). Responses were regarded as beneficial or noxious stressors or both. The greatest number of respondents, 22 (27%), provided data that was categorized as the subtheme, Shared Responsibility [Equally]—"They are willing to do whatever it takes. We all work together collectively as a team." The least number of responses, four (5.06%), was for the subtheme, Everything—"I make all the doctor appointments and take the parent, give emotional support, providing shelter, comfortable bed and secure, proper environment, is kept safe and warm. . . ."

From Ngangana et al. (2016). Intra-family stressors among adult siblings sharing caregiving for parents. *Journal of Advanced Nursing, 72*, 3169–3181. doi:10.1111/jan.13065. Reprinted with permission of John Wiley & Sons.

Present Main Findings First

After describing the subjects, the author presents the main findings, followed by secondary findings based on exploratory follow-up analysis. The order used to present this information should be consistent with the organization of the introduction and the way the purposes, questions, and/or hypotheses were listed earlier in the paper. This makes it easy for readers to relate the findings to the original questions for the study. If there were subgroups in the study, the findings for the entire sample should be reported first, then the data and related analyses for the subgroups.

Use Subheadings

Subheadings in the results section clarify the relationship of the findings to each research question or hypothesis. This is particularly important when the results are complex and extensive. If the section is short, though, subheadings are not necessary.

A good example of using subheadings that help the reader organize the findings is from the research report by Ngangana et al. (2016). Excerpts from the quantitative and qualitative results of that mixed-methods study are found in Exhibit 5.10.

Be Accurate and Precise

Although all researchers acknowledge the need for accuracy in conducting the research and reporting the findings, the author must be careful that the writing conveys the true results. Analysis results from every variable described in the measures subsection and every model or other analysis described in the analysis section should be described in the results section. Missing information confuses the readers and may suggest the unreliability of the overall report. While some evidence may support the hypotheses, other data may not. The author is responsible for presenting the comprehensive analysis and discussing any conflicting evidence in the discussion section of the manuscript. Data presented in the text should be consistent with the tables and figures and should be presented as ordered in the table, from left to right and top to bottom.

Scholarly writing requires accuracy, lack of bias, and completeness (APA, 2010). Accuracy is essential in carrying out the research and in presenting the results. Missing information about subsets of the subjects and strategies used to minimize the impact of missing data should be clearly shown, such that readers can evaluate the potential effects.

The author should also be precise in reporting the data. Rather than indicating that the data showed "promising trends in the directions hypothesized" or the findings "tended to support the model," the author should state exactly what were the findings of the study.

Report Data With Related Analyses

The data and the related statistical analyses are reported together. For means and other descriptive statistics, the author includes the standard deviations; for inferential statistics, the use of confidence intervals is strongly recommended and often required by journal editors (APA, 2010). The author should always check a manual of style if unsure what information to include when reporting statistics in the paper. Two helpful style manuals are *Publication Manual of the American Psychological Association* (APA, 2010) and the *American Medical Association Manual of Style* (AMA, 2007). Both of these references provide numerous examples of how to report statistics in a manuscript.

Most manuscripts are prepared using word-processing software. Statistical symbols are prepared with standard type, **boldface**, and *italics* (APA, 2010, p. 118). For example, Greek letters, such as α (alpha) and β (beta), subscripts, and superscripts use standard type. Symbols for vectors and matrices are bold, and the symbols N, n, M, and p are in italic type. Appendix A lists common statistical abbreviations and symbols.

There are a few other points that should be noted when reporting statistics in the results of research papers. When citing a statistic in the narrative, the statistical term is used, not the symbol. For example, "The M score was 25" should be written as "The mean score was 25." Remember also in preparing the manuscript that an uppercase N refers to the total sample, whereas a lowercase n refers to a part of the sample. The actual p value should be reported (e.g., $p = .04$) rather than $p < .05$ or $< .01$, unless $p < .001$. In that case it should be reported as $p < .001$ (AMA, 2007). A p value should not be listed as nonsignificant (NS) since the actual value is needed for eventual meta-analyses (AMA, 2007).

Develop Tables for Numerical Data

Tables are an effective means of presenting detailed and complex information succinctly and clearly. In the text, the author can describe the main findings and then use a table to display specific quantitative or qualitative data that supplement the statements in the text. Tables *support* the text and therefore should not duplicate that information. For intervention studies, tables are particularly valuable in comparing groups and how differences across groups were analyzed.

As an example of how tables are useful in presenting the results, consider the need to report demographic data. Including this information in the text would require a large amount of space, would be cumbersome to report, and more than likely would not maintain the reader's interest. The author should provide numerical data with as much nuance as is available. For example, if data are available on exactly how many years of school the subjects completed, the author should show the mean, median, and range and then may want to report the number and percent of subjects who completed education at intuitively logical levels.

1. Less than 12th grade
2. High school graduate
3. Trade school (2 years or less after high school)/some college
4. College graduate (bachelor's or other 4-year degree)
5. Postgraduate or professional program (e.g., master's degree, law degree)

Data such as these can be reported more efficiently in the form of a table. If such data are subsequently rescaled for analytic purposes, the reader will have the most comprehensive understanding of the raw data to assess the eventual findings.

Tables and figures, which include graphs, charts, diagrams, and other illustrations, have the advantage of allowing readers to visualize trends and patterns in the data more easily than when written in the narrative. Figures are particularly useful to show trends, make general comparisons, and help readers understand complex data.

Tables and figures are expensive to produce in a publication and should be used wisely by authors. Many journals limit the number of tables and figures submitted with a manuscript. Although tables are valuable for presenting the findings of a study, they should not be used when the data may be presented more easily in the text. Chapter 13 explains how to develop tables, figures, and other illustrations. In that chapter, examples are provided of how best to design a table and figure and use them in a manuscript. The AMA (2007) and APA (2010) style manuals are also excellent references for development of tables and figures.

Do Not Report Individual Scores

In most research reports, the author should not include the scores of individual participants or the raw data. Instead, summary statistics such as the mean and standard deviation are reported. For example, researchers presented results from a palliative care study of eight patient caregivers and eight clinician focus groups in two tables. In one table, data for patients, caregivers, and caregivers' previous experience of death were tabulated in three columns: 88-year-old female with colon cancer, 55-year-old daughter, and daughter's husband who died of melanoma when she was 41 years old. In a second table, focus group data were presented in five columns: group number (e.g., 1–8), description (e.g., primary care providers), age range (e.g., 29–46), length of time qualified (e.g., 6–22 years), and number of participants (e.g., 8). Although the study was small and the geographical area identifiable, participants in the study would not be identifiable using the summary data reported.

An exception to this rule is the case report, which is discussed in Chapter 8. Principles of confidentiality and autonomy govern what data on individual participants may be published. The rights of research subjects to privacy are discussed further.

Discussion

The discussion section provides an opportunity to interpret the results and explain what the findings mean in relation to the purpose of the study. Discussion sections should begin by making a clear statement of the answer to the research question or support or lack thereof for the research (APA, 2010). The author should not repeat what was already described in the results section.

In this section, the author discusses whether findings were consistent or not with prior research. While it may be tempting to cite only studies that support the findings of the current research, it is equally important to report studies with different conclusions. In those cases, the discussion includes potential reasons for differences in findings. Perhaps there were varied subjects or settings, the instruments and measures may have differed, or the data may have been analyzed using different statistical methods. The responsibility of the author is to evaluate possible reasons for these conflicting findings in order to refine what is known about the problem. The author should not repeat what was stated in the introduction, but rather reflect on previous work in light of the new findings of the current study and how understanding of the problem is refined with new information.

The discussion also allows the researcher to present implications of the study for clinical practice, teaching, administration, and others. What do these findings mean in terms of nursing practice? How can readers use this information in their work in nursing? Some journals have a separate section that discusses the implications of the research for practice.

It may be tempting for novice authors to overstate the implications of the study. The author should avoid unqualified statements and conclusions that are not completely supported by the data analysis, such as making comments about social, economic, health, or cost benefits, unless these outcomes were measured as part of the research (ICMJE, 2017).

The author should clarify for readers if the findings can be generalized to specific populations and settings. The findings are likely to be applicable only to patients or populations similar to the subjects in the research. If a study was conducted with acutely ill adults in a hospital setting, the findings may have limited or no implications for healthy adults; research on teaching methods for use with basic students may not be applicable to teaching graduate students or staff nurses. Many other examples could be cited. Although the implications are an important part of the discussion, they need to be based on the results of the study, considering its methods and limitations.

Limitations of the research should be addressed along with needs for further study. It is useful to suggest how the research should be extended.

As shown in Exhibit 5.11, Benjamin et al. (2016) use their discussion section to locate their findings in the context of recent work on gate-control theory and pain relief in children. Then they describe limitations of their study and recommendations for next steps in a research agenda.

EXHIBIT 5.11

Sample Discussion

DISCUSSION

The gate control theory suggests that physical interventions should interfere with the ascending pain signal, reducing perceived pain. However, as suggested by Cobb and Cohen (2009), who found the ShotBlocker ineffective with immunization pain, perhaps some physical interventions are insufficient to effectively stimulate the nerves, and therefore, close the "gate." Previous research supports the idea that vibration in conjunction with another treatment might be necessary, such as vibration and cold therapy, which in combination have been shown to be effective in reducing pediatric venipuncture pain (Baxter et al., 2011; Inal & Keileci, 2012). Cobb and Cohen (2009) also suggest that the overriding emotional and cognitive factors of an anticipated immunization might reduce the effectiveness of a physical intervention. This could explain the increased pain experienced by the older age group (4 to 7 years old), the more cognitively aware group. . . .

Several limitations to this study exist. First, blinding of the researchers was not possible because the vibration therapy was both visually and audibly apparent, potentially creating bias in scoring of pain, although the inter-rater reliability was good. . . . The FLACC score measures each nurse's perception of the patient's pain, rather than pain itself, and this proxy may contain error measurement. Another limitation is variability in the types of immunizations given to each child. . . . Another important limitation is that two clinical sites were used, with 10 nurses participating. Different immunization administration techniques existed between the clinics.

Further research is recommended on pain reduction techniques with childhood immunizations. New research might focus on a specific type of vaccination, such as influenza, to avoid the varying pain levels inherent with different vaccinations. A study that includes more research sites and a larger sample size would probably capture a more diverse patient population while still retaining the power to detect potential effects of the therapy. Including an older population with individuals who could assess their own pain would provide an actual measure of pain from the person experiencing the pain. Additionally, a cardio-respiratory monitor could be used to record heart and respiratory rates, providing an objective measure of distress or pain.

From Benjamin et al. (2016). Effects of vibration therapy in pediatric immunizations. *Pediatric Nursing*, 42, 124–129. Reprinted with permission of Anthony J. Jannetti Inc.

Many research papers end with the discussion section, but the author may choose to include a short summary paragraph at the end highlighting major findings and what they mean for readers. This can be labeled "conclusions."

Other Parts of a Research Paper

For some research papers, the author includes an acknowledgment section to recognize the support of others in the research and preparation of the manuscript. Every research paper, and nearly every other manuscript written, has a reference list. This is an important section in a research paper because it represents the literature used to establish why the study was conducted and its importance; a good reference list provides the critical work done previously on the topic.

Acknowledgments

For funded research, the acknowledgment specifies the financial and material support provided for the project, as discussed in Chapter 3. The acknowledgments section also expresses appreciation for individuals who assisted with preparation of or feedback on the manuscript but who did not meet the criteria for authorship, also described in Chapter 3. When an acknowledgment is included in print copy, it is placed between the text and references. For online submissions, directions will often specify a data-entry field where the acknowledgements should be cut and pasted.

References

As discussed in Chapter 4 on reviewing and reporting the literature, the references should be current, except for classic works that may be cited in the paper, and should be primary rather than secondary sources. The reference list is not exhaustive but instead represents the most recent and relevant work on the topic.

The format for the reference list varies with the journal. The journal's information for authors indicates the format to use for the journal and usually contains examples for preparing different types of references. When unsure, the author should refer to the manual of style used for that journal. Varied reference formats are discussed in Chapter 12, with examples of common ones the author might use when writing for nursing and healthcare journals.

The reference list should be consistent with the references cited in the paper. All citations in the text should be on the reference list, and every reference on this list should be cited in the paper. With APA format, the author should check that the names and years of publication cited in the manuscript are the same as on the reference list. With numbered references, the author should check that the number cited in the paper correctly matches the corresponding publication on the reference list.

Exhibit 5.12 provides a summary of the parts of the research manuscript discussed in this chapter and their order. Not every manuscript, however, will have each of these sections, but the order is consistent across journals. Use Exhibit 5.12 as a checklist when submitting a research paper.

QUALITATIVE RESEARCH REPORTS

The IMRAD format may be used as a structure for organizing qualitative research papers similar to quantitative studies. With this format the author begins with an introduction to the study, establishing the need for and importance of the study. As with quantitative studies, the choice of a qualitative design should be a logical extension of the state of the science on the topic, as presented in the review of background literature. The literature review might establish an unmet need to generate, modify, or extend a theory; describe, interpret, or understand some phenomenon; or describe a group, culture, or community. Other sections of the manuscript are methods, which include the setting, participants, procedures, and how data were collected and analyzed; results; and discussion. These components can be seen in the abstract of the qualitative study in Exhibit 5.1.

Presenting Findings of Qualitative Studies

By nature, qualitative findings involve thick interpretation of complex data from multiple sources, requiring a simplified explanation for actionability. In this chapter, we focus on the presentation of (or the author's way of communicating) the content of qualitative findings. First, findings of qualitative studies should be presented thematically, not as piecemeal quotations. As well, authors should present implications of their findings for specific clinical situations and settings. Finally, authors should discuss the context of settings or systems that might affect the appropriateness of implementation of their findings (Flannery, 2016).

EXHIBIT 5.12

Order of Sections of Research Manuscript

Cover letter
Copyright transfer (usually web based)
Title page (with acknowledgements, if any)
Abstract (and keywords if requested by journal)
Text
  Introduction
  Methods
  Results
  Discussion
  References
Tables (with titles and notes)
Figures (with captions)

In a qualitative research study, Adams et al. (2016) reported on in-depth interviews of 15 multiple myeloma or non-Hodgkin's lymphoma patients receiving outpatient treatment. Baseline interviews began with a definition of loneliness, based on loneliness theory, and explored experiences of loneliness, precipitating factors, and what protected against loneliness. Precipitating factors included being criticized and having unmet expectations for visits; protective factors included having a normal routine, believing that discomfort with another's illness is normative, and that time alone is desirable. The article concluded with specific recommendations for nursing assessment of social environment and cognitive interventions in clinical settings.

Organizing Qualitative Research

Qualitative research generates a lot of data that must be synthesized for readers. There are some studies for which multiple manuscripts might be written, and this decision should be made before the first manuscript is prepared. The author may have conducted a study on what it is like to care for a child with a chronic illness and its effect on the family system. One manuscript might present the experiences from the parents' point of view and a second on how children cope with a chronic illness.

Decisions on target journals for submission should directly influence manuscript preparation. Authors are urged to scrutinize not only a journal's guidelines for authors but also the content of recent issues of target journals, in order to prepare to present qualitative data according to the expectations of its editors, reviewers, and readers.

Recent studies have suggested that reports of qualitative research do a poor job communicating their methodological rigor and generalizability. These studies have implications for writing specific sections of a qualitative research manuscript. In the methods section, full disclosure of the participants, setting, and time frames is required. Furthermore, the specific analytic strategy should be clearly defined and referenced. In the results section, the perspectives of the participants, as distinct from the researcher's point of view, should be made apparent to readers, and the relationship of emergent themes to themes or research previously published should be made clear. Finally, qualitative research manuscripts should discuss a theoretical perspective amenable to transferability to whatever setting or population is the most clinically relevant data to the participants.

When organizing a manuscript that describes a qualitative research study, avoid rigid dependence on checklists that have proliferated, such as the Consolidated Criteria for Reporting Qualitative Research (COREQ; Tong, Sainsbury, & Craig 2007) or the Critical Appraisal Skills Programme (CASP, 2013). Sandelowski (2015) recommends the application of principles of good taste when building an argument from a body of qualitative research: "Connoisseurship in assessing the quality of qualitative research is not the mindless consumption of any single set of criteria but rather the selection from a stock of knowledge and prior experience with studies those considerations relevant to the study at hand" (p. 91).

MIXED-METHODS RESEARCH REPORTS

Scientific manuscripts that describe findings based on substantive quantitative and qualitative data have become increasingly prevalent, including in the nursing literature, and are valued for their promise of more comprehensive understanding of health-related experiences and practice (Huntley et al., 2017). However, reports that were unclear in their stated purpose and analysis strategies had limited usefulness for research, practice, and theory development.

O'Cathain, Murphy, and Nicholl (2008) proposed a set of six guidelines for Good Reporting of a Mixed Methods Study (GRAMMS).

1. Describe the justification for using a mixed-methods approach to the research question
2. Describe the design in terms of the purpose, priority, and sequence of methods
3. Describe each method in terms of sampling, data collection, and analysis
4. Describe where integration has occurred, how it has occurred, and who has participated in it
5. Describe any limitation of one method associated with the presence of the other method
6. Describe any insights gained from mixing or integrating methods

Building on this work, Pluye, Gagnon, Griffiths, and Johnson-Lafleur (2009) proposed that the best reports of mixed-methods studies justify their mixed-methods designs, combine the data collection and analysis procedures, and integrate the two types of data when reporting their results (Pluye et al., 2009).

HOW MANY MANUSCRIPTS ARE TOO MANY?

The author should avoid writing several manuscripts when one would be sufficient. Each paper should make its own unique contribution to the literature and should not overlap with one already published. The scientific evidence base is harmed when multiple manuscripts report on the same data, and readers must be able to assume that what they are reading in their journals are original ideas.

While some projects may lend themselves to writing more than one paper, most do not. An example of dividing a research study into separate manuscripts when one would suffice is with a study on the effectiveness of pressure ulcer treatments. In the study the researcher collected data on clinical outcomes, such as the location, stage, and size of the ulcer; hours of nursing care each patient received and level of education of nursing staff; and treatment costs. Separate manuscripts would not be appropriate in presenting the findings of this research because the author measured the effectiveness of the treatments based on clinical outcomes, staff variables, and cost. These measures are closely related and as a whole describe the treatments' effectiveness.

Some research studies and other projects, though, may be divided legitimately into more than one manuscript. The author may report the findings of research in one journal and a critical analysis of the literature in another. The implications of the findings for nursing practice may even be reported in yet a third article, as long as each of the manuscripts has an original message and presents original data and analysis not previously presented in the other articles.

When writing about a clinical project or an innovation in practice, a professional issue, and other nonresearch topics, the same question should be asked: Is it legitimate to divide the topic into separate manuscripts, or would one suffice? The author may be planning on writing a manuscript about nursing care for patients following a new surgical procedure recently initiated in the acute care setting. Separate manuscripts about care of these patients in the immediate postoperative period and home care would be appropriate for readers of two journals each with a focus on a distinct care setting. On the other hand, a single manuscript would be appropriate for a journal focused on the clinical population, read by nurses who care for these patients across the continuum of care settings.

Duplicate or Redundant Publication

The publication of essentially the same material in two or more publications is termed *duplicate* or *redundant publication*. Duplicate publication can range from disseminating the same content to different audiences in different forms to submitting duplicate manuscripts with identical content to different publishers (AMA, 2007). The Committee on Publication Ethics (COPE) defines redundant publication as any time that "a published work (or substantial sections from a published work) is/are published more than once (in the same or another language) without adequate acknowledgment of the source/cross-referencing/justification or when the same (or substantially overlapping) data is presented in more than one publication without adequate cross-referencing/justification, particularly when this is done in such a way that reviewers/readers are unlikely to realize that most or all the findings have been published before" (COPE, 2017).

The ethical issues associated with duplicate publication include the wasteful use of resources and the originality of scientific work. When an author submits the same material to two or more journals simultaneously, or attempts to divide a unified project into several publications, the resources of scientific publication are used inappropriately. The time and energy of peer reviewers and editors and the financial resources of publishers are invested in reviewing and preparing manuscripts for publication. A manuscript cannot be published in more than one journal due to copyright considerations; when the manuscript is accepted for publication in one journal and the author must withdraw it from consideration by others, the resources of the other journals are wasted, contributing to the ever-increasing costs of scientific publication (AMA, 2007).

Duplicate publication can also result in double-counting or wrongly weighting data in meta-analyses and suggesting more evidence of replication than is actual, which distorts the scientific evidence (APA, 2010).

Publishers, editors, and readers of scientific papers assume that published material is original. Editors are more concerned about redundant publications than any other breach of authorial ethics (Wager, 2007). Therefore, editors typically require authors of manuscripts to certify that their submitted manuscripts are not under consideration for publication elsewhere, and that if accepted for publication, the materials would not be published elsewhere in the same form without the consent of the editors (ICMJE, 2017).

Authors should guard against two specific forms of redundant and duplicate publication: shotgunning and salami slicing. Each practice has associated ethical issues.

Shotgunning

Shotgunning is submitting the same manuscript for review by two or more journals. An author who engages in shotgunning typically intends to wait until the manuscript is accepted for publication by one journal, and then withdraw it from consideration by others. However, the author has no control over the timing of review procedures, and at worst, this practice could lead to publication of the same material in more than one journal, violating the standard of originality of scientific publication. At a minimum, the author has inconvenienced the editor and reviewers of the journal from which the manuscript was withdrawn.

Shotgunning may be sanctioned as an inappropriate act according to the *Recommendations for the Conduct, Reporting, Editing, and Publication of Scholarly Work in Medical Journals* (ICMJE, 2017) or specific journal policy. The *Recommendations* suggest that, if duplicate publication occurs, a notice of redundant publication be published by the journal editor with or without the author's explanation or approval (ICMJE, 2017). Additional sanctions also may apply, such as notification of the author's dean, director, or supervisor (AMA, 2007). Notice of confirmed duplicated publications is placed on a numbered journal page and in the table of contents to facilitate linkage to the original articles in online searches.

Salami Slicing

Salami slicing (divided or fragmented publication) is the practice of breaking down findings from a single research study or project into a series of papers (known as "least publishable units") submitted to different journals or to the same journal at different times (APA, 2010). The intent of salami slicing usually is to increase the number of publications attributable to an author. Journal editors consider it to be unacceptable, wasteful, and an abuse of scientific publication (Gray & Baker, 2016; Pierson, 2015).

Divided publication can obscure the true value of the findings of a research study, making them appear more important than they really are; may confound meta-analyses of research findings; and may misrepresent the true incidence of reported phenomena. Divided publications may also blur the distinction between original research and secondary analysis and may lead to overgeneralization of implications for interventions that may adversely affect health outcomes of at-risk populations.

Acceptable Duplicate Publication

Duplicate publication does not include sending a manuscript rejected by one journal to another. When an author receives a notice that the manuscript was rejected, it may then be submitted to another journal for review. Other forms of publication not considered redundant include when a full manuscript follows (a) an abstract published as part of conference proceedings, (b) news media reports of study findings, or (c) detailed reports distributed to narrowly defined audiences (AMA, 2007; ICMJE, 2017).

The key to whether duplicate publication is acceptable or not is disclosure (AMA, 2007). It is unethical when authors do not notify editors about duplicate publications and do not include references to them. Authors should inform editors about duplicate publications, and copies of these articles should be sent with the submission. If there is any question about whether a manuscript reflects duplicate publication, the author should include a statement to the editor describing similar work. If the manuscript is based on the same subjects as one or more earlier publications, the author should cite the publications that inform the reader most completely about the data or report findings of relevance to the current manuscript. Earlier articles should always be referenced in a subsequent manuscript in both the text and reference list. Some journals, such as *Nursing Research*, require that when two or more papers based on a shared dataset are referenced or under review, the author must submit all relevant citations to the editor and describe adequately the relevant content in the text of the paper under review.

Roig (2015) discusses plagiarism and redundant publishing in detail in his *Guide to Ethical Writing* and provides guidelines for authors in a wide range of circumstances. Scientific writers who publish and present their research are urged to heed his general warning that "the provenance of data must never be in doubt" (Roig, 2015, p. 21).

Secondary Publication

Secondary publication is the republication or parallel publication of an article in more than one journal with consent of the involved editors (AMA, 2007, p. 149). An example of a secondary publication is when an article is translated for publication in a journal of a different language than the original. Typically, secondary publications, released at least 1 week after the primary publication, are intended for a different audience than the original paper, do not modify the data nor the conclusions of the original paper, and include a footnote on the title page that informs readers that the paper was previously published (ICMJE, 2017). The footnote should contain the full reference to the primary paper.

PROTECTING THE RIGHTS OF INDIVIDUALS IN PUBLICATIONS

In preparing a manuscript, the author needs to protect the rights of individuals to privacy and to avoid harming the reputations of others by defamation.

Privacy Rights

Publications in nursing, medicine, and other healthcare disciplines must protect the rights of certain individuals to privacy. Historically, this effort included omitting patient names, initials, and case numbers from published case reports; removing identifying information from x-ray films, digital images, and laboratory slides; deleting certain identifying details from the descriptions of patients or participants in research studies; and concealing certain facial features of patients in published photographs (e.g., placing black bars over the eyes). However, masking facial features does not always disguise identities sufficiently, and since the late 1980s, its use has not been recommended. If a patient's or legally authorized representative's written informed consent to publish a photographic likeness has not been obtained, the photograph should not be published (AMA, 2007). Authors who have obtained such written consents should, of course, include them with other permissions when the manuscript is submitted.

To prevent patients and participants in research studies from recognizing descriptions of themselves in published reports, some authors omit certain descriptive data from the manuscript, including age, sex, and occupation. However, omitting such details may hinder future investigations and meta-analyses. For example, occupational information might be useful to a researcher who is conducting a study of occupational injuries. Altering some demographic details about patients or research participants may appear to be a harmless way to protect the identities of these individuals, but doing so allows falsified data to be published, a serious breach of scientific integrity (ICMJE, 2017). Altered or falsified data can also affect a subsequent investigation or meta-analysis; for example, changing the name of a city can contribute error to an epidemiological analysis of disease outbreak locations (AMA, 2007). The recommendations suggest that identifying information about patients should not be published unless it is essential for scientific purposes, and that the patient or legally authorized representative should be allowed to review the manuscript before giving informed consent for the information to be published (ICMJE, 2017).

Defamation

Although every citizen is guaranteed freedom of expression by the First Amendment to the Constitution of the United States, this right is balanced against the right to protect one's personal reputation. Therefore, authors, editors, and publishers must take care not to harm the reputations of others by defamation, thereby exposing them to public ridicule, contempt, hatred, or financial loss. Defamation can take the form of libel or slander, but it always includes a false public statement concerning another (AMA, 2007).

Libel is a false, negligent, or malicious statement about another person or existing entity, made in print, images, or signs; *slander* is defamation by oral expression or gestures. With the increasing use of digital publication that includes mixtures of print, audio, and video content, the distinction between libel and slander has become increasingly blurred (AMA, 2007).

The laws concerning defamation are complex, and it is beyond the scope of this book to offer specific advice about how to avoid defamation in the process of writing for publication. Authors are advised to consult the editors of the publications to which they submit manuscripts for specific guidance.

MOVING FROM THESIS AND DISSERTATION TO MANUSCRIPT

Generally, sections of previously written theses, capstones, and dissertations need to be rewritten to comply with expected manuscript formats, with references carefully selected. Rarely can these other written forms be used "as is" for manuscripts. Problems with such submissions are widespread and often include failure to adhere to a journal's author guidelines, such as word counts or table/figure requirements, or to match topic to the scope of the journal; other problems are inappropriate referencing, excessive use of theory, and the absence of synthesis or new conclusions (Kennedy, Newland, & Owens, 2017).

Thus, a thesis and dissertation cannot be "cut and pasted" as a manuscript; they need to rewritten as such. A common reason for manuscript rejection is that it "reads like a thesis," often containing inappropriately long and extensive literature reviews. Even experienced researchers may find it difficult to revise a research grant into a manuscript.

Problematic manuscripts developed from theses and dissertations usually contain exhaustive literature reviews, extensive reference lists, and such a broad focus on the topic as to be inappropriate to the information needs of the audience of the journal to which submitted. They also may extend well beyond the page limits and may contain too many tables and figures. Dissertations and theses may also omit any implications for clinical practice.

What can be done to prepare a manuscript from a project that has a good chance of acceptance rather than a good chance of rejection? First, the author must decide what is the focus of the one or more manuscripts appropriate to the thesis, capstone, or dissertation. Is the goal to present the findings of the study to advance research on the topic, to describe the clinical implications of the research for practitioners, or both? If the author can write more than one paper, how many and what types of manuscripts are planned? Second, the author needs to choose a journal that would provide an avenue for publishing the first intended manuscript. Clinical journals want manuscripts with practice implications. Research journals want manuscripts that describe the study methods and findings even if implications are also discussed. Third, think about the target audience so the manuscript is geared to the readers of the journal.

Once these preliminary decisions are made, the next steps involve adapting the research project to a manuscript format. Some techniques follow.

- Shorten the title if needed
- Develop a new outline that reflects the required format of the journal
- Write new subheadings to reflect the goals of the manuscript rather than using the subheadings required for the thesis or dissertation
- Shorten the background of the study and introduce the purpose of the manuscript early in the introduction
- Synthesize the literature review, present the most important and relevant studies, and consider integrating the literature within the introduction (depending on the journal's format)
- Review sample research articles in the journal to determine if they include a separate section on the theoretical framework. If not, integrate a brief statement of the framework in the literature review. If articles include a section for the theoretical framework, shorten the one from the thesis and describe it briefly in the manuscript
- Shorten the methods section, omit the rationale for the methods, and shorten the discussion of psychometric properties of the measures unless submitting the manuscript to a research journal
- Revise the description of the sample and presentation of the demographic data to fit the journal being considered for submission
- Consider the extent of statistical analysis described in the manuscript and write for the audience
- If submitting to a clinical journal, emphasize practice implications
- Shorten the reference list to the most recent and relevant references
- Include only essential tables and figures, up to a maximum of four
- Rewrite the manuscript consistent with the writing style of the journal and for its readers who need the information
- Shorten the manuscript to comply with the page limits specified by the journal

Comparisons between manuscripts reporting various types of capstone projects may be helpful to students and new graduates at this career stage (Oermann, Turner, & Carman, 2014). For further assistance in revising a Doctor of Nursing Practice (DNP) capstone paper into a publishable manuscript, see Chapter 7.

SUMMARY

Nursing research is of little value if the findings are not made available for use by clinicians and others who need the research results for their work. Nurses who conduct research are responsible for reporting the results in journals that are read by nurses who can use the information in their practice, teaching, management, and other roles. By publishing the findings of research, nurses advance the body of knowledge of nursing and contribute to the scientific basis of nursing practice. Communicating the findings of research promotes the critique and replication of studies and is essential for EBP in nursing. Nurses also need research data to establish evidence for their decisions and interventions.

The conventional format for writing research papers is the IMRAD format: Introduction, Methods, Results, and Discussion, or an adaptation of this depending on the journal and type of research. IMRAD provides a way of organizing the paper and specifies in advance the headings for it.

The first section of the manuscript is the introduction, which is the author's opportunity to explain the nature and background of the study, its purpose, and its importance. The author begins the introduction with a discussion of the specific problem the research addressed and its significance. This discussion provides a framework for reading the related literature; determining how the study builds on previous research on the topic; and understanding the relationship of the purposes, questions, and/or hypotheses to the problem.

The literature review describes what is already known about the topic and what should be studied, thereby justifying the current project. Gaps in knowledge and limitations of prior studies are emphasized to provide support for the study. The literature review may be incorporated into the introduction or presented as a separate section in the manuscript. The literature review may contain the discussion of the conceptual or theoretical framework that guided the study, or the framework may be included in a separate section.

The last part of the introduction includes the purposes of the study, questions the research was designed to answer, and/or hypotheses that were tested. The author should review sample articles in the target journal before beginning the manuscript.

The next part of the manuscript is the methods section. In this section, information is presented about the study design, subjects, measures, intervention or procedures, and data analysis, in that order.

In the results section, the author presents the findings of the study. The findings should answer each of the research questions and address the original purposes of the study. This is the section in which the author presents the data and its analysis but without discussion of the findings.

The discussion section provides an opportunity to interpret the results and explain what the findings mean. In the discussion section, the author begins by stating the main conclusion that can be drawn from the results. The discussion allows the researcher to present implications of the study for clinical practice, teaching, administration, and other areas. Limitations of the research should be addressed along with needs for further study.

The IMRAD format also may be used as a broad structure for organizing qualitative research papers. With this format the author begins with an introduction to the study, establishing the need for and importance of the study. Other sections of the manuscript are methods, which include the setting, participants, procedures, and how data were collected and analyzed; results; and discussion. The content in each section, however, reflects the purpose of the study, qualitative method, and data.

Ethical considerations when writing research papers include deciding the appropriate number of articles to write from a single study and avoidance of redundant or duplicate publications, except as approved by journal editors. Authors should take care to protect the privacy rights of their subjects and to avoid defamation of other members of the research community.

A thesis or dissertation needs to be rewritten as a manuscript; they cannot be used as is. Often manuscripts developed from theses and dissertations are too long and are not relevant for the journal to which submitted. Strategies for preparing a manuscript from a thesis and dissertation were included in this chapter.

REFERENCES

Adams, R. N., Mosher, C. E., Abonour, R., Robertson, M. J., Champion, V. L., & Kroenke, K. (2016). Cognitive and situational precipitants of loneliness among patients with cancer. *Oncology Nursing Forum, 43*, 156–163. doi:10.1188/16.0NF.156-163

American Medical Association. (2007). *AMA manual of style: A guide for authors and editors* (10th ed.). New York, NY: Oxford University Press.

American Psychological Association. (2010). *Publication manual of the American Psychological Association* (6th ed.). Washington, DC: Author.

Benjamin, A. L., Hendrix, T. J., & Woody, J. L. (2016). Effects of vibration therapy in pediatric immunizations. *Pediatric Nursing, 42*, 124–129.

Benton, M. J. (2014). Dissemination of evidence: Writing research manuscripts for successful publication. *Clinical Nurse Specialist, 28*, 138–140. doi:10.1097/NUR.0000000000000040

Committee on Publication Ethics. (2017, October 13). Redundant publication. Retrieved from https://publicationethics.org/category/keywords/redundant-publication

Critical Appraisal Skills Programme. (2013, May 31). Qualitative research checklist: 10 questions to help you make sense of qualitative research. Retrieved from http://media.wix.com/ugd/dded87_29c5b002d99342f788c6ac670e49f274.pdf

Flannery, M. (2016). Common perspectives in qualitative research. *Oncology Nursing Forum, 43*, 517–518. doi:10.1188/16.ONF.517-518

Gray, R., & Baker, C. (2016). Salami-slicing. *Journal of Psychiatric and Mental Health Nursing, 23*, 541–542. doi:10.1111/jpm.12290

Hicks, R. (2014). I write, therefore, I cite: Why and how tools can help the author. *Journal of the American Association of Nurse Practitioners, 26*, 177–178. doi:10.1002/2327-6924.12115

Hudson, J. (2016). An analysis of the titles of papers submitted to the UK REF in 2014: Authors, disciplines, and stylistic details. *Scientometrics, 109*, 871–889. doi:10.1007/s11192-016-2081-4

Huntley, A. L., King, A. J. L., Moore, T. H. M., Paterson, C., Persad, R., Sharp, D., & Evans, M. (2017). Methodological exemplar of integrating quantitative and qualitative evidence— Supportive care for men with prostate cancer: What are the most important components? *Journal of Advanced Nursing, 73*, 5–20. doi:10.1111/jan.13082

International Committee of Medical Journal Editors. (2017). Recommendations for the conduct, reporting, editing, and publication of scholarly work in medical journals. Retrieved from http://www.icmje.org/urm_main.html

Jirge, P. R. (2017). Preparing and publishing a scientific manuscript. *Journal of Reproductive Sciences, 10,* 3–9. doi:10.4103/jhrs.JHRS_36_17

Jull, A., & Aye, P. S. (2015). Endorsement of the CONSORT guidelines, trial registration, and the quality of reporting randomised controlled trials in leading nursing journals: A cross-sectional analysis. *International Journal of Nursing Studies, 52*(6), 1071–1079. doi:10.1016/j.ijnurstu.2014.11.008

Kapu, A. N., Wheeler, A. P., & Lee, B. (2014). Addition of acute care nurse practitioners to medical and surgical rapid response teams: A pilot project. *Critical Care Nurse, 34,* 51–59. doi:10.4037/ccn2014847

Kennedy, M. S., Newland, J. A., & Owens, J. K. (2017). Findings from the INANE survey on student papers submitted to nursing journals. *Journal of Professional Nursing, 33,* 175–183. doi:10.1016/j.profnurs.2016.09.001

Kessler, R. S., Purcell, E. P., Glasgow, R. E., Klesges, L. M., Benkeser, R. M., & Peek C. J. (2012). What does it mean to "employ" the RE-AIM model? *Evaluation & the Health Professions, 36,* 44–66. doi:10.1177/0163278712446066

Moher, D., Hopewell, S., Schulz, K. F., Montori, V., Gøtzsche, P. C., Devereaux, P. J., . . . Altman, D. G. (2010). CONSORT 2010 explanation and elaboration: Updated guidelines for reporting parallel group randomised trials. *British Medical Journal, 340,* c869. doi:10.1136/bmj.c869

Newman, K. M., McGrath, J. M., Salyer, J., Estes, T., Jallo, N., & Bass, W. T. (2015). A comparative effectiveness study of continuous positive airway pressure-related skin breakdown when using different nasal interfaces in the extremely low birth weight neonate. *Applied Nursing Research, 18,* 36–41. doi:10.1016/j.apnr.2014.05.005

Ngangana, P. C., Davis, B. L., Burns, D. P., McGee, Z. T., & Montgomery, A. J. (2016). Intra-family stressors among adult siblings sharing caregiving for parents. *Journal of Advanced Nursing, 72,* 3169–3181. doi:10.1111/jan.13065

O'Cathain, A., Murphy, E., & Nicholl, J. (2008). The quality of mixed methods studies in health services research. *Journal of Health Service Research Policy, 13,* 92–98. doi:10.1258/jhsrp.2007.007074

Oermann, M. H., Nicoll, L. H., Chinn, P. L., Conklin, J. L., McCarty, M., & Amarasekara, S. (2018). Quality of author guidelines in nursing journals. *Journal of Nursing Scholarship.* Advance online publication. doi:10.1111/jnu.12383

Oermann, M. H., Turner, K., & Carman, M. (2014). Preparing quality improvement, research, and evidence-based practice manuscripts. *Nursing Economic$, 32,* 57–63, 64, 69. Retrieved from https://www.nursingeconomics.net/ce/2016/article32025769.pdf

Pierson, C. A. (2015). Salami-slicing—How thin is the slice? *Journal of the American Association of Nurse Practitioners, 27,* 65. doi:10.1002/2327-6924.12210

Pluye, P., Gagnon, M. P., Griffiths, F., & Johnson-Lafleur, J. (2009). A scoring system for appraising mixed methods research, and concomitantly appraising qualitative, quantitative and mixed methods primary studies in mixed studies reviews. *International Journal of Nursing Studies, 46,* 529–546. doi:10.1016/j.ijnurstu.2009.01.009

Roig, M. (2015). Avoiding plagiarism, self-plagiarism, and other questionable writing practices: A guide to ethical writing. Retrieved from https://ori.hhs.gov/images/ddblock/plagiarism.pdf

Sandelowski, M. (2015). A matter of taste: Evaluating the quality of qualitative research. *Nursing Inquiry, 22,* 86–94. doi:10.1111/nin.12080

Steege, L. M., & Rainbow, J. G. (2017). Fatigue in hospital nurses—"Supernurse" culture is a barrier to addressing problems: A qualitative interview study. *International Journal of Nursing Studies, 67,* 20–28. doi:10.1016/j.ijnurstu.2016.11.014

Thornton, P., McFarlin, B. L., Park, C., Rankin, K., Schorn, M., Finnegan, L., & Stapleton, S. (2017). Cesarean outcomes in U.S. birth centers and collaborating hospitals: A cohort comparison. *Journal of Midwifery & Women's Health, 72,* 40–48. doi:10.1111/jmwh.12553

Tong, A., Sainsbury, P., & Craig, J. (2007). Consolidated criteria for reporting qualitative research (COREQ): A 32-item checklist for interviews and focus groups. *International Journal for Quality in Health Care, 19*, 349–357. doi:10.1093/intqhc/mzm042

Tweed, S. A., D'Lima, G., Schnieder, P. V., & Zimbro, K. (2016). Achieving nursing excellence through research and evidence-based practice. *American Nurse Today (September)*. Retrieved from http://americannursetoday.mydigitalpublication.com/publication/frame.php?i=33 3240&p=&pn=&ver=html5&view=articleBrowser&article_id=2569214

U.S. Department of Health and Human Services, National Institutes of Health, National Library of Medicine. (2017a). MEDLINE®/PubMed® data element (field) descriptions. Retrieved from http://www.nlm.nih.gov/bsd/mms/medlineelements.html#ab

U.S. Department of Health and Human Services, National Institutes of Health. (2017b). The Omnibus Appropriations Act of 2009 makes the NIH Public Access Policy permanent (NIH Notice No. NOT-OD-09-071). Retrieved from http://grants.nih.gov/grants/guide/notice-files/NOT-OD-09-071.html

Wager, E. (2007). Do medical journals provide clear and consistent guidelines for authorship? *Medscape General Medicine, 9*, 16. Retrieved from https://www.ncbi.nlm.nih.gov/pmc/articles/PMC2100079

6

REVIEW AND EVIDENCE-BASED PRACTICE ARTICLES

Nurses in all clinical settings require the most current and complete evidence of effective approaches to guide their decision making and practice. The evidence should be based on a critical appraisal of studies that answer a specific clinical question or examine best practices and the synthesis of findings from across these studies. The preferential use of such approaches is known as evidence-based practice (EBP). With EBP, nurses rely on the review and synthesis of evidence from multiple studies rather than the report of one original research study. EBP is the application of that evidence in nursing practice.

EBP though is broader than only the use of research findings to guide clinical decisions. In EBP, nurses integrate the research with their own clinical expertise and the patient's preferences and values. An EBP approach allows nurses and other healthcare providers to use evidence to answer clinical questions (Melnyk & Fineout-Overholt, 2015). The process begins by identifying a clinical question on which the nurse needs more information to guide practices, searching for evidence to answer that question, critiquing and rating the strength of the evidence (and if appropriate deciding on a change in practice), integrating the evidence with the nurse's clinical expertise and patient preferences, evaluating the outcome of the practice change, and disseminating the EBP results (Halm et al., 2017; Melnyk & Fineout-Overholt, 2015; Stevens, 2013).

Nurses need to use a systematic process for reviewing and integrating individual studies and summarizing the evidence to answer a clinical question or explore a topic of interest. These review methods include integrative reviews, systematic reviews, meta-analyses, and qualitative syntheses. There are other types of reviews, such as scoping and mixed-method reviews, and authors are advised to search for available guidelines for reporting those reviews or to adapt the principles in this chapter. Translating the results of EBP reviews into clinical practice is the final step in research dissemination. Manuscripts on EBP address the effectiveness of new approaches or changes in practice as well as the resources needed for implementation and the process used by nurses in a clinical setting to engage in EBP.

This chapter describes various types of reviews and EBP manuscripts. The chapter also presents guidelines for preparing articles that disseminate the outcomes of those reviews. Only well-designed and conducted reviews should be used as evidence for practice. A detailed description of the methods used by the authors should characterize review articles, such that nurses may evaluate the quality of the review and whether its findings are robust enough for implementation into practice or, if not, what additional research is needed.

TYPES OF REVIEW AND EBP ARTICLES

Integrative Review

An integrative or narrative review provides a summary of empirical and theoretical literature to improve understanding of a particular topic. If comprehensive, this type of review presents the state of the science about the topic. Integrative reviews include both experimental and nonexperimental studies (Whittemore & Knafl, 2005). An integrative review tends to be broader in its description and understanding of a topic than a systematic review, which addresses a specific clinical question and combines evidence of multiple research studies. Because integrative reviews include diverse sources of information, they provide a holistic understanding of the topic (Hopia, Latvala, & Liimatainen, 2016).

In addition to summarizing evidence and presenting the state of the science on a topic, integrative review papers are also written to define concepts and explore theories. Whittemore, Chao, Jang, Minges, and Park (2014) described integrative reviews as reviews that focused on methodology, theory, or research. They suggested that an integrative review is the best method when the articles being synthesized include research and methods or theories. When the review is only of primary research papers, then a systematic review or meta-analysis is a better approach (Whittemore et al., 2014).

Whittemore and Knafl (2005) provided a framework for conducting an integrative review that includes five stages: problem formulation, literature search, data evaluation, data analysis, and presentation of the findings. This framework is useful as a guide for preparing manuscripts of integrative reviews for journals and other types of publications.

Problem Formulation

An integrative review begins with a clear purpose for the review and description of the problem addressed in it. A well-specified purpose and identification of variables of interest guide other stages of the review (Whittemore & Knafl, 2005). This same purpose statement can be used in the introduction of an integrative review manuscript to define its scope and explain why the review was done. A clearly articulated purpose statement or aim of the review is essential and guides the development of the search criteria. For example, in an integrative review of multimorbidity in older adults, the introduction begins with a description of multimorbidity as a significant public health concern because of its negative impact on functioning, quality of life, and use of healthcare resources (Northwood, Ploeg, Markle-Reid, & Sherifali, 2018). The authors use the background to explain the difficulties for older adults with multiple chronic conditions and diseases. This background leads into the purpose or aim of the integrative review: to examine how the social determinants of health have been considered in conceptualizations of multimorbidity in older adults in the literature and to identify implications for nursing practice, research, and healthcare policy.

Literature Search

An integrative review is a review of research and theoretical literature. It should be comprehensive, especially if used as evidence for practice, because if a review is incomplete and only some studies are considered, the findings may be biased and conclusions may be inaccurate. Multiple bibliographic databases should be searched, as described in Chapter 4, combined with other strategies such as ancestry searching (systematically reviewing citations from studies included in the review and from review articles) and searching the table of contents of relevant journals, among others (Bonnel & Smith, 2014; Polit & Beck, 2014). The search strategy used for the review should be described clearly for readers, including the search terms and how they were combined in the search, the specific databases used, and any additional search strategies employed for locating articles.

The Preferred Reporting Items for Systematic Reviews and Meta-Analyses (PRISMA) were developed to guide a systematic review or meta-analysis and to ensure that all essential information was included in the manuscript. Although not developed for integrative or literature reviews, PRISMA can be used as a framework in conducting the review and writing a thorough report of the review process and findings. PRISMA is discussed in more detail later in this chapter with the section on systematic reviews. Although ideally nurses would review all the relevant literature on a topic or problem and present the literature in the paper, for many reviews this would be a difficult, if not impossible, task because of the extent of available literature. When authors need to restrict the number of studies included in a review for it to be manageable, the rationale and criteria for deciding which papers to include and exclude in the review should be presented in the manuscript. Frequently this is done by restricting the years of the search or narrowing the focus of the review.

Data Evaluation

In this stage of an integrative review, the quality of each of the studies is evaluated. How this is done depends on the types of studies in the review. If only one type of research design was included, then the methodological quality of those studies could be assessed, and scores could be generated to represent different levels of quality. For reviews that include empirical and theoretical articles, different strategies are possible. For example, primary sources might be evaluated based on their methodological quality, informational value, and representativeness of available primary sources; theoretical reports might be assessed using techniques of theory analysis; and multiple instruments might be developed for each type of primary source (Whittemore & Knafl, 2005).

Regardless of the method used for evaluating the studies in the review, the manuscript should describe the method and how it was used to include or exclude papers from the review and evaluate those contained in it. It is important in any type of review paper for the author to explain the method or tool used to evaluate the quality of each included study. Typically, authors include a table that summarizes the studies in the review with the rating of their methodological quality.

Data Analysis

In integrative reviews, the data from the primary sources need to be interpreted and synthesized. The method used should be identified prior to beginning the review. Whittemore and Knafl (2005) suggested that research methods used for analyzing mixed-method and qualitative designs are applicable for integrative reviews and allow for comparisons across different types of studies included in the review.

Presentation of Findings

In the final stage, the findings of the review are presented. Conclusions should be supported by evidence from the review. In some manuscripts, details about each of the studies and findings are presented in a table format, but before developing this type of table for a manuscript, authors should check the journal guidelines and review similar articles published in the journal. Exhibit 6.1 provides an example of the methods and results sections of an integrative review. In this article, the authors included a table that summarized studies in the review and their main results. Table 6.1 provides an example of this table, which is in a typical format for a table of included studies.

Systematic Review and Meta-Analysis

Systematic reviews identify and critically appraise studies to answer a specific clinical or research question. With systematic reviews, authors attempt to identify all relevant studies to answer the question, use an explicit and reproducible methodology for searching for studies and selecting them for inclusion in the review, adhere to methodological standards for critically appraising studies, and synthesize findings across them. Systematic reviews combine evidence from multiple studies that are first critically evaluated.

EXHIBIT 6.1

Sample Sections From an Integrative Review Article[*]

AIM

The aim of this review was to examine how the social determinants of health have been considered in conceptualizations of multimorbidity in older adults in the literature and to identify implications for nursing practice, research, and healthcare policy.

METHODS

Search Methods

A comprehensive search of the literature was completed in the Ovid (Medline and Embase), CINAHL, HealthStar, Ageline, and PsycINFO databases. The primary keywords were "multimorbidity" and "multimorbid.". . . . Articles were included if they focused on older adults aged >60 years, were peer-reviewed, were published in English, included randomized controlled trials (RCTs) or cohort or qualitative studies, and defined multimorbidity. Articles were published between the years 2000 and 2015. Articles were excluded if . . .

Search Outcome

The search yielded 22 appropriate articles: 16 quantitative studies (3 RCT and 13 cohort), 4 qualitative studies, and 2 gray literature reports . . .

Quality Appraisal

The quality of the studies was assessed using the Cochrane Risk of Bias 2.0 Tool for the RCTs and the Critical Appraisal Skills Programme Checklists for the cohort and qualitative research . . .

Data Abstraction and Synthesis

Four critical questions were identified . . . Whittemore and Knafl's process of data analysis was used . . .

Results

This integrative review synthesized the evidence from the 22 included articles to answer four main questions. A summary of included articles is provided in Table 6.1. The RCTs had a high risk of bias. The cohort studies met most of the quality criteria but follow-up was incomplete. . . . Multimorbidity was viewed as a medical problem requiring healthcare system redesign, or a physician or interdisciplinary team response. . . . Another view was that managing multimorbidity was the responsibility of the older adult. . . .

[*]Selected parts of each section.
Source: From Northwood, M., Ploeg, J., Markle-Reid, M., & Sherifali, D. (2018). Integrative review of the social determinants of health in older adults with multimorbidity. *Journal of Advanced Nursing, 74,* 47–50. doi:10.1111/jan.13408. Reprinted by permission of John Wiley & Sons.

TABLE 6.1 EXAMPLE OF TABLE OF INCLUDED STUDIES

Authors, Year, Country	Design	Purpose	Sample	Results
Bayliss et al. (2008), United States	Qualitative	To explore patient perspectives on best processes of care for persons with multimorbidity	14 men and 14 women with diabetes, depression, and arthritis. Aged 65–84 Members of not-for-profit Health Maintenance Organization	Older adults desire clear communication of care plan, support, and continuity from single care coordinator, and "to be heard"
Bayliss et al. (2015), United States	Cohort (retrospective)	To assess effects of interpersonal continuity of care on rates of hospital utilization in population of older adults with multimorbidity in integrated healthcare system	9927 men and women Aged >65 years With three or more chronic conditions and three or more visits to primary or specialty care clinician between admission and index dates	Greater primary care continuity and greater specialist care continuity were each associated with lower risk of inpatient admission (respective HR = 0.97, 95% CI [0.96, 0.99] and HR = 0.95, 95% CI [0.93, 0.98]) and lower risk of emergency room visits HR = 0.97, 95% CI [0.96, 0.98] and HR = 0.98, 95% CI [0.96, 1.00])
Boyd et al. (2009), United States	Cluster randomized controlled trial	To evaluate the effects of "Guided Care" on patient-reported quality of chronic illness care in older adults with multimorbidity	904 men and women at risk for incurring high healthcare costs Aged ≥65 Urban and suburban primary care practices in Baltimore–Washington, DC, area	Compared with usual care, after 18 months, guided care recipients had twice greater odds of rating their chronic care highly (OR = 2.13, 95% CI [1.30–3.50], $p = .003$)

(continued)

TABLE 6.1 EXAMPLE OF TABLE OF INCLUDED STUDIES (*continued*)

Authors, Year, Country	Design	Purpose	Sample	Results
Ekdahl et al. (2015), Sweden	Randomized controlled trial	To examine costs and effects of ambulatory geriatric care unit on older adults with multimorbidity	844 men and women who had three or more hospitalizations in past 12 months Aged ≥75 Rural and urban municipality in southeastern Sweden	Compared with usual care, the number of hospitalizations did not differ, but the number of inpatient days was lower in the treatment group (11.1 compared to 15.2, $p = .035$)

CI, confidence interval; HR, hazard ratio; OR, odds ratio.
Source: From Northwood, M., Ploeg, J., Markle-Reid, M., & Sherifali, D. (2018). Integrative review of the social determinants of health in older adults with multimorbidity. *Journal of Advanced Nursing*, 74, 51. doi:10.1111/jan.13408. Reprinted by permission of John Wiley & Sons.

Two of the key characteristics of systematic reviews are that they use a structured approach to the review (that can be reproduced by others) and are based on a comprehensive search strategy.

A meta-analysis extends the critique of the research studies to include statistical analysis of their outcomes. With a meta-analysis, statistical techniques are used to integrate the results of studies included in the systematic review. By combining information from all relevant studies on a topic, meta-analyses provide a more precise estimate of the outcome of the intervention than an individual study.

Essential components of a systematic review and meta-analysis are the following:

- A clearly stated set of objectives and predefined criteria for including studies in the review
- An explicit and reproducible methodology
- A systematic search with the goal to identify all studies that meet the eligibility criteria
- An assessment of the validity of the findings of studies included in the review
- A systematic presentation and synthesis of the characteristics and findings of the studies (Higgins & Green, 2011; Higgins, Lasserson, Chandler, Tovey, & Churchill, 2016; Stovold, Beecher, Foxlee, & Noel-Storr, 2014)

The key to conducting a systematic review or meta-analysis is the use of a protocol. The protocol ensures that the review follows an explicit plan, with the aim of minimizing bias, and specifies the methods to be used. It is a template to guide the review and subsequent updates as new research findings become available. There are many resources to guide authors in developing these protocols and conducting systematic reviews, with or without meta-analyses, and authors should consult one of those before beginning. Two of these resources, among others, are the *Cochrane Handbook* (Higgins & Green, 2011) and the Joanna Briggs Institute *Reviewers' Manual* (Aromataris & Munn, 2017). Systematic reviews begin with a problem and specific questions to be answered and proceed through identifying inclusion criteria for studies, searching for and selecting studies for review, extracting data from the included studies, assessing their quality, synthesizing the findings either quantitatively through techniques such as meta-analysis or using a narrative approach, and summarizing the evidence. For many journals, the author also will provide implications for clinical practice, education, administration, and/or policy.

PRISMA Guidelines

The PRISMA guidelines should be used when reporting a systematic review or meta-analysis. Use of PRISMA improves the quality of the reporting of the review (Oermann, 2017; Tam, Lo, & Khalechelvam, 2017). By following PRISMA, authors ensure that the report of the review in the manuscript is comprehensive, and the methods are transparent and described with enough detail to be replicated. PRISMA also provides consistency across reviews for comparisons (Moher, Liberati, Tetzlaff, Altman, & the PRISMA Group, 2009). Robertson-Malt (2014) reported that PRISMA has become the international standard for reporting systematic reviews and meta-analyses.

The PRISMA Statement is a 27-item checklist of information to include in the manuscript with a brief description of each item. The Statement also includes a flow diagram to show the different phases of the review, number of articles identified in each phase, number included and excluded, and reasons for the exclusions (Moher et al., 2009). At the PRISMA website (www.prisma-statement.org/Default.aspx), authors can download a template of the PRISMA Checklist and use it as a guide when writing the manuscript. It also can be used as a framework for conducting the review. A template of the flow diagram can be downloaded from the website. The flow diagram can be seen in Figure 6.1. This diagram should be submitted as a figure with the manuscript. Although the use of PRISMA is recommended to improve the quality of reporting systematic reviews and meta-analyses, two studies of nursing journals revealed that few nursing journals were requiring use of PRISMA when submitting these manuscripts (Oermann et al., 2018; Tam et al., 2017).

Rationale for Review and Questions

Similar to an integrative review, a systematic review begins with a description of the problem and issues related to the questions being addressed. The background provides the rationale for the review in the context of what is

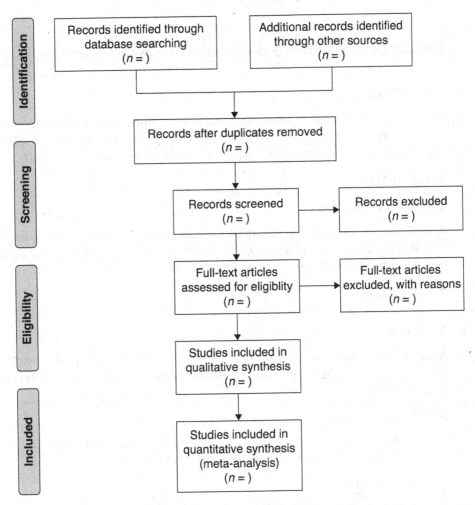

FIGURE 6.1 Flow diagram to show number of studies remaining at each stage of systematic review.

Source: From Moher, D., Liberati, A., Tetzlaff, J., Altman, D. G., & the PRISMA Group. (2009). Preferred reporting items for systematic reviews and meta-analyses: The PRISMA statement. *PLOS Medicine, 6*(7), e1000097. doi:10.1371/journal.pmed.1000097. The PRISMA Statement is distributed under the terms of the Creative Commons Attribution License, which permits unrestricted use, distribution, and reproduction in any medium.

already known. If other reviews have been done related to the question, the background includes a critique of those reviews and why a new one is necessary. The systematic review in Exhibit 6.2 provides an example of the main sections of the article conducted in line with the PRISMA guidelines.

Systematic reviews are intended to answer specific questions, and they are often developed using the PICOS framework: participants, interventions, comparison interventions, outcomes, and study designs. The question is then used to develop an objective or multiple objectives for the review.

EXHIBIT 6.2

Sample Sections From a Systematic Review Article

1. INTRODUCTION

The objective of this systematic review was to assess the prevalence of depression and anxiety reported in the literature, and the presence or absence of the experience of stigma among HIV-positive people on antiretroviral therapy . . .

2. METHODS

2.1 Review question

A systematic review of the literature was conducted to answer the question "What is the prevalence of anxiety, depression, and the experience of stigma in people with HIV infection on antiretroviral therapy?"

2.2 Definitions

2.3 Design

A systematic literature review was performed in line with the PRISMA (Moher et al., 2009) Statement and guidelines from the NHS Centre for Reviews and Dissemination.

2.3.1 Search strategy

Five databases were searched in August 2013: Embase, PsycINFO, Ovid MEDLINE, Web of Science, and the British Nursing Index . . .

2.3.2 Search terms

Group 1: (targeting HIV-positive patients): HIV, human immunodeficiency virus, AIDS, HIV/AIDS (combined using "OR"), Group 2: (targeting patients on antiretroviral therapy) antiretroviral therapy, highly active antiretroviral therapy, ART, ARV, HAART (combined using "OR"). Groups 1 and 2 were then combined using AND to make group 3 . . .

2.4 Inclusion and exclusion criteria

Inclusion and exclusion criteria are presented in Table . . .

2.5 Data extraction

Common tables were used to extract author name, year of publication, country in which the study was conducted, study aim, study design . . .

2.5.1 Analysis

Each paper was critically appraised using the Loney data quality appraisal tool to identify these sources of bias . . .

(continued)

EXHIBIT 6.2

Sample Sections From a Systematic Review Article (*continued*)

2.5.2 Quality assessment

The eight-item tool allocates a point based on the presence or absence of each criterion . . .

2.5.3 Reporting

First, study designs, outcome measurement tools, and country of research were summarized. Second, prevalence data were presented by mean and weighted mean point prevalence . . .

3. RESULTS

The search flowchart following PRISMA guidelines is presented in the Figure. The characteristics of retained citations are presented in Table . . ., with a Loney score of data quality (8 = best, 0 = worst).

3.1 Characteristics of eligible papers

Sixty-six citations were retained after application of the inclusion and exclusion criteria; 48% ($n = 32$) of papers . . .

3.2 Data quality

The quality of the included papers is summarized in Table . . . Over one half (57.5%) of the papers scored 6 or more out of a possible score of 8, indicating a generally high level of data quality.

3.3 Study design, tools, and measures

Among the retained citations, four reported baseline data from randomized controlled trials, nine were data from cohort studies, and 53 (80%) were cross-sectional studies . . .

4. DISCUSSION

This review has synthesized the data for depression, anxiety, and stigma among HIV-positive patients on antiretroviral therapy. The literature available was of high quality, although heterogeneous with respect to methodologies, sample characteristics, and assessment tools. Despite these limitations, the data presented provide a broader understanding of depression, anxiety, and stigma in HIV-positive people on antiretroviral therapy. [Discussion continues with limitations and conclusions.]

Source: From Lowther, K., Selman, L., Harding, R., & Higginson, I. J. (2014). Experience of persistent psychological symptoms and perceived stigma among people with HIV on antiretroviral therapy (ART): A systematic review. *International Journal of Nursing Studies, 51,* 1171–1189. doi:10.1016/j.ijnurstu.2014.01.015. Reprinted by permission of Elsevier.

Methods

Systematic reviews follow a specific methodology, which is planned in advance and outlined in a protocol. These methods are described in the manuscript, generally in this order:

1. Eligibility criteria for studies included in the review, for example, their relationship to the PICOS, years considered, if only English language, and others.
2. Search strategy, including the databases that were searched, years included, other limits, search terms, and other search strategies used.
3. Study selection, beginning with an initial screening of titles and abstracts to identify potential studies and then a full review of the articles.
4. Data extraction, which is the process used for collecting information about the study characteristics and findings (for example, forms tailored to the review question, if reviewed independently, process for confirming data from investigators, etc.).
5. Risk of bias in individual studies, including the methods for assessing this and how it was used in data synthesis.
6. Synthesis of results, which includes a description of how the results of individual studies were combined—with a meta-analysis or narrative approach.

Results

The results of the review provide details of included and excluded studies with numbers of studies screened, assessed for eligibility, included at each stage, and excluded with the rationale. Authors can develop a flow diagram to show the number of studies remaining at each stage of the review (Figure 6.1).

In presenting the findings of the systematic review or meta-analysis in a manuscript, authors include:

- A report of the study selection (numbers of studies screened, assessed for eligibility, and included in review) and study characteristics (e.g., PICOS, sample size)
- Results of the analysis of risk of bias in the studies
- Findings of the individual studies (including summary data and meta-analysis results)
- Synthesized findings across the studies
- Results of any additional analyses (e.g., sensitivity or subgroup analyses)

Tables are the preferred method for presenting the findings, for example, to describe the included studies and their characteristics and to summarize the extracted data. As with other tables, the main findings should be presented in the text and readers referred to the table for details and additional information. Table 6.1 is an example of a tabular display of the key characteristics of the studies in the review; the summary of findings table also allows authors to document the level of evidence for each study. A table of the studies in the review might be included within the text of the article, if the table is not too long, or as supplemental digital content, available via a link in the article. The results of meta-analyses are often displayed using forest plots, a graphical representation to illustrate the relative strength of treatment effects. The author can prepare a figure of the forest plots.

Discussion

In the discussion, authors summarize the main findings of the study with the strength of the evidence. Considering prior reviews, how do the findings from the systematic review or meta-analysis add to the evidence or raise new questions? The discussion should include the limitations of the review; for example, bias in the studies, difficulties in retrieving studies, and other factors that influence use of the findings in practice. It is important to identify the limitations that affect the quality of the data reported in the study and interpretation of the findings. For example, if there were a limited number of studies reviewed, which will affect the generalizability and applicability of the findings, this should be stated in the paper (Robertson-Malt, 2014). In the systematic review article in Exhibit 6.2, the authors wrote: "There were several methodological limitations encountered in this review. As described previously, sample characteristics such as gender, age, education level, socioeconomic status, and virus transmission route all affect life experience, and therefore the prevalence of depression, anxiety, and the experience of stigma. The reported data do not differentiate between these characteristics, and therefore the prevalence values reported encompass many different sub-populations within the HIV population" (Lowther et al., 2014, p. 1185). Authors should include a section in the discussion on implications of the findings for clinical practice, education, administration, and/or policy. Can the findings be used in clinical practice? What are the considerations for clinicians prior to adopting the evidence in their own settings? Is more study needed, and if so, what types of questions remain unanswered? The final section is a brief conclusion about the results of the review.

Systematic reviews and meta-analyses are increasingly important in EBP in nursing and other areas of healthcare. They provide strong evidence to guide clinical decisions and are often the basis for developing clinical guidelines (Moher et al., 2009). Reviews need to be continually updated to incorporate new evidence as it becomes available and to ensure the findings are current. Elliott et al. (2017) developed an approach to updating systematic reviews, labeling these as "living systematic reviews." Across all types of reviews, the value of the review depends on "what was done, what was found, and the clarity of reporting" (p. 1).

Qualitative Synthesis

Reviews of qualitative research can also be prepared as manuscripts. The purpose of conducting a synthesis of qualitative studies is to gain a deeper understanding of the phenomenon (Whittemore et al., 2014). Multiple methods for synthesizing qualitative research have been reported and choice of a method depends on the purpose of the review and questions to be answered. *Metasynthesis* is a synthesis of qualitative research. There are a number of different methods and approaches that have been proposed for this type of review and synthesis (Britten, Garside, Pope, Frost, & Cooper, 2017). The phases of a metasynthesis are similar to other systematic reviews, beginning with a problem and question, identifying types of studies and inclusion criteria, searching for and selecting studies for review, extracting and coding data, and assessing the quality of studies. Another qualitative synthesis method is *meta-ethnography*, the synthesis of interpretive research. Similar to reporting primary qualitative studies, for a synthesis of qualitative research, it is important to be transparent in the methods used to synthesize the studies (Whittemore et al., 2014). Selected guidelines for reporting a qualitative synthesis are in Appendix C.

Other Types of Review

There are other types of reviews that can be done and published. For example, a *scoping review* is a preliminary review of the research on a topic. Khalil et al. (2016) defined this type of review as one that examines the extent of literature on a particular topic. Another type of review is an *umbrella review*, which is a synthesis of existing systematic reviews (Aromataris et al., 2015). A *mixed-methods review* combines quantitative, qualitative, economic, and other types of research. By including evidence generated from diverse forms of research, mixed-methods reviews maximize the findings on a given topic (Aromataris & Munn, 2017). With the need to summarize evidence for busy clinicians, authors also might prepare synopses of high-quality systematic reviews. Editors of journals with broad clinical readerships often seek synopses to disseminate evidence to clinicians. These synopses are typically streamlined reviews of the evidence with recommendations for clinical practice.

EBP Applications

As nurses implement EBP in their clinical settings, manuscripts can be prepared on these initiatives and their outcomes. Many settings have adopted models of EBP to guide nurses in implementing this process in their clinical practice. An EBP model guides nurses in understanding various aspects of EBP (Stevens, 2013). Papers can be prepared on how nurses selected a model, its implementation, outcomes, and implications for other settings. Other potential topics for manuscripts are types of clinical questions asked by nurses that led to a search for evidence, strategies used in clinical settings to facilitate EBP, educating nurses with knowledge and competencies for EBP, methods that worked and were not effective for integrating evidence into the practice setting, and creating a culture of EBP, among many other topics.

A critical need is for nurses to disseminate their evaluations of evidence they implemented in their settings and outcomes of changes in practice. Dissemination of this information is essential to establish the effectiveness of an intervention or approach and determine if it is better than standard practice. Findings of EBP projects implemented in a clinical setting can inform nurses in other settings *if* those outcomes are disseminated.

WRITING REVIEW ARTICLES

This section of the chapter provides additional guidelines for writing all types of review papers. Some journals have their own format for preparing different types of reviews, and authors are advised to check those prior to writing the manuscript.

Title

The title of the paper should include the type of review. This will facilitate searching for specific types of reviews for EBP, research, and other purposes. Indicating the type of review in the title also alerts researchers performing meta-analyses about the paper (Oermann & Leonardelli, 2013). Authors should use established labels for their reviews, for example, integrative review, systematic review, meta-analysis, or type of qualitative synthesis. The first two examples that follow are the titles of the sample reviews in Exhibits 6.1 and 6.2, and the third example is from a metasynthesis.

Integrative Review of the Social Determinants of Health in Older Adults with Multimorbidity

Experience of Persistent Psychological Symptoms and Perceived Stigma Among People With HIV on Antiretroviral Therapy (ART): A Systematic Review

A Qualitative Metasummary on Caregiving at End-of-Life

Abstract

The abstract should specify the background for the review, objective, data sources, review methods, results, and conclusions. It should provide information for readers to assess the validity and relevance of the review (Oermann, 2014). Beller et al. (2013) developed a checklist for writing abstracts for systematic reviews, which also can be used for other types of review papers. The checklist is based on PRISMA guidelines. For some journals, authors also will include a statement on the relevance of the review findings for clinical practice. Two examples of abstracts for review articles are in Exhibit 6.3. The structure of the abstract and its length depend on the journal requirements.

The information for authors at the journal website specifies the type of abstract to prepare, format to use, and maximum word length. In the first example, from the systematic review on the prevalence of depression and anxiety and the experience of stigma among HIV-positive people on antiretroviral therapy, the abstract is prepared using a structured format. Some journals use unstructured abstracts written in paragraph form, as seen in Example 2 in Exhibit 6.3.

Introduction

The introduction presents the background of the problem and why a review was needed to understand the problem or answer the question. If prior reviews were done, authors should critique those reviews and explain why an additional review was indicated, for example, prior reviews may have included only one age group, one type of clinical setting, or patients with certain problems. It also may be that prior reviews were inconclusive or that recent research has changed what we know about the topic.

EXHIBIT 6.3

Examples of Structured and Unstructured Abstracts for a Systematic Review

---

EXAMPLE 1: STRUCTURED ABSTRACT

Background

Advances in HIV care have resulted in increasing numbers of HIV patients receiving antiretroviral therapy and achieving viral control. This has led to a focus on the biomedical aspects of care, leaving the data on psychological and social problems relatively neglected; in fact they have never before been systematically reviewed. If present and unmanaged, psychological and social problems are associated with unnecessary suffering and nonadherence to medication, with potentially serious clinical and public health consequences.

Objective

To assess the prevalence of depression and anxiety reported in the literature, and the presence or absence of the experience of stigma among HIV-positive people on antiretroviral therapy.

Design and Review Methods

A systematic review based on PRISMA guidelines. The prevalence data from retained studies were analyzed by study location and data quality.

(continued)

EXHIBIT 6.3

Examples of Structured and Unstructured Abstracts for a Systematic Review (continued)

Data Sources

Five databases were systematically searched (Embase, PsychINFO, MEDLINE, Web of Science, and British Nursing Index) from 1996 (first availability of highly effective antiretroviral therapy) to August 2013 using a predefined search strategy.

Results

Sixty-six original studies identified the prevalence of depression, anxiety, and presence or absence of the experience of stigma. The mean point prevalence of depression was 33.60% (SD 19.47) with lower reported point prevalence in high-income countries (25.81% [15.21]) compared to low- and middle-income countries (41.36% [21.42]). The 1- to 4-week period prevalence of depression was 39.79% (21.52), similar in high-income countries and low- and middle-income countries. The point prevalence of anxiety was 28.38% (17.07), with a higher prevalence in low- and middle-income countries (33.92% [10.64]) compared with high-income countries (21.53% [22.91]) with wide variability. The mean point prevalence of stigma was 53.97% (22.06) and 1-year period prevalence 52.11% (25.57). Heterogeneity in both sampling and methodology prevented meta-analysis of this data.

Conclusion

HIV-positive patients on antiretroviral therapy report a higher prevalence of depression and anxiety than the general population, which nursing assessment and practice should address. Over half of HIV-positive people report experiencing stigma. The difficulties with heterogeneous studies should be addressed through the development of a cross-culturally validated, multidimensional assessment tool in this population, and an increase in data disaggregated by risk groups.[1]

EXAMPLE 2: UNSTRUCTURED ABSTRACT

This study was a systematic review intended to assess the prevalence of depression and anxiety, and the experience of stigma among HIV-positive people on antiretroviral therapy. Five databases were searched; 66 original studies were included in the review. The mean point prevalence of depression was 33.60% (SD 19.47) with lower prevalence in high-income countries. The point prevalence of anxiety was 28.38% (17.07), with a higher prevalence in low- and middle-income countries of 33.92% (10.64). The mean point prevalence of stigma was 53.97% (22.06). HIV-positive patients on antiretroviral therapy report a higher prevalence of depression and anxiety than the general population, and over half experience stigma.

Source: [1]From Lowther, K., Selman, L., Harding, R., & Higginson, I. J. (2014). Experience of persistent psychological symptoms and perceived stigma among people with HIV on antiretroviral therapy (ART): A systematic review. *International Journal of Nursing Studies, 51,* 1171–1189. doi:10.1016/j.ijnurstu.2014.01.015. Reprinted by permission of Elsevier.

The objectives of the review, or specific questions addressed in it, should be included at the end of the introduction or immediately following it. These should be stated clearly for readers, as seen in the following examples:

- The objective was to assess the prevalence of depression and anxiety reported in the literature, and the presence or absence of the experience of stigma among HIV-positive people on antiretroviral therapy (Lowther et al., 2014, p. 1171)
- The aim of this systematic review was to evaluate the effects of practice on retention of cardiopulmonary resuscitation skills

Review Methods

The earlier discussion in the chapter on different types of reviews can be used as the framework for writing the methods section of these papers. This part of the manuscript should specify the inclusion criteria for studies, databases searched and dates of coverage, search strategies, process for selecting studies, methods of data extraction, variables for which information was collected, how the quality of individual studies was assessed, and how data were synthesized. Authors should use subheadings to indicate these parts of the methods section. Exhibit 6.2 provided an example of the methods section of a systematic review article showing the specific subheadings used by the authors.

Results

In reporting the results, authors should provide details of studies included in and excluded from the review. As indicated earlier, a flow diagram should be used to show the numbers of studies remaining at each stage of the review. In the results section, authors report the characteristics and results of individual studies (often done with tables) and the synthesis of the findings. The results of meta-analyses can be displayed using forest plots, which graphically show the results.

Discussion

In the discussion section of the manuscript, the main findings of the review are examined, considering the strengths and weaknesses of the review methods, quality of the studies included in the review, how bias was controlled and its potential impact on the results, and strength of the evidence for each outcome of the study. The discussion section should include an interpretation of the results and whether they are applicable to clinical practice, education, administration, and/or policy. Limitations of the review should be considered when drawing conclusions about use of the evidence in practice. Reviews are future oriented; they identify gaps in the research and make suggestions for further research. Reporting the gaps in the research is as important as reporting the findings (Robertson-Malt, 2014).

Authors should write a brief conclusion that summarizes the major findings from the review with implications for practice and where additional study is needed. The conclusion may be the final paragraph in the discussion section or a separate section that follows the discussion section.

SUMMARY

This chapter presented different types of review papers that authors can prepare. An integrative review provides a summary of empirical and theoretical literature to better understand a particular topic. With an integrative review, both experimental and nonexperimental studies are included. These are broad reviews to more fully describe and understand the topic, in comparison with a systematic review that addresses a specific clinical question. An integrative review progresses through five stages: problem formulation, literature search, data evaluation, data analysis, and presentation of the findings. This framework is useful as a guide for preparing manuscripts of integrative reviews for nursing journals.

Systematic reviews identify and critically appraise studies to answer a specific clinical or research question. With systematic reviews, authors attempt to identify all relevant studies to answer the question, use an explicit methodology for searching for studies and selecting them for inclusion in the review, adhere to methodological standards for critically appraising studies, and synthesize findings across studies. For these reasons, systematic reviews are useful for EBP.

Many systematic reviews include meta-analyses. A meta-analysis uses statistical techniques to integrate the results of studies included in the review, resulting in a more precise estimate of the effectiveness of an intervention or practice than an individual study.

Essential components of a systematic review and meta-analysis are a clearly stated set of objectives and predefined criteria for including studies in the review, an explicit and reproducible methodology, a systematic search intended to identify all studies that meet the eligibility criteria, an assessment of the validity of the findings of studies included in the review, and a synthesis of the characteristics and findings across studies in the review.

Reviews of qualitative research can also be prepared as manuscripts. There are varied methods for conducting a qualitative synthesis, and the choice of method depends on the aims of the synthesis.

As nurses implement EBP in their clinical settings, manuscripts can be prepared on these initiatives and their outcomes. Many settings have adopted models of EBP to guide nurses in implementing this process in their clinical practice. Papers can be prepared on how nurses chose a model, its implementation, outcomes, and implications for other settings. Other papers can provide a summary of the evidence and describe how nurses used the evidence to change practice. A critical need is for nurses to disseminate their evaluations of evidence implemented in their settings and outcomes of changes in practice. Dissemination of this information is essential to establish the effectiveness of an intervention or approach and determine if it is better than standard practice.

REFERENCES

Aromataris, E., Fernandez, R., Godfrey, C. M., Holly, C., Khalil, H., & Tungpunkom, P. (2015). Summarizing systematic reviews: Methodological development, conduct and reporting of an umbrella review approach. *International Journal of Evidence Based Healthcare, 13*(3), 132–140. doi:10.1097/xeb.0000000000000055

Aromataris, E., & Munn, Z. (Eds.). (2017). *Joanna Briggs Institute reviewer's manual.* South Australia: The University of Adelaide, The Joanna Briggs Institute. Retrieved from https://reviewersmanual.joannabriggs.org

Beller, E. M., Glasziou, P. P., Altman, D. G., Hopewell, S., Bastian, H., Chalmers I., . . . PRISMA for Abstracts Group. (2013). PRISMA for abstracts: Reporting systematic reviews in journal and conference abstracts. *PLOS Medicine, 10*(4), e1001419. doi:10.1371/journal.pmed.1001419

Bonnel, W., & Smith, K. V. (2014). *Proposal writing for nursing capstone and clinical projects.* New York, NY: Springer Publishing.

Britten, N., Garside, R., Pope, C., Frost, J., & Cooper, C. (2017). Asking more of qualitative synthesis: A response to Sally Thorne. *Qualitative Health Research, 27*(9), 1370–1376. doi:10.1177/1049732317709010

Elliott, J. H., Synnot, A., Turner, T., Simmonds, M., Akl, E. A., McDonald, S., . . . Thomas, J. (2017). Living systematic review: 1. Introduction-the why, what, when, and how. *Journal of Clinical Epidemiology, 91*, 23–30. doi:10.1016/j.jclinepi.2017.08.010

Halm, M. A., Alway, A., Bunn, S., Dunn, N., Hirschkorn, M., Ramos, B., & Pierre, J. (2017). Intersecting evidence-based practice with a Lean improvement model. *Journal of Nursing Care Quality.* Advance online publication. doi:10.1097/ncq.0000000000000313

Higgins, J. P. T., & Green, S. (Eds.). (2011). *Cochrane handbook for systematic reviews of interventions Version 5.1.0* [updated March 2011]. London, UK. The Cochrane Collaboration. Retrieved from http://handbook.cochrane.org/handbook

Higgins, J. P. T., Lasserson, T., Chandler, J., Tovey, D., & Churchill, R. (2016). *Methodological expectations of Cochrane intervention Reviews (MECIR).* London, UK: Cochrane.

Hopia, H., Latvala, E., & Liimatainen, L. (2016). Reviewing the methodology of an integrative review. *Scandinavian Journal of Caring Scieneces, 30*(4), 662–669. doi:10.1111/scs.12327

Khalil, H., Peters, M., Godfrey, C. M., McInerney, P., Soares, C. B., & Parker, D. (2016). An evidence-based approach to scoping reviews. *Worldviews on Evidence-Based Nursing, 13*, 118–123. doi:10.1111/wvn.12144

Lowther, K., Selman, L., Harding, R., & Higginson, I. J. (2014). Experience of persistent psychological symptoms and perceived stigma among people with HIV on antiretroviral therapy (ART): A systematic review. *International Journal of Nursing Studies, 51*, 1171–1189. doi:10.1016/j.ijnurstu.2014.01.015

Melnyk, B. M., & Fineout-Overholt, E. (2015). *Evidence-based practice in nursing & healthcare: A guide to best practice* (3rd ed.). Philadelphia, PA: Wolters Kluwer.

Moher, D., Liberati, A., Tetzlaff, J., Altman, D. G., & the PRISMA Group. (2009). Preferred reporting items for systematic reviews and meta-analyses: The PRISMA statement. *PLOS Medicine, 6*(7), e1000097. doi:10.1371/journal.pmed.1000097

Northwood, M., Ploeg, J., Markle-Reid, M., & Sherifali, D. (2018). Integrative review of the social determinants of health in older adults with multimorbidity. *Journal of Advanced Nursing, 74*, 45–60. doi:10.1111/jan.13408

Oermann, M. H. (2014). Writing the abstract of your manuscript. *Nurse Author & Editor, 24*(1), 7. Retrieved from http://naepub.com/writing-basics/2014-24-1-7

Oermann, M. H. (2017). Reporting guidelines: Tools for preparing your manuscript. *Nurse Author & Editor, 27*(4), 2. Retrieved from http://naepub.com/reporting-research/2017-24-4-2

Oermann, M. H., & Leonardelli, A. (2013). Make the title count. *Nurse Author & Editor, 23*(3), 9. Retrieved from http://naepub.com/writing-basics/2013-23-3-9

Oermann, M. H., Nicoll, L. H., Chinn, P. L., Conklin, J. L., McCarty, M., & Amarasekara, S. (2018). Quality of author guidelines in nursing journals. *Journal of Nursing Scholarship.* Advance online publication. doi:10.1111/jnu.12383

Polit, D. F., & Beck, C. T. (2014). *Essentials of nursing research: Appraising evidence for nursing practice* (8th ed.). Philadelphia, PA: Lippincott Williams & Wilkins.

Robertson-Malt, S. (2014). Presenting and interpreting findings. *American Journal of Nursing, 114*(8), 49–54. doi:10.1097/01.NAJ.0000453044.01124.59

Stevens, K. R. (2013). The impact of evidence-based practice in nursing and the next big ideas. *Online Journal of Issues in Nursing, 18*(2), 4. doi:10.3912/OJIN.Vol18No02Man04

Stovold, E., Beecher, D., Foxlee, R., & Noel-Storr, A. (2014). Study flow diagrams in Cochrane systematic review updates: An adapted PRISMA flow diagram. *Systematic Reviews, 3,* 54. doi:10.1186/2046-4053-3-54

Tam, W. W. S., Lo, K. K. H., & Khalechelvam, P. (2017). Endorsement of PRISMA statement and quality of systematic reviews and meta-analyses published in nursing journals: A cross-sectional study. *BMJ Open, 7*(2). doi:10.1136/bmjopen-2016-013905

Whittemore, R., Chao, A., Jang, M., Minges, K. E., & Park, C. (2014). Methods for knowledge synthesis: An overview. *Heart & Lung, 43,* 453–461. doi:10.1016/j.hrtlng.2014.05.014

Whittemore, R., & Knafl, K. (2005). The integrative review: Updated methodology. *Journal of Advanced Nursing, 52,* 546–553. doi:10.1111/j.1365–2648.2005.03621.x

ARTICLES REPORTING QUALITY IMPROVEMENT STUDIES

Many of the current projects in clinical settings are intended to improve the quality of patient care and can be published in nursing and healthcare journals. Quality improvement (QI) is a systematic and continuous process that leads to improvements in patient care and delivery of healthcare. The goal of QI is to make changes that will promote better patient outcomes and system performance. Dissemination of QI studies provides a way for nurses to share problems addressed in their clinical settings, interventions they evaluated, and the effectiveness of different approaches. For nurses and others to use the findings from QI, articles need to describe the problem that led to the need for the study, setting, population, intervention, and outcomes. Accurate and complete reporting of QI is essential to convey this information to readers.

STANDARDS FOR QUALITY IMPROVEMENT REPORTING EXCELLENCE GUIDELINES

Guidelines have been developed to improve the reporting of QI studies. These guidelines are the Standards for QUality Improvement Reporting Excellence (SQUIRE). Similar to other guidelines presented in this book, SQUIRE provides a checklist of information that authors should include when reporting QI to ensure the manuscript is complete (Holzmueller & Pronovost, 2013; Mosher & Ogrinc, 2016; Oermann, 2017; Oermann, Turner, & Carman, 2014; Ogrinc, Davies, Goodman, Batalden, Davidoff, & Stevens, 2016). The quality of evidence from a QI study depends not only on the design of the study but also on how well it is reported in an article. By using the SQUIRE guidelines, authors can prepare manuscripts that adequately describe the problem that led to the QI study, setting and other local conditions, intervention that was developed to solve the problem, and outcomes. Readers need complete information to determine if the intervention might be useful in their own settings. For this reason, QI manuscripts include a clear description of the context of the study: the local setting and conditions.

The current guidelines (SQUIRE 2.0) build on an earlier version from 2008. There are 18 sections, and each of these has a list of items to consider when preparing a manuscript or another type of report on QI. The SQUIRE guidelines, the checklist, and a description of the items are available at squire-statement. org. Some papers submitted to nursing and healthcare journals may not include each of the items listed, for example, because of restrictions on the length of manuscripts. With short manuscripts, it is difficult to include all of the items in the SQUIRE checklist. However, if the journal specifies that SQUIRE be used when reporting QI, then authors should attempt to follow the checklist of items to the extent possible. Authors are advised to review QI articles published in the target journal to gain a sense of how SQUIRE is used in those papers.

SQUIRE not only serves as a guide for reporting QI, but the checklist also can be used when planning a QI study (Oermann, 2017). By referring to SQUIRE during the design of the study, authors ensure that they are considering important elements of QI and collecting the information they will need when publishing their work.

SQUIRE was developed to improve reporting of QI in healthcare, and the examples in this chapter are patient oriented. However, the guidelines and principles in the chapter also can be applied to reporting quality initiatives in nursing education and other areas. The SQUIRE website (squire-statement .org) has many resources for authors on reporting QI studies.

FORMAT OF MANUSCRIPTS REPORTING QI

Principles for writing articles on QI follow; these principles are consistent with the SQUIRE 2.0 guidelines. The guidelines provide a format for organizing the content and headings to use in the manuscript (Oermann, 2017). Authors should remember that items in the SQUIRE checklist can be combined rather than reported as separate components in a manuscript.

Title

Developing the title is an important step in preparing the QI manuscript. Similar to other papers, the title should be informative and clear (Hartley, 2012). This is important because titles are used for screening potential articles during a search (Oermann & Leonardelli, 2013). Because of that, the title should indicate that the paper is a report of QI. Otherwise, individuals searching for publications on QI may not locate the article. Two examples of titles from articles that report QI follow. In both of the examples, it is clear that the paper describes a QI study.

Reducing Hospital-Acquired Pressure Ulcers: A Quality Improvement Project Across 21 Hospitals

Quality Improvement Study to Reduce Noise in the Neonatal Intensive Care Unit

Abstract

As described in other chapters, the format and length of the abstract depend on the journal guidelines. Some abstracts are structured, specifying each of the items to include, and other abstracts are unstructured. For QI manuscripts, the abstract should contain the words "quality improvement" or related terms that communicate the paper is on QI (Oermann, Turner, & Carman, 2014). Similar to the title, abstracts are used for searching, and those terms can lead readers to the article during a search.

Introduction

Similar to other manuscripts, the introduction describes the background of the problem and literature review. QI reports, however, also include information about the local problem or system issue that created the need for the study. The introduction should explain the gap in quality care in the setting and the standard to be met. For example, authors might explain that the current average total patient visit time in their clinic was 110 minutes, but the standard in their setting was 60 minutes or less from beginning to end.

In addition to describing the local problem, authors should report the intended improvement and include a rationale as to why a particular intervention was selected and is expected to work (SQUIRE, 2017). The SQUIRE guidelines suggest that the rationale for the intervention can often be provided by describing the framework or model that guided the study and development of the intervention. For example, in a QI study on improving pain management, the authors described how they used human-centered design for the study and development of the pain management interventions (Trail-Mahan, Heisler, & Katica, 2016).

The last item in the introduction should describe the specific aims of the study and goals of the manuscript. An example is: The aim of the QI study was to examine if falls and fall-related injury rates would improve by using a Virtual Breakthrough Series (VBTS) collaborative. This article describes the VBTS collaborative, processes developed for the QI study, and outcomes (Zubkoff et al., 2017).

The example in Exhibit 7.1 includes QI in the title and abstract, and the introduction provides a summary of knowledge about the problem addressed in the study, reducing pressure ulcer rates across 21 hospitals. The authors describe the local problem and its severity, and identify the specific aim.

EXHIBIT 7.1

Sample Title, Abstract, and Introduction of QI Manuscript

TITLE

Reducing Hospital-Acquired Pressure Ulcers: A Quality Improvement Project Across 21 Hospitals

(continued)

EXHIBIT 7.1

Sample Title, Abstract, and Introduction of QI Manuscript (*continued*)

ABSTRACT

A quality improvement initiative across 21 hospitals incorporated a multidisciplinary approach, breakthrough collaborative methods, evidence-based improvement methods and care guidelines, frontline rapid improvement cycles, consistent process-of-care documentation, and real-time incidence data. Statistically significant decreased rates in both all-stage and stages III, IV, and unstageable hospital-acquired pressure ulcers have been sustained for 5 years.

INTRODUCTION

Hospital-acquired pressure ulcers (HAPUs) are a costly and largely preventable condition. All-stage HAPU prevalence among hospitalized patients in the United States is approximately 5%, and estimated prevalence of full-thickness HAPUs is approximately 1.4%.[1–5] An estimated 3 million U.S. inpatients are affected by HAPUs of all stages each year at an estimated aggregate annual cost of $11 billion.[6]

Patient-level risk factors associated with HAPUs are documented, as are evidence-based practice guidelines for their prevention.[4,7–12] Preventing HAPUs improves quality and reduces costs. . . .

THE PROBLEM

Within Kaiser Permanente Northern California (KPNC), regional quality improvement (QI) efforts to reduce HAPU rates had met with limited success, failing to achieve substantial and rapid improvement or produce sustained quality gains. In 2007, the average baseline HAPU incidence at 21 hospitals was higher than the state average reported by CALNOC (California Collaborative Alliance for Nursing Outcomes).[15]

SPECIFIC AIM

KPNC aimed to achieve breakthrough performance in the incidence of HAPUs in all 21 hospitals. The initial target was an 18% reduction in the incidence of stage III, IV, and unstageable HAPUs per 1,000 patient-days in 2009.

Source: From Crawford, B., Corbett, N., & Zuniga, A. (2014). Reducing hospital-acquired pressure ulcers: A quality improvement project across 21 hospitals. *Journal of Nursing Care Quality, 29,* 303–310. doi:10.1097/NCQ.0000000000000060. Reprinted with permission of Wolters Kluwer Health, Lippincott Williams & Wilkins.

Methods

The methods section of a QI manuscript is similar to a research report. This section typically includes the following descriptions.

1. Context of the study, including information about the setting, patient population and size, staffing, relevant processes in place at the start of

the intervention, and other characteristics that might influence the effective-ness of the intervention (SQUIRE, 2017).

2. Description of the intervention, which presents the intervention and its components with enough details for others to reproduce it.
3. Study of the intervention, including the approach used for evaluating the impact of the intervention.
4. Measures and instruments for studying the processes and outcomes, why selected, their validity and reliability, scoring, measures to ensure the complete-ness and accuracy of the data (e.g., blinding, training data collectors, and others).
5. Data analysis, identifying the methods (both quantitative and qualitative) for analyzing the data.
6. Ethical aspects of the study with a statement about whether QI study was reviewed and approved by the institutional review board (IRB) or had another type of review.

In most healthcare settings, QI studies are no longer reviewed by the IRB. The author can include a statement in the manuscript similar to one of these examples: This project was QI in nature and not subject to IRB oversight, or this was a QI project, which are not reviewed by the IRB in our setting.

Excerpts from the methods section of the QI study introduced earlier, in Exhibit 7.1, are shown in Exhibit 7.2. The authors begin with a description of the setting and then present the interventions: (a) a SKIN bundle and (b) the Hospital and Emergency Department Reliability and Operational Excellence for Safety (HEROES), which uses the Institute for Healthcare Improvement breakthrough collaborative model and performance improvement methods. After describing these two interventions, the authors report the primary outcome measures: (a) the rate of all-stage hospital-acquired pressure ulcers (HAPUs; stages I–IV and unstageable ulcers) per 1,000 patient days and (b) the rate of stage III, IV, and unstageable HAPUs per 1,000 patient days, and finally, how the data were analyzed. The final section in methods details the implementation of the intervention involving a collaborative learning summit, action teams that implemented the SKIN bundle, multidisciplinary teams and collaboration, and use of Plan–Do–Study–Act (PDSA) cycles.

In the methods section, authors should describe any specific QI approaches used, such as the PDSA cycle. This information often can be included in the manuscript in the section on intervention. In reporting these approaches, authors should describe them in sufficient detail consistent with the key prin-ciples of the approach.

Results

The results section of a QI report is similar to a research paper. This is the sec-tion in which the findings are presented, relating back to the specific aims. In a QI report, though, the results section also includes the implementation of the intervention, for example, the steps or phases of the study and what happened during each one, often presented with a timeline or flowchart, and the partici-pants in various phases; extent to which the intervention was implemented and if modified; and changes in processes of care and outcomes associated with the intervention (SQUIRE, 2017). Figure 7.1 provides an example of using a figure to convey the implementation of a QI initiative and changes in outcomes over time.

EXHIBIT 7.2

Methods Section of QI Manuscript

METHODS

Setting

Kaiser Permanente . . . provides healthcare for 3.4 million members in settings that include 21 hospitals. . . .

Interventions

The QI effort was a collaborative initiative between regional risk management and patient care services. Called HEROES (Hospital and Emergency Department Reliability and Operational Excellence for Safety), it used the Institute for Healthcare Improvement breakthrough collaborative model and performance improvement methods that included the rapid improvement methodology. . . .

A regional group of multidisciplinary experts identified evidence-based content to assist frontline teams to reduce HAPUs. . . . The group, which included physicians, clinical services managers, quality and wound care nurses, respiratory therapists, nutritionists, and health information managers, conducted an evidence review to refine and enhance the SKIN bundle first described by Ascension Health.[18] The resulting KPNC SKIN bundle consisted of four elements: (a) skin assessment and correct surface, (b) keep turning, (c) incontinence management, and (d) nutrition. Bundle performance targets are as follows. . . .

Measurement

The primary outcome measures were (a) the rate of all-stage HAPUs (stages I–IV and unstageable ulcers) per 1,000 patient days and (b) the rate of stage III, IV, and unstageable HAPUs per 1,000 patient days. . . .

To assess incidence, wound, ostomy, and continence (WOC) nurses or assistant nurse managers maintained a daily log of HAPUs on individual nursing units, which enabled staff, managers, and leadership to access real-time HAPU data for all units in their hospital. . . .

On a monthly basis, hospitals submitted these data to regional risk management and patient care services leaders, who collated and distributed them. All 21 hospitals were able to view their performance relative to other sites. After the initiative began, each nursing unit also conducted process-of-care audits on five charts each week to ensure that the components of the SKIN bundle were being consistently implemented.

Analysis

A segmented linear regression model with a seasonality effect separately analyzed rates for all-stage HAPUs and stages III, IV, and unstageable HAPUs

(continued)

EXHIBIT 7.2

Methods Section of QI Manuscript (*continued*)

for two time periods: the first 2 years of the program (2008 and 2009) and subsequent years (2010–2012). . . . This project was carried out as a QI initiative and did not meet KPNC institutional review board criteria for oversight.

Implementation

Before implementation, all medical centers sent a multidisciplinary team to the first collaborative learning summit, at which performance improvement methods and the SKIN bundle were introduced. Afterward, action teams at medical centers implemented the SKIN bundle. . . . Unit-specific implementation occurred through Plan–Do–Study–Act cycles [continues]

Source: From Crawford, B., Corbett, N., & Zuniga, A. (2014). Reducing hospital-acquired pressure ulcers: A quality improvement project across 21 hospitals. *Journal of Nursing Care Quality, 29,* 303–310. doi:10.1097/NCQ.0000000000000060. Reprinted with permission of Wolters Kluwer Health, Lippincott Williams & Wilkins.

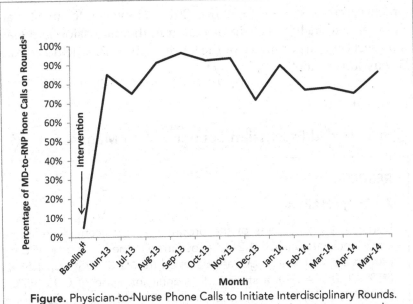

Figure. Physician-to-Nurse Phone Calls to Initiate Interdisciplinary Rounds.
[a]Calculating by dividing the number of completed physician-to-nurse phone calls by the number of total possible encounters during the audit period.

FIGURE 7.1 Sample figure depicting of implementation and outcomes of QI initiative and effects over time.

Source: From Young, E., Paulk, J., Beck, J., Anderson, M., Burck, M., Jobman, L., & Stickrath, C. (2017). Impact of altered medication administration time on interdisciplinary bedside rounds on academic medical ward. *Journal of Nursing Care Quality, 32,* 218–225. doi:10.1097/ncq.0000000000000233. Reprinted with permission of Wolters Kluwer Health, Lippincott Williams & Wilkins.

The order of information in the results section should be the same as presented in the methods section. Typically, it is best to first present the demographic characteristics of participants in the study and other characteristics of the setting, often in a table, and then the findings. Consistent with research papers, the text highlights the main results with the tables and figures presenting details. Exhibit 7.3 provides an example of the results section.

Discussion

Similar to research reports, the discussion section presents the meaning of the findings, linking them to prior studies (Oermann, Turner, & Carman, 2014). The discussion also should relate back to the aims and rationale for the intervention. SQUIRE 2.0 guidelines recommend that in the discussion authors provide reasons for differences between the anticipated outcomes, presented earlier in the manuscript, and what they found (SQUIRE, 2017). Limitations include factors that might have affected the study outcomes, issues with the implementation of the intervention, and features of the local setting that might influence using the intervention elsewhere. SQUIRE 2.0 recommends that the conclusions, the last section of the manuscript, include plans for sustainability, potential for spreading the innovation to other settings, implications for practice, and next steps (SQUIRE, 2017). However, for most manuscripts, it is preferable to include that information in the discussion and leave the conclusion section as a summary of the study. Exhibit 7.3 includes excerpts from the discussion section of a QI report.

EXHIBIT 7.3

Results and Discussion Sections of QI Manuscript

RESULTS

All-Stage HAPUs

During the first 2 years of the program, a significant decrease of 1.37 (95% confidence interval [CI], 1.2–1.54) occurred in the all-stage HAPU rate per 1,000 patient days. The average rate declined from 2.03 (95% CI, 1.88–2.17) to 0.66 (95% CI, 0.54–0.78), a statistically significant slope of 0.05 (95% CI, –0.06 to –0.04). By 2012, it decreased further to 0.59. Although it was not included in the regression analysis, the 2013 annual rate of all-stage HAPUs per 1,000 patient days was 0.47.

Stage III, IV, and Unstageable HAPUs

During the first 2 years of the program, a significant decrease of 0.13 (95% CI, 0.09–0.18) also occurred in the rate of stages III, IV, and unstageable HAPUs per 1,000 patient days. . . . All medical centers reduced the incidence of HAPUs,

(continued)

EXHIBIT 7.3

Results and Discussion Sections of QI Manuscript (*continued*)

with the majority of medical centers performing better than the regional targets from December 2008 onward. . . .

DISCUSSION

This QI initiative reduced the incidence of all-stage and stage III, IV, and unstageable HAPUs to a statistically significant degree across 21 hospitals. Strengths of this work include improvements occurring throughout a multihospital system and sustained over time. An additional strength is the use of surveillance data, which identify a higher proportion of HAPUs than do administrative data.[21] Limitations include the fact that the generalizability of this experience is unknown. . . .

Two barriers initially interfered with fully implementing the SKIN bundle. The first was a lack of appropriate surfaces. Before launching the QI initiative, the HEROES steering committee created a business case for purchasing the correct surfaces. KPNC subsequently invested more than $2 million in pressure redistribution mattresses and surfaces. . . . Although the effect of any single element of the initiative cannot be determined, the reduction in HAPU incidence and published evidence suggest that this investment was money well spent.[24]

A second barrier was the limited availability of nurses with expertise on skin assessment, because an accurate Braden score is required to trigger the SKIN bundle appropriately for at-risk patients. WOC nurses have this expertise, but not all KPNC hospitals had one on staff. . . .

An early challenge was that original HAPU incidence logs were not standardized across hospitals before regional reporting. The overall reporting burden increased significantly with the implementation of regional reporting, eliciting negative reactions from regional and local hospital leaders. [discussion continues]

QI, quality improvement.
Source: From Crawford, B., Corbett, N., & Zuniga, A. (2014). Reducing hospital-acquired pressure ulcers: A quality improvement project across 21 hospitals. *Journal of Nursing Care Quality, 29,* 303–310. doi:10.1097/NCQ.0000000000000060. Reprinted with permission of Wolters Kluwer Health, Lippincott Williams & Wilkins.

The final section of the manuscript is the conclusion, which summarizes the outcomes of the study and the value of the intervention. The conclusions can be a subsection at the end of the discussion or a separate section at the end of the manuscript.

SUMMARY

The goal of QI is to make changes that will promote better patient outcomes and system performance. Dissemination of QI studies provides a way for nurses to share problems addressed in their clinical settings, interventions they evaluated, and the effectiveness of different approaches. For nurses and others to use the findings from QI, articles need to describe the problem that led to the need for the study, local setting, population, intervention, and outcomes. Accurate and complete reporting of QI is essential to convey this information to readers.

When preparing papers on QI, nurses can follow the SQUIRE guidelines. These guidelines provide a format for the manuscript, ensuring that it includes sufficient information about the QI study for readers to understand it and evaluate its applicability to their own setting. Not all items in the guidelines are included with most manuscripts, but referring to them while planning and outlining the paper will ensure major principles for complete and accurate reporting are addressed in the manuscript.

REFERENCES

Crawford, B., Corbett, N., & Zuniga, A. (2014). Reducing hospital-acquired pressure ulcers: A quality improvement project across 21 hospitals. *Journal of Nursing Care Quality, 29*, 303–310. doi:10.1097/NCQ.0000000000000060

Hartley, J. (2012). New ways of making academic articles easier to read. *International Journal of Clinical and Health Psychology, 12*, 143–160. Retrieved from http://www.aepc.es/ijchp/articulos_pdf/ijchp-405.pdf

Holzmueller, C. G., & Pronovost, P. J. (2013). Organising a manuscript reporting quality improvement or patient safety research. *BMJ Quality & Safety, 22*, 777–785. doi:10.1136/bmjqs-2012-001603

Mosher, H., & Ogrinc, G. (2016). Between the guidelines: SQUIRE 2.0 and advances in healthcare improvement practice and reporting. *BMJ Quality & Safety, 25*, 559–561. doi:10.1136/bmjqs-2015-005039

Oermann, M. H. (2017). Writing manuscripts about quality improvement: SQUIRE 2.0 and beyond. *Author Resource Review*. Trevose, PA: Wolters Kluwer. Retrieved from http://wkauthorservices.editage.com./resources/author-resource-review/2017/May-2017.html

Oermann, M. H., & Leonardelli, A. (2013). Make the title count. *Nurse Author & Editor, 23*(3). Retrieved from http://naepub.com/writing-basics/2013-23-3-9

Oermann, M. H., Turner, K., & Carman, M. J. (2014). Preparing quality improvement, research and evidence-based practice manuscripts. *Nursing Economic$, 32*, 57–63, 69.

Ogrinc, G., Davies, L., Goodman, D., Batalden, P., Davidoff, F., & Stevens, D. (2016). SQUIRE 2.0 (Standards for QUality Improvement Reporting Excellence): Revised publication guidelines from a detailed consensus process. *Journal of Nursing Care Quality, 31*, 1–8. doi:10.1097/ncq.0000000000000153

SQUIRE. (2017). *Explanation and elaboration of SQUIRE 2.0 guidelines*. Retrieved from http://www.squire-statement.org/index.cfm?fuseaction=page.viewpage&pageid=504

Trail-Mahan, T., Heisler, S., & Katica, M. (2016). Quality improvement project to improve patient satisfaction with pain management: Using human-centered design. *Journal of Nursing Care Quality, 31*, 105–112; quiz 113–104. doi:10.1097/ncq.0000000000000161

Young, E., Paulk, J., Beck, J., Anderson, M., Burck, M., Jobman, L., & Stickrath, C. (2017). Impact of altered medication administration time on interdisciplinary bedside rounds on academic medical ward. *Journal of Nursing Care Quality, 32*, 218–225. doi:10.1097/ncq.0000000000000233

Zubkoff, L., Neily, J., Quigley, P., Delanko, V., Young-Xu, Y., Boar, S., & Mills, P. D. (2017). Preventing falls and fall-related injuries in State Veterans Homes: Virtual Breakthrough Series Collaborative. *Journal of Nursing Care Quality*. [E-pub ahead of print]. doi:10.1097/ncq.0000000000000309

8

CLINICAL PRACTICE ARTICLES

This chapter presents strategies for writing articles about clinical practice. There are many opportunities for preparing these manuscripts. Nurses can write about their innovations in practice, unit-based initiatives and projects, updates on clinical topics, and new directions in patient care. Lectures and presentations on clinical topics can be adapted into manuscripts for clinical journals, disseminating this new information to readers. Considering the wealth of clinical journals in nursing, these publications provide a venue for nurses to share their work with others.

WRITING FOR CLINICAL JOURNALS

There are many nursing journals that address topics in clinical practice. Most of the journals in nursing are clinical specialty journals. The articles in these journals disseminate new knowledge and skills for patient care, enabling nurses to stay current in clinical practice. With these types of articles, nurses in one setting can describe their practice innovations for use and testing by nurses in other settings. Dissemination of innovations is needed to advance nursing practice, but they often do not get shared with other nurses because of barriers to writing for publication (Tyndall, Scott, & Caswell, 2017). In clinical articles, nurses can discuss issues they encountered in patient care and how they resolved those issues, and they can share nursing approaches that worked and ones that did not work. Readers can then build on the experiences of others rather than starting from the beginning. Writing for publication provides a way for staff nurses and nurse leaders to share innovative advances in practice, leadership, education, and research (Batcheller, Kirksey, VanDyke, & Armstrong, 2012; von Isenburg, Lee, & Oermann, 2017). To remain competent, professionals need to continually expand their own knowledge base and skills; clinical practice articles provide a source of information for meeting this need.

Idea for Clinical Article

The process for writing a manuscript on clinical practice begins with an idea, similar to other manuscripts. This idea may come from a patient experience the author had or a clinical situation in which the author was involved, from activities in the clinical setting in which the author participated, and from discussion with nursing staff and other providers. Projects, innovations, and initiatives implemented on the unit, in the clinical setting, and in the community lend themselves to publication, which is essential to disseminate this information to other nurses for use in their own settings. The idea for a manuscript may evolve from a frustrating experience the author had or an issue in clinical practice that the author eventually resolved. Clinical articles often result from the nurse's own experiences with patients, families, and staff and later reflection on those experiences. Thus, one primary source of ideas for manuscripts for clinical journals is the author's clinical practice and interactions with other nurses and healthcare providers.

Lectures and presentations provide another source of ideas for manuscripts for clinical journals. Nurse educators in academic and clinical settings are continually preparing lectures and other types of presentations, many of which pertain to clinical practice or are intended to keep nurses up to date. If the presentation relates to new knowledge and interventions for patient care, a change in practice that will benefit patients across clinical settings, a trend in nursing and healthcare, an issue involving patients and consumers, and so forth, these lectures may be rewritten as manuscripts. Lectures and other types of presentations can be developed into manuscripts for journals that publish papers across clinical practice areas, such as the *American Journal of Nursing*, or journals in specialty areas of practice, depending on the topic.

One technique used to generate publications is to write the manuscript first and then develop the lecture or presentation. That strategy encourages nurses to write for publication and use wisely their limited time for writing. Course materials that nurse educators develop also might be adapted for publications. It is critical, however, to think about possible manuscripts before beginning to develop the lecture or presentation. By planning the paper as the first step, educators can identify possible journals and conduct a literature review that would be appropriate for that journal and audience.

Another strategy is to expand conference presentations (oral and poster) into manuscripts. Unfortunately, many abstracts developed for conferences and presentations at conferences are never turned into manuscripts. The same strategy can be used as recommended for lectures: write the manuscript prior to preparing the abstract for submission to or presentation at the conference. The author should review the conference guidelines to ensure that abstracts can be submitted on work that has been published or should time the submission of the manuscript to allow first for presentation at the conference and then subsequent publication of the project.

Ideas for clinical articles also may evolve from research studies, literature reviews, educational experiences, and other activities that lead to new information or a different perspective about nursing practice. When deciding if the idea is worth pursuing for a manuscript for a clinical journal, the author should answer these questions.

- Is the idea new and innovative?
- If the idea is not new, does it provide a different perspective to current practice?
- Is the content relevant to clinical practice? If so, is it applicable to nursing practice in a specialty area or in general?
- Do nurses *need* this information for their practice, and will it improve patient care?
- Will the information be valuable in keeping nurses up to date about trends in nursing and healthcare?
- Will the content inform readers about the types of activities and work nurses are doing in other settings and places?

These questions give authors a framework for deciding if the clinical topic is worth pursuing for publication.

Purpose of Article

From the initial idea, the author specifies the purpose of the manuscript. This is an important step because manuscripts for clinical journals can have many different perspectives. What is the goal of the paper? Is it to present new nursing care practices and interventions? Will the rationale and related research other evidence be emphasized? Is the intent to describe nursing interventions and their effectiveness, to present a clinical guideline and how well it worked with a specific patient population, or to describe an interdisciplinary plan of care? Or, is the goal to present a personal experience with a patient? Answering questions such as these enables the author to clarify the purpose of the paper.

Intended Readers

The next step is to identify the intended readers of the manuscript. These readers may be staff nurses, advanced practice nurses, managers, and nurses in other roles. Who will read the article dictates the content included in it.

Manuscripts about clinical practice may be written for a general nursing audience, providing information to help nurses across specialties and settings stay current. Other clinical articles address nurses who practice in a particular specialty area. These articles focus on specific health problems and patient populations or communities. This is an important difference when deciding on the journal for submission because it determines the complexity of the content and types of examples used in the discussion. Clinical articles written for a general nursing audience may describe the content more broadly and use more common examples. In planning the content, the author takes into consideration the knowledge and background of the intended readers. This is another reason that selecting the target journal for submission is an early step in the writing process.

In preparing the manuscript, the author also determines the prerequisite knowledge needed by readers to understand the content. This guides the author in deciding on the background material to include in the paper to make the new information clear. For example, in preparing a manuscript on clavicle fractures in children for the journal *Orthopaedic Nursing*, limited background information would be needed about the general care of patients with fractures. However, if the manuscript is written for nurses across specialties as a means of updating them and for general interest, more discussion would be required about common mechanisms of injury, care of patients with fractures, anatomy and function of the clavicle, and other background information.

FORMAT OF MANUSCRIPTS ABOUT CLINICAL PRACTICE

The format for writing manuscripts about clinical practice depends on the purpose of the article and journal chosen for submission. Some journals have departments, columns, or sections for different types of clinical articles. The author decides prior to beginning the paper if it will be developed for a department in a journal because often these manuscripts have different requirements; for example, they may be shorter and more focused than the main articles. Research and clinical practice manuscripts submitted to the *Journal of Emergency Nursing* are limited to a maximum of 15 pages, but papers submitted for publication in one of the departments or sections in the journal are no more than five pages including references. The allowed length is important to know before beginning to write to plan the content.

There is no standard format for writing manuscripts on clinical topics. A manuscript that presents nursing interventions for patients with a particular health problem will be organized differently than one that reviews pharmacology. In contrast to research articles, which follow a standard format, clinical manuscripts vary because of the wide range of topics addressed in them.

Some general guidelines for writing clinical articles follow. However, the author should remember that these guidelines may not pertain to every manuscript, depending on its focus.

Title

As with other manuscripts, every clinical paper needs a title. The purpose of the title is to inform readers what new information will be presented in the paper. Keywords that represent the content should be used in the title, and the title should be concise.

Nurses are busy professionals, and with a series of articles to read in a journal and limited time, the title needs to draw the attention of readers. For example, "Screening Patients for Alcohol Abuse: *No More Surprises*" is more of an attention-getter than the title "Assessment of Patients for Alcohol Abuse."

Similar to research articles, only one title may be written, or the article may be developed with a subtitle that provides more specific information about the paper. When subtitles are used, the terms that represent the main focus of the article should be placed first in the title. For example:

Single Title

Physical and Communication Problems in Feeding Patients With Dysphagia Following a Stroke

Title With Subtitle

Feeding Poststroke Patients With Dysphagia: Physical and Communication Problems

Abstract

Not all clinical manuscripts are submitted with an abstract, but when an abstract is required, it should concisely present the content included in the paper and its clinical implications. The abstract is the author's first chance to convince readers that the paper is important to read. Because abstracts are indexed and available in an electronic search, the abstract is critical to guide readers to the paper. Four to five of the most important points, findings, or implications should be integrated in the abstract, using specific terms that others might include in a search (American Psychological Association [APA], 2010).

Abstracts vary in length. A study of nursing journals indicated that abstracts ranged from as short as 40 words to 500 words, with a median of 200 words (Oermann et al., 2018). How to prepare the abstract for a particular journal and the maximum number of words allowed are described in the author guidelines.

Examples of abstracts for clinical articles are provided in Exhibit 8.1. These examples show that the abstracts inform readers about the content in the article and its practical implications.

Introduction

The first section of the manuscript is the introduction. In the introduction the author presents the purpose of the paper, an overview of the topics in it, the relevance of the content for clinical practice, and the value of the article to nurses.

The first or lead paragraph of the introduction is the most important one because if it is unclear or poorly written, the readers will not continue with the article. The lead-in paragraph also needs to capture the reader's interest. The author can use the lead-in paragraph to indicate the purpose, topics, and relevance to clinical practice. For example:

Many patients are unable to report the pain they are experiencing. This places them at risk for pain that is undertreated because of communication problems. This article describes how to assess a patient's pain using the basic measures of pain intensity as a framework and following six other steps. The information is important for nurses when caring for patients who are unable to report their pain.

Other types of lead-in paragraphs introduce the topic but focus more on getting the readers' attention. There are three types of opening paragraphs that attempt to get the attention of the readers as their primary purpose: anecdotal opening, placing the reader in the clinical situation, and using statistics.

EXHIBIT 8.1

Sample Abstracts for Clinical Articles

EXAMPLE 1

Preeclampsia, one of four hypertensive disorders of pregnancy, has traditionally been characterized as new-onset hypertension and proteinuria developing after 20 weeks' gestation. It is, however, now understood to be a complex, progressive, multisystem disorder with a highly variable presentation and a number of potentially life-threatening complications. The American College of Obstetricians and Gynecologists Task Force on Hypertension in Pregnancy has refined preeclampsia diagnostic criteria accordingly, and as the disorder's pathogenesis has been more clearly defined, new targets for screening, diagnosis, prevention, and treatment have emerged. This clinical update provides a review of current practice related to preeclampsia risk assessment, prediction, and management. It discusses preeclampsia pathophysiology and points readers to valuable healthcare resources on the topic.[1]

EXAMPLE 2

Hyperglycemia occurs in more than 30% of hospitalized patients. The condition has been associated with higher mortality and poor outcomes. Systems to effectively treat dysglycemia have been put into place, although many focus on critical care areas. The purpose of this article is to provide an overview of the challenges for glycemic control in noncritical care areas. Standardized order sets, critical pathways, professional education, and collaborative systems can support improved control.[2]

EXAMPLE 3

Galactosemia is an inborn error of galactose metabolism that results from a deficiency in one of three enzymes, uridine diphosphate galactose 4'epimerase, galactokinase, or galactose-1-phosphate uridyltransferase (GALT). This article focuses on classical, clinical variant, and biochemical variant (Duarte) galactosemias caused by GALT enzyme deficiency. A brief overview of galactosemia and newborn screening is presented, followed by detailed

(continued)

EXHIBIT 8.1

Sample Abstracts for Clinical Articles (*continued*)

information about each of the conditions. Confirmatory testing, acute and long-term management, and outcome for these galactosemia types are discussed as well as the importance of genetic counseling and testing for the infant and family to refine reproductive risk.[3]

Sources: [1]From Anderson, C. M., & Schmella, M. J. (2017). CE: Preeclampsia current approaches to nursing management. *American Journal of Nursing, 117*(11), 30–38. doi:10.1097/01.NAJ.0000526722.26893.b5
[2]Gerard, S. O., & Ritchie, J. (2017). Challenges of inpatient glycemic control. *Journal of Nursing Care Quality, 32*, 267–271. doi:10.1097/ncq.0000000000000257
[3]Anderson, S. (2018). GALT deficiency galactosemia. *MCN: The American Journal of Maternal/Child Nursing, 43*(1), 44–51. doi:10.1097/nmc.0000000000000388

Anecdotal Openings

Anecdotal openings share a real or simulated clinical experience or present a case scenario that readers can identify with professionally or personally. The opening may describe a patient and his or her health problems, begin with a case scenario, or describe nurses' experiences in caring for patients and their own feelings. Anecdotal openings capture readers' interest by indicating the professional or personal relevance of the information to them as nurses.

The following is an example of an anecdotal opening to an article on adrenal crisis, related physiology, how to differentiate it from other conditions, nursing care and related medical management, and averting future episodes.

> Ms. S, age 52, is brought to the ED with severe abdominal pain, fever, and rapid pulse. She walks slowly and is unsteady. Ms. S has been vomiting for more than 2 days, and she has had no appetite for the last week. Her past medical history includes surgery for an adrenal gland tumor. You realize this is not the flu.

This example also shows the contrast in writing style from research articles, which tend to be more formal and use an academic style of writing. Often clinical journals prefer a more informal writing style, as seen in this example.

Placement in Clinical Situation

A similar type of lead-in paragraph is when the reader is placed in the clinical situation. In this introduction, the nurse is involved in the scenario as a realistic participant who needs to make decisions and act in response to the situation. The question for the reader is, "What would you do in this clinical situation?" An example of this type of attention-getter is as follows:

> You have been working in the clinical agency for nearly 10 months. Recently you noticed a colleague having difficulty completing her

assignments on time. She is often late for work and asks you to
cover for her. Today you notice her moving from one patient to the
next without washing her hands.

This example provides the clinical context for the article and engages the reader as a participant in it. Here the reader "becomes" the nurse involved in this dilemma, which the article analyzes and provides options for how the nurse might handle the situation. A personal experience of the nurse, positive or negative, also serves to "connect with readers" who may have had similar experiences and to engage them in the topic.

Use of Statistics

Another attention-getter is using statistics that demonstrate the impact of the information on patient care, the nurse's own practice, or healthcare in general. In this type of introduction, statistics are presented to show the magnitude of the problem and its implications, signifying the importance of the article. For example, this lead-in paragraph to an article on screening patients for alcohol abuse uses alarming facts to illustrate the magnitude of the problem:

The next time you attend a social event, look around the room
and consider this: about 6.2% of adults in the United States have
an alcohol use disorder. Nearly 26.9% of people aged 18 or older
engaged in binge drinking in the past month, and 7.0% admitted to
heavy drinking.

Text

The text or body of the paper following the introduction varies depending on the content. Because clinical manuscripts can address a wide range of topics, from general practice updates to specific interventions for one type of patient problem, there is no one outline that can be used. The following principles guide development of the text for clinical articles.

- Organize the content from simple to complex and from known to unknown.
- Provide background information, rationale, and evidence, for readers to understand the problems, interventions, and outcomes.
- Focus on what nurses need to learn about assessment of patients, significant data to collect, related diagnostic tests, and interpretation of data, considering alternate perspectives and possibilities.
- Focus on what nurses need to learn about patient responses, problems, and diagnoses; interventions; and outcomes. Emphasize related research, evidence, and implications for clinical practice.

- Focus on nursing management rather than medical management even though this content also may be included in the paper. The goal is to help nurses assess patients and effectively manage their problems.
- If using a scenario as an attention-getter, relate the content in the paper to the scenario for readers to see how this new information can be used in clinical practice.
- Use examples from clinical practice in the paper to assist readers in applying the new information to patient care. Consider using one scenario throughout the paper as a way of demonstrating how the concepts relate to assessment, diagnoses, interventions, and outcomes. In this way, the scenario provides a model of how the new information is actually used in clinical practice.
- Answer questions of "Why?" "What if . . .?" "What are other options and possible decisions?" "How?" Answering these questions promotes the nurses' higher level thinking and clinical judgment about the content.
- When using an acronym, write it out the first time it is mentioned in the paper, but from that point on use only the acronym for the remainder of the manuscript. For example: "This paper describes the outcomes of a nurse-managed clinic for patients with heart failure (HF). Nurse practitioners care for patients with HF both inpatient and in the clinic."
- Use a writing style consistent with the journal. Some of the clinical journals use "I" and "you" rather than "the nurse." The author should gather information about writing style before beginning the draft by reading through some of the articles in the target journal.
- Use frequent and specific subheadings that clearly describe the content in that section. The author should review a few articles in the journal for submission because types of subheadings often vary. Some journals use more formal subheadings than do others. This difference can be seen in Table 8.1.

The extent of background information to include is based on the author's professional judgment and an understanding of the readers' needs. When presenting new information not available in nursing textbooks or through other resources, the author includes more background material than would be necessary for a manuscript on a common patient problem known by most readers. For example, if writing an article on congenital hyperinsulinism, the author would include

TABLE 8.1 COMPARISON OF SUBHEADINGS FOR CLINICAL ARTICLE

Formal	Informal
Venous Thromboembolism	What Is VTE?
Pathophysiology	Why Does VTE Occur?
Incidence of Venous Thromboembolism	How Common Is VTE?
Risk Factors of Venous Thromboembolism and Evidence	Assessment of Risk Factors: Be Alert
Nursing Care and Clinical Guidelines	Caring for Your Patient With VTE

VTE, venous thromboembolism.

a thorough description of this condition and its etiology because most readers would not be familiar with it, in contrast to a manuscript on hypoglycemia.

Other considerations in planning the content for a clinical paper are the journal and the readers of that journal. The author needs to understand the background of readers because the content should be at an appropriate level for them. A paper on management of hypertension written for a cardiovascular nursing journal would present limited background information because readers of that journal know about this condition and typical treatments. However, that same paper prepared for a general nursing journal would explain the pathophysiology and progression of hypertension, usual treatments, and other basic information so that readers will understand the new approaches to managing hypertension discussed in the article. The content, therefore, needs to reflect the emphasis of the journal and background of readers.

The organization of the content is based on the purpose of the manuscript and the style of the journal. Authors should organize the content logically, for example, beginning with the background for readers to understand the problem, and then progressing to the care of patients or other focus of the paper. In clinical journals, it is important for authors to present the evidence supporting their interventions and identify where further evidence is needed to make decisions about clinical practice.

Conclusion

Every clinical article, similar to other papers, ends with a conclusion. The conclusion summarizes the information and its value to nurses in their own clinical practice. It also may suggest areas where further work is needed, such as testing of an intervention across settings, but the conclusion should not introduce new information. The conclusion is generally one to two paragraphs in length.

Many of these same principles can be used in writing other types of articles. The author is reminded to follow the format of the journal for submission and gear the paper to intended readers.

WRITING RESEARCH REPORTS FOR CLINICAL JOURNALS

Chapter 5 explained how to write research reports, and while those principles apply to preparing papers on original research studies for clinical journals, there are some additional guidelines to consider when writing these manuscripts. Findings from research need to be disseminated in the clinical nursing literature to reach nurses who can implement them in their own practices and to build the evidence base for nursing. Clinical journals are an effective mechanism for accomplishing these goals. Through citation analysis, Oermann, Shaw-Kokot, Knafl, and Dowell (2010) explored the dissemination of original research reports with clinical relevance into clinical nursing journals. The 28 research articles had a total of 759 citations, and 717 (94.5%) of those were in clinical articles. In addition to clinical articles keeping readers up to date on practice changes, this study confirmed the important role of clinical journals in disseminating research findings to readers.

Guidelines for Writing

The IMRAD format presented in more detail in Chapter 5—Introduction, Methods, Results, and Discussion—can be used for a research report intended for a clinical journal. This structure provides a way of organizing the manuscript, and for some clinical journals, these headings can be used with an additional section on clinical implications. In the introduction, the author should identify the clinical problem that led to the study, gap in the research, and why this study was essential to better understand the problem, develop interventions for it, and improve patient outcomes, among other reasons. A good introduction in a clinical journal links the significance of the study to the nurse's own clinical practice. This writing not only sets the stage for the remainder of the manuscript, but also captures the reader's interest.

When writing research reports for clinical journals, the literature review is generally less extensive than for a research journal. The review of the literature can be incorporated into the introduction, consistent with the IMRAD format, or presented separately. Reviewing research articles in the target clinical journal gives the author a sense of how these manuscripts are developed in terms of the literature review and other parts of the manuscript.

The next section of the manuscript presents the methods that the researcher used to carry out the study. In a research journal, the methods section provides detailed information about the design, subjects, measures, procedures, and data analysis, in that order. Generally, each subsection is labeled similarly. When preparing manuscripts on research studies for clinical journals, the methods section may not be as complex or detailed as in research journals. The principle is to present enough information for clinicians to understand the findings and consider how they might be used in their own clinical setting, and then to replicate the study. Authors should also keep in mind that clinicians may not have the background to understand the methods and statistical analysis. Instead, clinicians want to know how the research findings can guide their practice and work in nursing.

Exhibit 8.2 provides two examples of methods sections written for clinical specialty journals. Example 1 describes the clinical research methods for a quantitative study and Example 2 describes them for a qualitative study.

Another type of method that clinical authors often need to present in a manuscript is their underlying literature search strategy, especially when developing a clinical protocol, document, or innovation and writing about evidence-based practice. For these projects, clinicians search not only the empirical literature but also practice and professional documents from various nursing organizations. For readers to evaluate the value and applicability of the proposal,

EXHIBIT 8.2

Examples of Methods Section From Articles Published in Clinical Journals

EXAMPLE 1

Method

Design and Sample

This was an exploratory study on patients' perspectives of quality healthcare. A convenience sample was used of 116 patients who received healthcare in the past 6 months in a wound clinic associated with a large health system in the Midwest.

Instruments

Subjects completed the Quality Health Care Questionnaire (QHCQ) on which they rated the personal importance of 16 attributes of health care and nursing care quality. Three of those attributes related to patient education by the nurse: (a) teaching patients about their wounds, treatments, related health problems, and medications; (b) teaching patients how to maintain their health; and (c) providing access to a wound care nurse for teaching after a clinic visit. A Likert scale of 1 (not at all important) to 5 (very important) was used. Patients also completed a demographic data sheet.

Procedures

The QHCQ and demographic data sheet were mailed to patients within 48 hours after receiving care at the wound clinic.

Data Analysis

Data were analyzed using descriptive statistics. Means and standard deviations were calculated for each of the attributes on the QHCQ. Pearson correlation was used to examine the correlations between demographic characteristics of the patients and their scores on the QHCQ.

EXAMPLE 2

Patients and caregivers were recruited at a large suburban hospital Level I trauma center during their initial hospitalization to participate in the research. Target subjects were caregivers of patients aged 20 to 60 years who sustained one or more extremity fracture and/or pelvic fractures and were hospitalized at least 5 days. Patients with a diagnosis of TBI or SCI were excluded from the study . . . . Approval for the study was obtained from the hospital's institutional review board.

Subjects met with the researcher for three private, in-depth, semistructured, face-to-face interviews: during the initial hospitalization; upon returning home; and 4 to 5 months postinjury. Interview questions were designed to identify the most salient concerns to family members at the time of the interview . . . . The interviews ranged between 1 and 2 hours and were de-identified, recorded, and transcribed.

(continued)

EXHIBIT 8.2

Examples of Methods Section From Articles Published in Clinical Journals (*continued*)

A qualitative approach was chosen for this project . . . . A community advisory board (CAB) consisting of caregivers, patients, and a nurse was engaged throughout the project to offer guidance and feedback from project design, interview guide development, and data analysis . . . .

An initial set of themes was derived from the first several transcripts of interviews conducted in the hospital . . . . Themes, such as "system barriers" or "community support," were then refined iteratively and collectively: The CAB members developed additional codes in a review of the same transcripts. . . . The resulting final codebook was applied to each remaining transcript. . . . Coding fragments relevant to each theme were extracted from individual transcripts and compiled into separate data sets for further analysis of themes and patterns across and between cases. These data sets were analyzed to identify the range of experiences and common themes regarding burdens, stressors, facilitators, barriers, coping, and impact.[1]

Note: Selected parts of each section.
Source: [1]From Newcomb, A. B., & Hymes, R. A. (2017). Life interrupted: The trauma caregiver experience. *Journal of Trauma Nursing, 24,* 125–133. doi:10.1097/jtn.0000000000000278

the search strategy needs to be presented succinctly but convincingly as to its comprehensiveness. This process was described and illustrated in Chapter 6.

As with any research paper, the aim of the results section is to present the findings. However, when the readers are clinicians, authors should avoid reporting complex statistics and for qualitative studies detailed discussions of the theoretical perspective, method, and data analysis. Clinicians may not have the background to understand these and are primarily interested in the clinical implications of the study. Easy-to-read tables and figures that demonstrate visually the outcomes of the study are valuable to promote understanding of the results (Exhibit 8.3).

The discussion section is one of the most important. It allows the author to explain the implications of the findings for clinical practice. In this section, the author should explain why the findings are important. The author should be explicit about how the findings can or cannot be used in practice and identify considerations in implementing the results in one's own setting. For example, a study on the relationship between blood culture contamination rates and workload perceptions done in a children's hospital may not be applicable to adult patients. In the discussion section, authors should guide readers in identifying how and under what conditions the findings could be used in practice, for example, by describing types of patients and conditions under which the findings could be used. The implications for practice can be integrated in the discussion section or can be a subsection. Authors should check the guidelines of the journal, as some journals specify whether a separate section should be included on implications.

EXHIBIT 8.3

Example of Easy-to-Read Tables and Figure

Table. Differences in Importance Ratings Between Men and Women

Importance Ratings	Men M (SD)	Women M (SD)	t
Able to ask nurse questions	4.13 (.83)	4.12 (.85)	0.07
Having nurse teach me about illness and treatments	4.58 (.81)	4.51 (.89)	0.61
Having nurse teach me self-care for discharge	4.56 (.89)	3.91 (.98)	2.51*

*$p = .006$

Table. Comparison of Websites for Asthma Patient Education

Content Areas	Percent of Websites With Content	
	2016 study (N = 70)	2018 study (N = 145)
Asthma triggers	77.8	92.1
Asthma pathophysiology	72.0	84.4
Avoidance of triggers	67.6	71.2
Action of long-term control medications	62.9	55.6
Action of quick relief rescue medications	60.4	61.0
Self-care skills	36.9	52.8
Asthma action plan	32.0	41.2

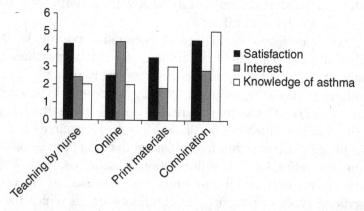

Figure. Satisfaction, interest, and knowledge gain of patients taught by different methods. Ratings from 0 (none) to 6 (high).

Writing About Pilot and Evaluation Studies

These same principles apply when preparing a paper on a pilot study or an evaluation of a project or initiative on the unit. These studies may have small samples and may not be as rigorous as other research, but nevertheless should be shared with clinicians who are considering similar projects in their own settings. The knowledge gained from evaluations done by nurses of interventions and new initiatives may be important for answering questions about clinical practice. Reports of clinical projects conducted and evaluated in one setting may guide the practice and activities of nurses in another setting.

There are other situations in which the nurse initiated a research study but because of problems in implementation was not able to carry it out as planned. In developing a manuscript about the study, the nurse might view it as a pilot to inform others about its purpose and provide a basis for subsequent research. The nurse also might develop a manuscript on the difficulties encountered in conducting this type of study and possible solutions.

Rather than the conventional format of a research report, manuscripts on pilot studies and evaluations of projects and initiatives can be developed based on the problem that led to the study or project, a description of the study or project and the data collected, the findings, and the implications for practice. If changes were subsequently made in practice, then the manuscript also may describe these changes and the evaluation planned to monitor them over time. In manuscripts such as these, the research process may guide authors in deciding on content to include and how to organize it, but they may decide not to use the IMRAD headings.

Some journals do not publish pilot and evaluation studies, so authors should review the journal guidelines and query the editor at the outset. With these studies, authors should weigh the conclusions and implications for practice against the sample size and quality of the study, being careful not to overstate them.

SUMMARY

Clinical practice articles disseminate new knowledge and skills for patient care, provide information for nurses to stay current in clinical practice, and update them on new technologies and advances in care. With this type of article, nurses in one setting can describe their practice innovations for use and testing by nurses in other settings. They can discuss issues they encountered in patient care and how they resolved those issues, and they can share nursing approaches that worked and ones that did not work.

The process for writing a clinical article begins with an idea. From this idea, the author specifies the purpose of the manuscript and then identifies the intended readers. Who will read the article dictates the content included in it. In planning the content, the author takes into consideration the knowledge and background of the intended audience.

There is no standard format for writing clinical articles, in contrast to research papers, because it depends on the purpose of the manuscript. Some general guidelines for writing clinical articles were presented in this chapter, including how to write the title, abstract, introduction and different types of lead-in paragraphs, and body of the paper. Every clinical article ends with a discussion section, with implications for practice and the value of the information to the nurse's own clinical practice, and a conclusion that summarizes the information in the paper.

The IMRAD format presented earlier can be used for a research report intended for clinician readers. This structure provides a way of organizing the manuscript; for some clinical journals, these headings can be used with an additional section on clinical implications.

In the introduction, the author should identify the clinical problem that led to the study, gap in the research, and why this study was essential to better understand the problem, develop interventions for it, and improve patient outcomes, among other reasons. A good introduction links the significance of the study to the nurse's own clinical practice. When writing research reports for clinical journals, the literature review is generally less extensive than for a research journal. The review of the literature can be incorporated into the introduction, consistent with the IMRAD format, or presented separately. In the methods section the authors should explain what was done, who participated, how they measured and interpreted the results, and how they carried out the study, keeping in mind that the main readers are clinicians, not researchers.

As with any research paper, the aim of the results section is to present the findings. Easy-to-read tables and figures that demonstrate visually the outcomes of the study are valuable to promote understanding of the results. The discussion section is one of the most important: it allows the author to explain what the findings mean for clinical practice. It is important to be explicit about how the findings can or cannot be used in practice and to identify considerations in implementing the results in one's own setting. These same principles apply when writing manuscripts about pilot and evaluation studies.

There are many clinical situations in which nurses find themselves that lend to writing for publication. Nurses need to take advantage of these opportunities to disseminate their ideas and innovations to others.

REFERENCES

American Psychological Association. (2010). *Publication manual of the American Psychological Association* (6th ed.). Washington, DC: Author.

Anderson, S. (2018). GALT deficiency galactosemia. *MCN: The American Journal of Maternal/Child Nursing, 43*, 44–51. doi:10.1097/nmc.0000000000000388

Anderson, C. M., & Schmella, M. J. (2017). CE: Preeclampsia current approaches to nursing management. *American Journal of Nursing, 117*, 30–38. doi:10.1097/01.NAJ.0000526722.26893.b5

Batcheller, J., Kirksey, K. M., VanDyke, Y., & Armstrong, M. L. (2012). Publish or perish: Writing clinical manuscripts suitable for publication. *Journal of Continuing Education in Nursing, 43*, 44–48. doi:10.3928/00220124-20111003-01

Gerard, S. O., & Ritchie, J. (2017). Challenges of inpatient glycemic control. *Journal of Nursing Care Quality, 32*, 267–271. doi:10.1097/ncq.0000000000000257

Newcomb, A. B., & Hymes, R. A. (2017). Life interrupted: The trauma caregiver experience. *Journal of Trauma Nursing, 24*, 125–133. doi:10.1097/jtn.0000000000000278

Oermann, M. H., Nicoll, L. H., Chinn, P. L., Conklin, J. L., McCarty, M., & Amarasekara, S. (2018). Quality of author guidelines in nursing journals. *Journal of Nursing Scholarship.* Advance online publication. doi:10.1111/jnu.12383

Oermann, M. H., Shaw-Kokot, J., Knafl, G. J., & Dowell, J. (2010). Dissemination of research into clinical nursing literature. *Journal of Clinical Nursing, 19*, 3435–3442. doi:10.1111/j.1365-2702.2010.03427.x

Tyndall, D. E., Scott, E. S., & Caswell, N. I. (2017). Factors facilitating publication by clinical nurses in a Magnet® hospital. *Journal of Nursing Administration, 47*, 522–526. doi:10.1097/nna.0000000000000525

von Isenburg, M., Lee, L. S., & Oermann, M. H. (2017). Writing together to get AHEAD: An interprofessional boot camp to support scholarly writing in the health professions. *Journal of the Medical Library Association, 105*, 167–172. doi:10.5195/jmla.2017.222

CHAPTERS, BOOKS, AND OTHER FORMS OF WRITING

9

OTHER TYPES OF WRITING

Although research and clinical practice articles are the primary formats for nurses to present knowledge to readers, other forms of writing are equally important. Some articles address emerging issues that affect nursing practice, education, or research. These articles may include case reports; descriptions of theory development; commentaries on policies, ethics, or legal aspects of nursing; innovative research methods; historical studies; editorials; and letters to the editor. Nurses also write book reviews and articles for consumer and nonprofessional audiences. These other types of writing differ in the purposes they are trying to achieve, their format, and often their writing style. Yet all are similar because they address nontrivial topics, provide original insight, and have implications for advancing health and well-being.

As with all scientific writing, the first part of any article must convince the reader that it addresses a topic of broad importance. Authors might ask themselves about their work, "So what?" If the article stands little chance of changing something important for the better, it is probably not worth the author's time to write! For editors and readers, the time and expense of reviewing, publishing, and reading the article would not be justified. The importance of the topic should be made quickly evident in all types of articles, that is, in the first or second paragraph.

In the first sentence, the author should identify a problem or knowledge gap. Then the reader will want to know how the problem is defined, and what are its dimensions and scope. For example, health problems should be described by their incidence, prevalence, and outcomes. At the conclusion of the brief introduction, the reader should understand how the article will address an important problem.

The paragraphs that follow the introductory paragraphs expand on the background material on the problem. Usually, the author summarizes other recent published articles that focus on the problem, describes how much progress has been made in solving the problem, and discusses the background issues that affect the problem. If there is disagreement among published authors, these should be highlighted. The author should identify gaps in the knowledge base in order to provide a rationale for the article. Who needs what in order to accomplish what goal? By the end of the first part of the article, the reader should clearly understand what the rationale for the article is and what are its intended objectives.

The middle part of an article presents the author's original contribution to addressing the problem or issue. When new data are not the focus as in research articles, the original material may include an analysis of the secondary material, application of previous material to a new setting, proposal of new dimensions to a problem, refinement of a concept or procedure, report of a new type of case, and other novel material. When presenting such material, authors should be specific and concrete about any new definitions, dimensions, relationships, or flow among the components of the material. Graphics are particularly useful for readers in order to visualize the nature or scope of new material. The author should also describe clearly the settings and circumstances in which the new material was developed or emerged or is relevant.

The last part of the article should summarize briefly how the aims and objectives of the article were met. The author can be specific about how the original material advances previously published work, as well as what limitations it has. Without overreaching the logical implications of the original material, the author should reflect on how the contents of the article might be used in patient care settings, educational institutions, research groups, or policy arenas. If additional work would be useful to extend the material, the author should describe the logical next steps. In the following sections, we describe how to approach the rationale and background, original material, and conclusions and implications in specific types of articles.

PROFESSIONAL ISSUES ARTICLES

What about the emerging issues in nursing? Information about trends and issues in nursing is becoming increasingly available in real time on the Internet. However, nurses still need publications that analyze issues in terms of why and how they developed, the varied positions that can be taken on them, and multiple strategies for resolving them. Many clinical journals publish this type of paper. Some specialty journals have a department or column on professional issues affecting nurses in that area of clinical practice, societal issues facing patients, and other opinion pieces. As well, the *Online Journal of Issues in Nursing (OJIN)* presents a variety of perspectives on issues in nursing across clinical specialties and settings. The journal recognizes that individuals have differing views on issues and provides a forum for readers to express their opinions and understand others' views (American Nurses Association, 2017).

Professional issues articles begin with a discussion of the issue and why and how it developed. Some articles address information needed to understand the issue itself, increasing nurses' knowledge about it. In these manuscripts, the goal is to improve understanding of issues in healthcare and nursing practice, not for nurses to assume a position about an issue. For example, a paper might provide an overview of prenatal testing, a historical perspective, and examples of prenatal tests, nursing views, and ethical considerations. Rather than taking a position about prenatal testing, the goal of the author is to present information about the issue and lay a foundation for better understanding related to ethical decisions.

In another approach, the author analyzes the issue from different points of view. In this type of article, the issue and the varied perspectives with rationales are presented for readers. For example, a manuscript on whether continuing education should be mandatory or voluntary might present both positions and the rationale for each, leaving the readers to decide on their position. Alternatively, the author might take one point of view and present a rationale to support it.

In issue papers, an author often specifies the assumptions on which thinking is based, the evidence used to guide the analysis of the issue, and how the author developed a position. In preparing these manuscripts, authors are advised to be clear about their own biases and perspectives so the content reflects an objective analysis of the issue rather than the author's view only.

CASE REPORTS AND HISTORIES

Case reports provide new information by focusing on a single patient, family, community setting, or organization, where in-depth knowledge of the specific case may be informative for understanding larger groups of patients or settings. These manuscripts often begin with why the case was selected and its importance to nursing practice and continue with a description of the case and related care by nurses and other disciplines. For example, authors presented a case report of a multiparous woman who presented at 34 weeks gestation with an intracranial hematoma (ICH) and subsequently underwent a successful emergency caesarean section and craniotomy (Stein-Fredbeck, Rosenberg, & Frank 2017). The case highlighted the critical need for the development of more inclusive best practices to reduce morbidity and mortality for all types of ICH in pregnancy.

Although a single case study and its findings cannot be generalized, these articles can be used to describe patient care; illustrate how concepts, theories, and research are used in practice; present issues in a patient's care and strategies for resolving them; and apply new information to a real or hypothetical case. Case reports also can be used for promoting the clinical judgment, decision making, and critical thinking skills of nurses and nursing students. A case can be presented as involving multiple possible decisions and options that the nurse might choose. Consequences of each decision can be examined, followed by the decision the nurse made in the case.

A case report typically includes the following content areas:

- Introductory discussion of why this case is significant and how it will help nurses to better understand their patients' problems and care. An effective introduction makes it clear why the case is worth reading.

- Description of the case. In this section, the author presents relevant data about the case and background information. The case presentation may follow a chronological sequence or may represent one particular phase of the health problem.
- Nursing care planned and implemented for the patient, family, or community; evaluation of its effectiveness; and implications for nursing practice. The author might include in this section changes in practice suggested as a result of this case.
- Alternate decisions possible in the case and consequences of each. This is an important section if the case is designed to promote nurses' clinical judgment and critical thinking skills. The author might also include in this section how nurses might approach the patient's care from different perspectives.
- Ethical considerations. Cases may be used to present ethical issues in a patient's care and strategies for resolving ethical dilemmas.
- Conclusions with implications for clinical practice or research. The manuscript should conclude with a discussion of the implications of this case for the nurse's own practice and what it means to care for other patients. If systematic research is needed to generalize to populations, the author should specify research questions (American Psychological Association, 2010).

Publications in nursing, medicine, and other healthcare disciplines must protect the rights of individuals to privacy, as discussed in Chapter 5. Except in rare cases, patient names, initials, and case numbers should be omitted from published case reports. The *Recommendations for the Conduct, Reporting, Editing, and Publication of Scholarly Work in Medical Journals* suggest that identifying information about patients should not be published unless it is essential for scientific purposes, the patient or legally authorized representative gives written informed consent for publication in print and on the Internet, and the patient or legally authorized representative is allowed to review the manuscript before giving informed consent for the information to be published (International Committee of Medical Journal Editors [ICMJE], 2017). When informed consent is obtained, it should be indicated in the published article. Only essential details should be provided (American Medical Association [AMA], 2007).

If interested in publishing a case report, the author is cautioned to query the editor or check the author guidelines regarding a journal's interest in case reports as articles. Some journals have a department for which the case would be appropriate. As an example, the *Journal of Obstetric, Gynecologic, and Neonatal Nursing* (Wiley Interscience, 2017a) has a category for manuscripts that are case reports, that is, reviews of cases that present new information for nursing and interprofessional care.

PHILOSOPHICAL AND THEORETICAL ARTICLES

Other topical articles may be philosophical in nature or deal with theory development or testing. The format used to develop these manuscripts should fit the goals of the paper, the philosophical theory used for its development or the position taken, or the structure of the theory or framework.

Manuscripts of this type might discuss the historical development of nursing theory, present the results of the testing of concepts and theories in a defined population, analyze an existing theory and propose an extension of it or an alternative theory, identify a flaw in a theory, or compare different theories. Varied philosophical perspectives can be analyzed and compared. In general, these papers should include a review of the literature that serves as the foundation for the author's thinking and perspective. The authors should discuss the internal consistency and external validity of the theory, and implications for nursing research and further development of the theory. In writing philosophical and theoretical manuscripts, the author should be careful to present ideas in an order that is logical and sequenced appropriately.

As an example, Blok (2017) developed a middle-range theory of patient self-management behavior. She began the paper by describing the limitations of current definitions and applications of the concept of self-management behavior and the eight-step procedure and underlying framework that would guide her concept analysis. Next, she detailed the data sources and flowchart that yielded the $n = 189$ referent articles from which antecedents, attributes, and consequences of self-management behaviors emerged, as well as a model case. Finally, she presented a graphic representation of her proposed middle-range theory and discussed its advantages for interdisciplinary research and practice. In this way, the content and its presentation reflected concepts of theory development in nursing.

Some journals in nursing are devoted to nursing science and theory development. For example, the primary purpose of *Advances in Nursing Science* (Lippincott Williams & Wilkins, 2017) is to develop nursing knowledge and promote integration of theory and practice. Elements of such manuscripts routinely include literature reviews of existing theories, their extensions and alternatives; comparative analyses of related theories; and implications for nursing practice, research, and future theory development (Lippincott Williams & Wilkins, 2017). *Nursing Science Quarterly* also publishes papers on nursing theory development, existing nursing frameworks, and person-centered models of care (Sage Publications, 2017b).

POLICY ARTICLES

Nurses shape organizational and public policies in a way that affects their practice, education, and research. Articles are needed that describe the circumstances in which the need emerged for new or revised policies, how the structure and processes of new policies developed, and the outcomes of policy review and evaluation. Authors should clearly describe how data were gathered to understand the problem. What stakeholders were consulted? How were resources coordinated? What decisions were implemented? What did the evaluation plan entail? The general purpose, scope, timeline, and responsibilities of the policy should be summarized with enough specificity that the reader can evaluate its applicability to one's own setting and circumstances.

Policy-related articles may be appropriate for several kinds of journals. Some journals, such as *Policy, Politics, and Nursing Practice* (Sage Publications, 2017c), are dedicated to publishing a broad range of articles that describe the impact of public policy, legislation, and regulation on nursing practice and, conversely, of nurses on health policy at the national, state, and organizational levels. For example, recent articles in that journal have focused on an analysis of Affordable Care Act reforms (Rambur, 2017), on findings that support expansion of maternal care policies in New Hampshire (Hamlin, 2017), and on use of agency nurses to fill vacancies in palliative care settings (Cozad, Lindley, & Mixer, 2016)

Journals with broad interest and influence in professional nursing regularly publish articles focused on policy-related issues. Some evaluate the relationship between nursing practice and specific policies in clinical segments of the healthcare system. For example, the *Journal of Advanced Nursing* published an article that focused on the relationship between the content of advanced care planning policies for dementia patients in nursing homes and the care planning behaviors of healthcare professionals (Ampe, Sevenants, Smets, Declerq, & Van Audenhove, 2016). *Nursing Outlook* published an article revalidating an intergenerational model of partner violence that suggested important policy-related actions for nurse professionals (Fredland et al., 2016).

Authors may also find that editors of specialty journals are interested in articles on relevant policies for education or practice, especially when new policies from national or local oversight groups appear. For example, noting that Minnesota mandated an antibullying policy in all school districts without guidance on content or enforcement, Gower and colleagues assessed the relationship between the quality of school antibullying policies and the reported victimization and subsequent adjustment among 6th, 9th, and 12th graders in that state (Gower, Cousin, & Borowsky, 2017). The article, published in the *Journal of School Health* (Wiley Interscience, 2017c), discussed the inadequacy of even high-quality policies to reduce bullying and the additional contextual factors within school environments that require additional evaluation research. Similarly, in a geriatric nursing journal, Quinn, Brassard, O'Brien, and Reinecke (2017) described both progress in achieving full access and prescriptive authority for nurse practitioners across all 50 states in the wake of the 2010 *Campaign for Action* and the resources available to nurses for policy enhancement at the state level.

ETHICS ARTICLES

Although many types of articles written by nurses will feature a brief discussion of the ethical implications of a topic, authors may also organize an article to focus specifically on ethical issues related to organizations or patient care.

A journal such as *Nursing Ethics* (Sage Publications, 2017a) features a broad range of such articles. Recent ones have focused on the nurses' performance on clinical ethics committees, everyday ethical problems of nurses in combat zones, and the ethics of nurse participation in assisted suicide. Specialty journals and organizations also publish articles that focus on ethical practice related to specific kinds of care. Recent examples of ethics articles in the nursing literature include an exploration of the ethics related to the Cancer Moonshot (Hammer, 2016), older persons' withdrawal from dialysis (Hain, Diaz, & Paixao, 2016), and administration of antipsychotic medications (Smith & Herber, 2015).

The organization of an ethics paper will be dictated by the type of information being presented. All of the ethics articles noted earlier begin with a description of the background of the ethical dilemma or concern and what is at stake in a thorough investigation of it. The middle section includes the specifics of the original cases or data, laid out in a logical framework that makes clear what the author has found. The articles conclude with a synthesis or analysis of what was learned in such a way that readers take away new insights into ethical development or practice.

Some ethics articles may be similar to a research article, with introduction, methods, results, and discussion sections. For example, Smith and Herber (2015) introduced their article by documenting the potential for conscientious objections among nurses to restraining or coercing patients to receive antipsychotic depot or long-acting intramuscular injections for their own safety and well-being. In the Methods section, they described their study of eight mental health nurses and the qualitative methods used for analyzing their responses. In the results section, they presented four themes: lack of alternatives, safety, feeling uncomfortable, and difficulty maintaining the therapeutic relationship. The authors concluded with a discussion of the gaps and tensions among nurses under these circumstances and the potential remedies.

ARTICLES ON LEGAL ISSUES

Nursing practice, education, and research are constrained and empowered by legislation and regulation. Therefore, articles on legal issues are of critical interest in generalist nursing and specialty journals.

Articles on legal issues are structured according to the material to be presented, often in the IMRAD format. For example, two nurses studied legislation nationwide that governed access to indoor tanning beds among adolescents with a focus on parental consent and enforcement (Driscoll & Darcy, 2015). The introduction included the physiology, legislative history, and epidemiology of indoor tanning. The authors analyzed public access data on state laws in 50 states using an established coding instrument and interviewed Department of Health employees. States diverged widely in access, consent, and enforcement, and the authors concluded by presenting strategies for school health and advanced practice nurses as well as legislators.

Legal implications for professional practice are also important areas for articles by nurses. These topics include the legal issues associated with discharge processes for patients receiving Schedule II and III pain medications in emergency departments (Wolf, Delao, & Perhats, 2015) and the feasibility of legislation requiring newly licensed associate degree and diploma nurses to earn a bachelor of nursing degree within 10 years (Sarver, Cichra, & Kline, 2015).

ARTICLES ON RESEARCH METHODS

Nurses often identify concepts from grounded theory studies or clinical practice for which valid and reliable assessment tools are not available. When developing and testing original tools and scales, authors must use a rigorous research protocol. Results should be presented using the IMRAD format described in Chapter 5. Even when refining tests of validity and reliability of scales in new demographic populations or when using a subset of the original questionnaire items, authors should use a research manuscript format for presenting the findings.

However, some methodological innovations can be presented using nonresearch formats. Authors might describe the need for a translation of a specific survey tool into the language of a high-risk group of patients, what translation and back-translation procedures were employed, where the new tool was pilot tested, and what kind of next steps would demonstrate reliability. Another author might have developed ethical and effective strategies either for recruiting subjects who are often underrepresented in research studies or for retaining patients in high-stress circumstances over time for longitudinal studies. These manuscripts should include the background on the lack of a suitable methodological strategy, the original contribution of the authors to filling the need, and implications for how to apply it in the practice of research or practice.

HISTORY OF NURSING ARTICLES

Articles on the history of nursing are found throughout scientific publications. A search of the Cumulative Index of Nursing and Allied Health Literature (CINAHL) database yielded more than 40 citations to articles published between 2014 and 2017 whose titles included "Florence Nightingale." *Nursing History Review* is the only peer-reviewed, scholarly journal that focuses on the history of nursing and healthcare, as well as offering a department for book reviews (American Association for the History of Nursing, 2017). However, the *Bulletin of the History of Medicine* (Johns Hopkins University, 2017) and the *Journal of the History of Medicine and Allied Sciences* (Oxford University Press, 2017) publish articles on the history of nursing. Some specialty journals also publish articles on the history of nursing. For example,

Public Health Nursing has a department for history manuscripts on "any aspect of the development of public health nursing or the role of nurses in the evolution of population-based care in any country, including original historical research, critical analyses of past events or trends, and oral histories or biographies" (Wiley Interscience, 2017b).

The structure and formatting of scientific articles on the history of nursing are subject to the same principles as those for all research studies, as described in Chapter 5. The primary source data for nursing history articles may include diaries, journals, correspondence, organizational records, photographs, manuscripts, audiovisual records of oral histories, and other original material. Data from such sources require the author to introduce the material with a description of the import of the knowledge gap that will be addressed by the article. The manuscript should also describe, analyze, and synthesize the data succinctly for the reader. The author should make clear to the reader how the particular historical record presented in the article would contribute to nurses' understanding of their roles and practice. Regardless of the order of presentation, all articles on the history of nursing address the significance, approach, and meaning of the research.

EDITORIALS

Some journals have editorials that are written only by the editor, but with other publications nurses may be asked to write a guest editorial. Preparing an editorial for a journal requires a different type of writing than that used for other manuscripts. Editorials are short essays that represent the official opinion of the publication or an invited guest editor (AMA, 2007). Often editorials are issue oriented, related to the theme of articles in the journal. For example, if the theme of the journal is genetic counseling, the editorial may focus on related ethical considerations.

An editorial may also be a critical review of an original paper in the journal or a summary of new developments in the field. Editorials that comment on papers in the journal may provide an alternative view of the issue or even a different interpretation of the data. New findings may have been presented recently that readers should be aware of when they read the article; editorials are a way of providing these other perspectives. An editorial might also emphasize the practice implications of articles in the journal.

Editorials are usually short, so the first task of the author is to plan the content within a limited number of words. In comparison to manuscripts that generally range from 15 to 18 pages of text, editorials may be only three to six typed pages.

Many editorials can be written using the following format: statement of the problem, issue, or opinion; possible solutions and approaches; supporting evidence for each; and the author's conclusion based on this evidence. In some situations, the author may indicate that there is a lack of evidence to support a decision or an action and that more study is needed.

LETTERS TO THE EDITOR

Letters to the editor are an essential component of holding authors accountable for what they write (AMA, 2007). Comments, questions, and criticism of previously published articles stimulate public debate that can be healthy for the common good. Letters to the editor usually comment on a recently published article and are sometimes accompanied by a brief response from the author, which is solicited by the editor. Letters to the editor engage a large audience, are often monitored by opinion leaders, and provide new information to the audience of the publication.

Although anyone can write a letter to the editor, not everyone can get it published. Journals, newspapers, and other types of publications receive many letters, only some of which they publish. Letters may be written to the journal's editor to provide an alternate perspective to an earlier article; they may be sent to a newspaper to explain a topic to the public or present a viewpoint about an issue.

Not every journal publishes letters to the editor, so the author should first check the "information for authors" page or scan copies of the journal. If commenting on an article published earlier in the journal, the author should make this clear in the beginning of the letter. The letter should focus on a scientific, clinical, or ethical implication of the original article and avoid personal attacks on the author (AMA, 2007). The writing style and format are similar to editorials. Because most journals limit the length of letters to the editor, the author should keep this in mind and prepare a letter that is short and to the point. Authors also can send letters to newspapers, magazines, and other types of publications.

REVIEWS OF BOOKS AND OTHER MEDIA

Nurses might write book or media reviews for journals describing what the work is about and addressing its quality. This is a good opportunity for nurses with limited writing experience. Book reviews are typically short pieces similar in length to editorials, and authors need to communicate their ideas clearly and succinctly.

The purpose of the review is to inform readers about the quality of the book and its content so they can decide whether to purchase or consult it. Authors should provide a substantive overview of the contents of the work, followed by a comparison to other similar products. For instance, a new instructional film or textbook may emphasize topics that were secondary or absent in older works. Praise or criticism should be supported with evidence from the work. Rather than saying the book is "too basic for experienced nurses and they should not buy it," the author can cite examples from the book that demonstrate the depth of content and then conclude that the "book is most useful to new graduates."

Evidence-based characteristics of a good book review include the following:

- Written in a professional and constructive manner
- Incisive pinpointing of the strengths and weaknesses of the book
- Comprehensive yet succinct
- Provides a good critique of theory in the field and the place of the book within it
- Criticism is substantiated and constructive
- Goes beyond criticisms to draw conclusions of much broader importance
- Judgment of the book against its competitors
- Addresses the potential book readers' needs and uses of the book
- Indicates how the reviewer's views changed as a result of reading the text
- Includes declaration or statement of conflict of interest
- Follows journal's guide/house style/requirements (Lee, Green, Johnson, & Nyquist, 2010, p. 64)

WRITING FOR CONSUMERS AND NONPROFESSIONAL AUDIENCES

Another type of writing is for consumers and nonprofessional audiences. Nurses have the background and education for writing health articles for the public, and they need to take the initiative to prepare articles of this nature. Consumer magazines are a major source of health education for the public, and these publications allow nurses to share their expertise with readers (Penrose & Katz, 2010). Examples include general news magazines, specialty magazines that target demographic interest groups (health and fitness, parents), company publications, and newspapers.

With this type of writing, the author needs to be clear about who reads the publication so the content and writing can be geared to them. Examples can be used that are relevant to the readers' knowledge level and needs. A manuscript on how to choose a primary care provider would have different examples if written for a magazine read by parents of young children compared with one geared to older readers.

Before starting to write, the author should be clear about what is important to the readers and how the readers might apply the information provided in the article. What does the author hope the reader will do with the information? Finally, it is important for the author to write the article in a way that relates to the direct experience of the readers. Be as specific and concrete as possible about the problems faced by the reader, the supporting evidence for its scope and impact, and any recommendations that are included in the article.

The format and content of articles for popular audiences differ from articles written for scientific or professional readers. The author should avoid using technical terms and develop the manuscript at a level that readers without any healthcare background can understand. Any terminology should be defined clearly. The author should use her expertise to provide an analysis of any complex issues using simple but accurate wording, as well as pictures wherever allowed by the publishers. Comparisons can often help the reader to understand important differences. For instance, instead of describing the symptoms of only the H1N1 virus, the author could compare and contrast them with symptoms of other viral diseases. Other effective writing strategies for popular audiences include storytelling, examples, and graphics.

The author can begin by writing health pieces for newsletters and local newspapers. This provides experience in gearing the writing to a nonprofessional audience and deciding what information is most important to communicate to the public. In general, the conventions for writing for popular audiences are not as formulaic as for professional audiences. Therefore, the nurse-author can improvise and be creative, to the benefit of the readers.

SUMMARY

What about issues in nursing? These papers analyze issues, why and how they developed, varied positions that can be taken, and multiple strategies for resolving them.

Other topics may be philosophical in nature or deal with theory development or testing. In writing philosophical and theoretical manuscripts, the author is careful with how ideas are presented and ordered so they are logical and sequenced appropriately. It is important to present a sound argument to support ideas and defend them using theory and research.

Nurse-authors may also write articles on public and organizational policies developed by nurses or that affect their role, ethical challenges that they confront, legal and regulatory precedents with implications for patient care and professional practice, and methodological innovations for research studies. History of nursing articles use primary source material to inform current readers about the roots of their professional identity, perspective of patients, and evidence-based practice. Case reports provide new information on nursing practice and the care of patients with particular health problems through the presentation of an actual case.

With some journals, nurses may be asked to write the editorial. Editorials may be issue oriented, summarize new developments in the field, or critically review an original paper in the journal. Nurses also might write book reviews describing what the book is about and addressing its quality, letters to the editor, and articles for consumers and nonprofessional audiences.

There are many situations in which nurses find themselves that lend to writing for publication. Nurses need to take advantage of these opportunities so their ideas are communicated to and used by others.

REFERENCES

American Association for the History of Nursing. (2017). *Nursing history review*. Retrieved from https://www.aahn.org/publications

American Medical Association. (2007). *AMA manual of style: A guide for authors and editors* (10th ed.). New York, NY: Oxford University Press.

American Nurses Association. (2017). About OJIN. *Online Journal of Issues in Nursing*. Retrieved from http://www.nursingworld.org/ojin/

American Psychological Association. (2010). *Publication manual of the American Psychological Association* (6th ed.). Washington, DC: Author.

Ampe, S., Sevenants, A., Smets, T., Declercq, A., & Van Audenhove, C. (2016). Advance care planning for nursing home residents with dementia: Policy vs. practice. *Journal of Advanced Nursing, 72*, 569–581. doi:10.1111/jan.12854

Blok, A. C. (2017). A middle-range explanatory theory of self-management behavior for collaborative research and practice. *Nursing Forum, 52*, 138–146. doi:10.1111/nuf.12169

Cozad, M. J., Lindley, L. C., & Mixer, S. J. (2016). Using agency nurses to fill RN vacancies within specialized hospice and palliative care. *Policy, Politics & Nursing Practice, 17*, 147–155. doi:10.1177/1527154416671711

Driscoll, D. W., & Darcy, J. (2015). Indoor tanning legislation: Shaping policy and nursing practice. *Pediatric Nursing, 41*(2), 59–63, 88. Retrieved from http://www.pediatricnursing.net/issues/15marapr/abstr1.html

Fredland, N., McFarlane, J., Symes, L., Maddoux, J., Pennings, J., Paulson, R., . . . Gilroy, H. (2016). Modeling the intergenerational impact of partner abuse on maternal and child function at 24 months post outreach: Implications for practice and policy. *Nursing Outlook, 64*, 156–169. doi:10.1016/j.outlook.2015.10.005

Gower, A. L., Cousin, M., & Borowsky, I. W. (2017). A multilevel, statewide investigation of school district anti-bullying policy quality and student bullying involvement. *Journal of School Health, 87*, 174–181. doi:10.1111/josh.12480

Hain, D. J., Diaz, D., & Paixao, R. (2016). What are ethical issues when honoring an older adult's decision to withdraw from dialysis? *Nephrology Nursing Journal, 43*(5), 429–434, 450.

Hamlin, L. (2017). Comparison of births by provider, place, and payer in New Hampshire. *Policy, Politics, & Nursing Practice, 18*, 95–104. doi:10.1177/1527154417720680

Hammer, M. J. (2016). Research ethics considerations regarding the Cancer Moonshot Initiative. *Oncology Nursing Forum, 43*, 428–431. doi:10.1188/16.ONF.428-431

International Committee of Medical Journal Editors. (2017). *Recommendations for the conduct, reporting, editing, and publication of scholarly work in medical journals*. Retrieved from http://www.icmje.org/urm_main.html

Johns Hopkins University. (2017). *Bulletin of the History of Medicine*. Retrieved from https://www.press.jhu.edu/journals/bulletin_of_the_history_of_medicine

Lee, A. D., Green, B. N., Johnson, C. D., & Nyquist, J. (2010). How to write a scholarly book review for publication in a peer-reviewed journal: A review of the literature. *Journal of Chiropractic Education, 24*(1), 57–69. Retrieved from https://www.ncbi.nlm.nih.gov/pmc/articles/PMC2870990

Lippincott Williams & Wilkins. (2017). Instructions for authors. *Advances in Nursing Science*. Retrieved from http://edmgr.ovid.com/ans/accounts/ifauth.htm

Oxford University Press. (2017). About the journal. *Journal of the History of Medicine and Allied Sciences*. Retrieved from http://www.oxfordjournals.org/our_journals/jalsci/about.html

Penrose, A. M., & Katz, S. B. (2010). *Writing in the sciences: Exploring conventions of scientific discourse* (3rd ed.). New York, NY: Pearson Longman.

Quinn, W. V., Brassard, A., O'Brien, M., & Reinecke, P. (2017). Health care and nursing policy: Impact of the Campaign for Action to increase consumer access to care. *Geriatric Nursing, 38*, 362–364. doi:10.1016/j.gerinurse.2017.06.013

Rambur, B. (2017). What's at stake in U.S. health reform: A guide to the Affordable Care Act and value-based care. *Policy, Politics, & Nursing Practice, 18*, 61–71. doi:10.1177/1527154417720935

Sage Publications. (2017a). About this journal. *Nursing Ethics*. Retrieved from http://nej.sagepub.com

Sage Publications. (2017b). *Nursing Science Quarterly*. Retrieved from http://www.sagepub.com/journals/Journal200789/manuscriptSubmission

Sage Publications. (2017c). *Policy, Politics, and Nursing Practice*. Retrieved from http://www.sagepub.com/journalsProdDesc.nav?prodId=Journal201332

Sarver, W., Cichra, N., & Kline, M. (2015). Perceived benefits, motivators, and barriers to advancing nurse education: Removing barriers to improve success. *Nursing Education Perspectives*, *36*, 153–156. doi:10.5480/14-1407

Smith, J. P., & Herber, O. R. (2015). Ethical issues experienced by mental health nurses in the administration of antipsychotic depot and long-acting intramuscular injections: A qualitative study. *International Journal of Mental Health Nursing*, *24*, 222–230. doi:10.1111/inm.12105

Stein-Fredbeck, L., Rosenberg, R., & Frank, R. (2017). A case report of maternal cerebral hemorrhage in preterm pregnancy. *Journal of Obstetric, Gynecologic & Neonatal Nursing*, *46*, 609–616. doi:10.1016/j.jogn.2017.04.135

Wiley Interscience. (2017a). Author guidelines. *Journal of Obstetric, Gynecologic, and Neonatal Nursing*. Retrieved from http://onlinelibrary.wiley.com/journal/10.1111/%28ISSN%291552-6909/homepage/ForAuthors.html

Wiley Interscience. (2017b). Author guidelines. *Public Health Nursing*. Retrieved from http://onlinelibrary.wiley.com/journal/10.1111/%28ISSN%291525-1446/homepage/ForAuthors.html

Wiley Interscience. (2017c). *Journal of School Health*. Retrieved from http://onlinelibrary.wiley.com/journal/10.1111/%28ISSN%291746-1561

Wolf, L. A., Delao, A. M., & Perhats, C. (2015). Emergency nurses' perceptions of discharge processes for patients receiving Schedule II and III medications for pain management in the emergency department. *Journal of Emergency Nursing*, *41*, 221–226. doi:10.1016/j.jen.2014.06.010

BOOKS AND BOOK CHAPTERS

Writing a book or book chapter is different from writing an article because the author has more opportunity, with more pages allowed, to provide background information and discuss related content than in a manuscript for a journal. While a journal manuscript may be 15 to 18 double-spaced pages, a chapter may be 30 to 50 pages, depending on the book length. Books also provide an opportunity for the author to develop strategies that guide readers in learning the content, such as including bulleted lists that emphasize the key points, case scenarios that demonstrate how the content applies to clinical practice, learning activities and questions for discussion at the end of each chapter, and so forth.

Whereas articles generally focus on one topic, books address multiple but related content areas. A book designed for use in an undergraduate maternity course contains the range of topics needed by students at that level to understand maternity nursing and gain knowledge and skills for safe and competent practice. Even a book with a more specific focus, such as case management, will contain the content areas needed to understand and implement case management in varied clinical settings.

One consideration for faculty members is that books and book chapters are generally not peer reviewed and often carry less weight in tenure and promotion decisions than publications in peer-reviewed journals. Although the publisher may have experts review the book proposal or prospectus, specific chapters, and sometimes the finished book manuscript, this review is generally done to identify missing content, suggest changes in organization, recommend a different emphasis among chapters, and assess other areas important to the publisher. These expert reviewers do not conduct a peer review of the rigor of the content. New and tenure-track faculty members need to understand the types of dissemination important in decisions about promotion in their school.

WRITING A BOOK

Nurses with experience in writing journal articles will have a sense of the time commitment required in writing a manuscript and following the paper through to publication. Yet, a journal manuscript takes a short time. A major consideration before embarking on a book is this time commitment: Books without contributed chapters can easily take 1 year or more to complete. Experienced authors will have an idea of how to approach a large writing project such as a book, their writing style and process established, and will have contacts with other experts who might contribute chapters to the book if it is an edited work. Nevertheless, writing a book requires an extensive time commitment that authors should weigh against their other responsibilities.

Some questions potential book authors should answer for themselves when deciding if they want to write a book follow:

- Is there a clear need for the book, and who might read it?
- What content would be in the book?
- Is there sufficient content for a book-length manuscript, which might be 450 pages or more? Those 450 pages are double-spaced manuscript pages in 12-point font, with 1-inch margins. For a book that is 6 inches by 9 inches in size, about 1.5 manuscript pages equal 1 book page. When considering that a journal article is often restricted to about 15 to 18 manuscript pages, the magnitude of writing a book becomes clear.
- Would the book be developed from chapters contributed by other authors or written by an author or coauthors?
- Are coauthors and contributors available, and what are their writing styles and habits; for example, do they submit manuscripts on time?
- Are there administrative and other resources available to assist with contacting contributors, managing their submissions, and handling other details?
- If approached by a publisher to serve as an editor of a book, what resources and assistance will be provided by the publisher, for example, contacting potential chapter authors, consulting with them on their individual chapters, communicating with them, monitoring their progress, reviewing drafts, and editing the final versions of the chapters?
- Is time available in one's own work schedule and personal circumstances to write the book?
- What are the benefits personally and professionally of writing the book?
- What is the quality of the publisher?

Types of Books

There are different types of books that nurses might write. These include textbooks for students, which may be written for particular courses; resource books for nurses in clinical practice, teaching, administration, and other roles; handbooks and manuals, which present abbreviated versions of content and are practical, such as a handbook on health assessment and manual on clinical nursing skills; case studies, usually in a specific clinical area, such as critical care; and edited books that contain chapters written by different authors that are coordinated by an editor or editors. Some nurses also write novels, short stories, essays, and poetry for the general public.

Authored Versus Contributed Book

When thinking about writing a book, an early consideration is whether the author or coauthors will write all of the chapters themselves or if the book will be a contributed text. An authored book is one in which the author or coauthors assume full responsibility for the content of the text, writing each chapter in it, the front matter (beginning pages), and other parts of the book, and completing all of the related activities required for its publication. In a contributed book, in contrast, authors or coauthors write individual chapters under the guidance of an editor who assembles those chapters into a book. With a contributed text, the heading of each chapter includes the authors' names and sometimes credentials; their affiliations are usually listed in a contributors' page in the front matter. The editor's name, or names of multiple editors, is on the title page, and the book's cover would indicate the editor, but not the contributors.

A contributed book allows the editor to invite experts to prepare chapters in their area of specialization. The editor may not have a background in those topics, which are important for the book to meet the readers' needs. Editing a book requires less time than writing all of the chapters, but the editor is responsible for ensuring accuracy of content, a similar format for presenting the content across chapters, transition between chapters, and that the chapters as a whole contain the relevant information for the aims of the book. Issues with a contributed book are the different writing styles of chapter authors, varying levels of details and specificity with how authors develop their content, authors not adhering to the format for chapters, and authors not submitting their chapters on time, according to the due dates set by the editor. All too often with edited books, contributing authors are delayed in completing their chapters, but it is the editor's responsibility to submit the book manuscript to the publisher on time. Working with chapter authors is sometimes challenging, and the editor should be clear about expectations when asking authors to contribute a chapter. With some books, contributors are paid an honorarium, but with others they are not compensated financially.

Initial Contact With Publisher

The idea for a book may be initiated by the author, often as a result of the author's inability to find a book for teaching a course or to meet a professional or personal need. Existing books in an area of specialization may be out of date or not available because of current advances in the field of practice. In those situations, the author will approach different publishers to find one interested in publishing the work.

Alternately, authors with known expertise may be asked by a publisher to write a book. In this instance, the publisher may not have a book in that content area to market to faculty for courses and for other readers. The publisher may be aware of the nurse's work based on journal articles and other publications or from suggestions of nurses and authors. Usually, the acquisitions editor contacts the author to inquire about the author's interest.

Publishers include commercial firms that publish books in nursing, medicine, allied health, and other fields; organizations such as the American

Nurses Association; and university presses. Commercial scholarly publishers such as Springer and Elsevier publish books for profit in nursing and other fields. Some commercial publishers focus on clinical nursing books and textbooks for undergraduate nursing students, while others publish more specialized books with smaller markets. It is important for authors to explore publishers that have experience marketing to the audience of the book being considered. Some of the publishers have more experience with nursing books than do others, and authors should have this information at hand when deciding on which publisher to contact about their ideas.

Professional organizations such as the American Nurses Association and Sigma have book publishing divisions. Often, these books meet specific needs of the members of the organization and are marketed primarily to that group.

University presses are another type of publisher but do not commonly publish nursing books. They tend to publish books in the arts and humanities that have a regional focus and that are of interest to a wider audience than nurses or nursing students.

Large commercial publishers of fiction and nonfiction books for the general public are not likely to be interested in books aimed at nurses or nursing students. If a nurse is thinking about writing a novel or series of short stories, those publishers might be interested. Some authors also publish their own work, but some of the issues with this are a lack of technical assistance through the publication process, need for a printer, and knowledge of how to advertise and market the book, among others. Authors often receive less recognition for a book published independently (Al-Ubaydli, Whitehurst, Koshy, Gundogan, & Agha, 2017). With self-publishing the author absorbs all of the costs.

Prospectus

Whether the author approaches the publisher with an idea or is contacted by the acquisitions editor or another representative of the publisher, the process begins with a literature search and completion of a prospectus. The prospectus is the proposal or plan for the book, outlining its goals and how the author envisions the development of content.

Publishers have their own formats for preparing the prospectus, which generally include the following:

- Purpose of the book and why it is needed
- List of chapters in the book and content of each
- Features of the book
- Contributors, if any, and chapters they will prepare
- Intended readers, including the level of nursing students if it is a textbook
- Courses the book could be used in and other market considerations
- Competition, including a review of every competing book on the market and statement as to why the proposed book would be better
- Timetable for completion
- Size of the book, including total number of pages
- Sample chapter

Exhibit 10.1 is an example of a prospectus that authors would complete for a book.

EXHIBIT 10.1

Example of Book Prospectus

BOOK PROPOSAL SUBMISSION GUIDELINES

Editorial Information

What is the tentative title of your book?

Who will be the authors and/or editors? Please provide a current CV or resume for each primary author/editor.

Will some chapters be contributed by others? If yes, please list those whom you plan to invite: include name, credentials, and affiliation for each within the table of contents.

Provide a description of the book's contents (3–4 paragraphs). Include what the book will contribute to the literature; its main themes and objectives; its distinctiveness in comparison to current competitor titles; and what pedagogical features it will include (e.g., if a textbook, will it include objectives, review questions, case studies, etc.?).

What are the key features of this book? (Please provide a list of why people will buy this book in list format.)

Who is your book's intended audience? (Please list specific education, specialty, or practice areas and/or professional associations, as appropriate.)

If this is a textbook, please indicate whether it is intended for the undergraduate or graduate-level audience. Include a list of programs and course titles where the book should be considered for adoption. If enrollment numbers per program or course are available, please include them.

Table of contents (Please provide an annotated list of sections and chapters, including authors per chapter, with degrees and affiliation for each.)

How long will the manuscript be? (Please include an estimate of the number of manuscript pages, illustrations, and photographs.)

What is your estimated completion date for the manuscript?

Please list what you think are the key sales features and benefits. (List the kind of information that should be highlighted, for example, on the book's back cover as well in print and web advertisements for the book.)

Professional associations to consider for marketing:

Journals that should receive copies for book review purposes:

What books provide the most direct competition to your book? (Your list should include the author's last name, title of book, publisher and year of publication, price, length in pages, and any special features such as an Instructor's Resource Guide. Please note how your book is different or better.)

Source: Springer Publishing (n.d.). Resources for authors. Retrieved from http://www .springerpub.com/authors. Reproduced with the permission of Springer Publishing.

Authors should contact a publisher first, and if there is interest in the proposal, then prepare a prospectus for that publisher. It is risky to begin writing the manuscript without a publisher in case none can be found. It may be that the market is too small, or there are too many books on the same content. While the topic may be important to the author, there may be minimal interest in it from the publisher's point of view. In other cases, the publisher may be interested only if the focus changes considerably. For these reasons the author is advised to contact publishers before beginning to write.

Responsibilities of Author and Publisher

The prospectus is then submitted to the publisher who reviews it and, if interested, sends the author a contract. The review of the prospectus may take from a few weeks to months depending on the publisher. It is likely that the prospectus will be sent to external reviewers for feedback as to whether the book should be published and for suggested changes in content or focus.

The contract is a legal document outlining the responsibilities of the author, or editor if a contributed book, and the publisher. The author is responsible for preparing the book and submitting it on time. The publisher is responsible for getting the book into production, copyediting the manuscript, designing the book, carrying out other details to produce it, and marketing it. Details of the book, such as its focus, due date, number of manuscript pages, and royalties, are commonly included in book contracts; some of the details can be negotiated while others cannot. The contract will include information about transfer of copyright similar to a journal article. Authors should read the contract carefully and consult with experts if unsure about some aspect of it.

Once the contract is signed, publishers will provide authors with detailed information about how to prepare and submit the book manuscript. This information will include guidelines on the overall format of the book and individual chapters; details on the format of the pages, such as size of the margins and spacing; use and preparation of displays, boxes, tables, figures, and illustrations; numbering and placement of those in the text; abbreviations and other style considerations; responsibilities for permissions; and format for submission of the final manuscript. The manuscript is likely to be submitted electronically, but some publishers may also request a hard copy.

Authors are generally responsible for preparation of figures and any artwork included in their book. Similar to journals, these need to be in a format ready for production. If the author intends on including multiple illustrations or artwork in the book, it would be good to discuss this with the publisher prior to signing the contract, because the author may need assistance in developing them.

Authors who serve as editors of contributed books have added responsibilities to define the content and length of each chapter for contributors, develop schedules for submission, and make sure that contributors adhere to them. With some books, contributed chapters may be peer reviewed to provide feedback on the quality of the content and its comprehensiveness;

contributors would need to consent to revise their chapters based on that feedback. With a contributed book, it is important that format and writing style are consistent across chapters. This may require rewriting by the editor.

Some publishers send the completed book manuscript for external review to identify omissions of content and possible redundancies. With journal manuscripts, authors do not receive copyedited pages to review but instead are sent the page proofs, with copy edits already included, to check prior to publication. The proofs are the pages as they will appear in the publication; Figure 16.1 in Chapter 16, provides an illustration of page proofs. For book manuscripts, however, authors may receive the edited versions and page proofs to review, or only the proofs. With contributed books, individual chapter authors may be asked to review the edited versions of their chapters and page proofs, or the editor may do this for all of the chapters in the book.

The publisher's responsibilities include copyediting the manuscript, designing the book, moving it through production, and marketing it. Authors may have different contacts with the publisher during this process, beginning with the acquisition editor who contacted the author about writing the book, reviewed the prospectus, and provided feedback on the book's contents. Once the contract has been signed, the author may interact with other editors, such as the managing editor, who will guide the author or editor in preparing the manuscript, answer questions, and ensure that the book is ready for production.

When the book manuscript has been submitted, the publisher is responsible for copyediting it, developing the manuscript pages into proofs of the pages, and completing other details. Authors will review the edited pages, which include changes suggested by the copy editor to improve understanding of the text, correct grammatical errors, and modify the text to adhere to the publisher's style. Except for style, other changes need to be read carefully and approved by the author: copy editors will not have expertise in the content and may suggest revisions that change the intent of the text. Copy editors also will include queries for the author to answer. With some publishers, authors will not receive the copyedited pages to review, but instead will receive the page proofs, the next phase, with the copy editors' changes incorporated in them, similar to journal manuscripts. While changes can be made in this phase of production, once the copyedited pages become page proofs, few corrections can be made. Exhibit 10.2 provides an example of a copyedited page, with the editing done using the "Track Changes" feature in Microsoft Word. Exhibit 10.3 shows the subsequent proof of that same page.

The other major responsibility of the publisher is marketing the book. At some point in the production phase, the author will be asked to complete a marketing questionnaire that provides detailed information to guide the publisher with these activities. Typically, authors describe the book's contents, most important sales features, and differences from other books in the same content area. Authors also may be asked to list professional associations and meetings where the book could be advertised and to identify colleagues and journals to be notified about its publication.

EXHIBIT 10.2

Sample Copyedited Page

<LRH> Part VI. Scholarship in Nursing Education around the World

<RRH> 18 Evidence-Based Teaching in Nursing

<CN> ~~Chapter~~ 18

<CT> Evidence-Based Teaching in Nursing: ~~Some Principles~~

Marilyn H. Oermann, ~~PhD, RN, ANEF, FAAN,~~ and Jamie L. Conklin, ~~MSLIS~~

<tct> Evidence-based teaching is ~~using~~ the use of research findings and other evidence to ~~make~~ guide educational decisions and practices. ~~Teachers should use~~ Available evidence should be used when developing the curriculum and courses, selecting teaching methods and approaches to use with students, planning clinical learning activities, ~~evaluating students in the simulation lab,~~ and assessing students' learning and performance. Yet many nurse educators rarely search for evidence when they make educational decisions. They update their courses by incorporating new evidence about the content but ~~may~~ they might not seek ~~strong~~ evidence on how those courses are best designed, taught, and evaluated. How much practice do students need to retain their motor skills? What are best practices with debriefing? What characteristics of online courses are critical to learning and retention? These are ~~some of~~ the types of questions that every educator should be raising no matter what course or level of learner they are teaching.

<p> Teachers can then search the literature for research studies and other evidence to answer these questions and guide their educational practices. By reviewing the literature, the . . .

EXHIBIT 10.3

Proof of the Page

18

Evidence-Based Teaching in Nursing

MARILYN H. OERMANN AND JAMIE L. CONKLIN

Evidence-based teaching is the use of research findings and other evidence to guide educational decisions and practices. Available evidence should be used when developing the curriculum and courses, selecting teaching methods and approaches to use with students, planning clinical learning activities, and assessing students' learning and performance. Yet many nurse educators rarely search for evidence when they make educational decisions. They update their courses by incorporating new evidence about the content, but they might not

(continued)

EXHIBIT 10.3

Proof of the Page (*continued*)

seek evidence on how those courses are best designed, taught, and evaluated. How much practice do students need to retain their motor skills? What are best practices with debriefing? What characteristics of online courses are critical to learning and retention? These are the types of questions that every educator should be raising no matter what course or level of learner they are teaching.

Teachers can then search the literature for research studies and other evidence to answer these questions and guide their educational practices. By reviewing the literature, the teacher can also learn about the experiences of other educators, to build on

Source: From Oermann, M. H., De Gagne, J. C., & Phillips, B. C. (2018). *Teaching in nursing and role of the educator: The complete guide to best practice in teaching, evaluation, and curriculum development* (2nd ed., p. 363). New York, NY: Springer Publishing.

Process of Writing Books

The purpose of the book guides the depth and complexity of the content. Similar to other types of manuscripts, the author needs to keep the goals of the book and the readers in mind when preparing the text. A book written for prelicensure nursing students will be more explanatory and may include multiple displays, tables, and summaries to guide their learning about the content than that same book written for readers who have a background in the content. Authors are experts in the content they are communicating to others, but need to think about readers as novices and plan how best to explain the ideas to them.

Table 10.1 lists the typical parts of a book in their order. The content of the book was outlined in the prospectus, and the author can start by developing a more detailed outline for each of the chapters. This should be done before beginning to write because the author may identify gaps in or overlapping content once the chapters are planned in more detail. For contributed texts, editors should provide guidelines for writing each chapter, including the use of displays, boxes, learning activities for readers, and other strategies, as well as the topics to be included.

Authors should receive the prospectus and outlines of their chapter and others in the book to better understand how their chapter fits into the book as a whole. It also is important in a contributed book for the editor to develop a realistic timetable for chapter authors to follow, requirements of each chapter, and information about the writing style (Oermann, 2013).

The process for writing a book is no different than other manuscripts, except for the length of the project and the need to stay within a strict time frame. When writing a book, the author must keep to deadlines and persevere or the book will never be completed. Techniques discussed in other chapters on preparing to write, organizing the writing project, and working with groups are important when writing a book. The author can view the writing project as a series of smaller "assignments," each with its own due date for completion. For large

TABLE 10.1 TYPICAL BOOK CONTENTS SUBMITTED BY AUTHOR

Part	Content
Front Matter	Title page with the book title and authors' names, credentials, and affiliations. There may be a half-title page (prepared by the publisher) with the book title only that precedes the title page.
	Copyright page including the copyright date, International Standard Book Number (ISBN), edition, and other publication data.
	Dedication
	Contributors (author names, credentials, and affiliations)
	Table of contents
	Foreword (statement by an expert, not the author or editor, about the book and its relevance)
	Preface (discussion by the author or editor about the content of the book, often with a summary of each chapter, how the book can be used, and intended readers). In some books, the preface serves as an introduction.
	Acknowledgments (this page might be earlier in the front matter following the dedication)
Text	Chapters of the book. They may be grouped into sections or parts, each with its own title. References are included at the end of each chapter. Displays, boxes, tables, figures, and other illustrations follow and are labeled with the chapter number and number representing the order in which each one was cited in the chapter.
Back Matter	Appendices
	Glossary if relevant (definition of terms in the book)
	Index (prepared when the book is completed). Although authors can index the text themselves, it is usually done by the publisher or indexer.

writing projects, deadlines must be met because lost time is difficult if not impossible to make up. Exhibit 10.4 provides tips for completing chapters, books, and other writing projects that extend over a period of time.

WRITING A BOOK CHAPTER

The process of writing a book chapter is the same as journal articles, although with chapters the author typically has more pages allowed; chapters might be from 30 to 50 manuscript pages depending on the book length and other chapters in it. With these additional pages, authors have an opportunity to explain their topics more thoroughly and develop the content in more depth. This is essential

EXHIBIT 10.4

Tips for Completing Books

Work on one chapter at a time.

Develop an outline of topics to be covered in the chapter.

Consider each topic on your outline as a separate writing project and assign a realistic due date to each of the topics.

Keep a running list of related activities that need to be completed for each chapter in the book; assign due dates to these.

Adhere to the due dates.

Finish a chapter in its entirety before beginning the next one.

Find your best time for writing and use it for writing the book.

Use other times of day for completing related activities, such as checking references.

Keep your focus on writing the book until you finish it.

for chapters in textbooks, which are primary sources of information for learning about a topic. Because chapters in a book meet a particular goal, chapter authors are guided by the editor as to content to include, format of the chapter, displays and other materials to include, and other requirements. Chapter authors need to be committed to preparing the chapter as specified and meeting the editor's due dates. Chapter contributors who are not clear about what they are supposed to do may create more work for the editor and for copy editors, proofreaders, indexers, and others in the production process (Nicoll, 2013).

Although chapters are not considered as evidence of scholarship in some schools of nursing, depending on the tenure and promotion criteria, writing a chapter in a leading book may be advantageous to the nurse's career. Writing a chapter is a good way of becoming known in a content area and getting mentoring on writing from the editor. Writing a chapter also provides a way of becoming immersed in a content area and developing expertise in it. An issue with chapters, in addition to their not carrying as much weight in tenure and promotion decisions as journal articles, is that chapters are not cited to the same degree as articles and thus do not "spread" ideas as effectively. In a study of pediatric nursing literature, journals were the most frequently cited sources, followed by books (Watwood, 2016).

SUMMARY

Writing a book requires time and commitment: Although experienced authors know how to write and may have contacts with experts who could contribute chapters to the book, nevertheless, preparing a book takes time. An early consideration is whether the author or coauthors will write all of the chapters themselves or if the book will be a contributed text. In a contributed book, authors or coauthors write individual chapters under the guidance of an editor who assembles those chapters into a book.

The idea for a book may be initiated by the author, often because of the author's inability to find a book for teaching a course or to meet a professional or personal need. Or, authors with known expertise may be asked by a publisher to write a book. Usually, the acquisitions editor contacts the author to inquire about the author's interest. Publishers include commercial firms that publish books in nursing, medicine, allied health, and other fields; organizations such as the American Nurses Association and Sigma; and university presses.

Whether the author approaches the publisher with an idea or is contacted by the publisher to write a book, the process begins with a literature search and completion of a prospectus. The prospectus is the proposal for the book outlining its goals and how the author envisions the development of content. Typical content in the prospectus was discussed in the chapter. The prospectus is then sent to the publisher, who reviews it and, if interested, sends the author a contract. The contract is a legal document outlining the responsibilities of the author, or editor if a contributed book, and the publisher.

The author is responsible for preparing the book according to the format of the publisher and submitting it on time. Editors of contributed books have added responsibilities to define the content and length of each chapter for contributors, develop schedules for submission, and make sure that contributors adhere to them. The publisher is responsible for getting the book into production, copyediting the manuscript, designing the book, carrying out other details to produce it, and marketing it.

The process for writing a book is no different than writing other manuscripts except for the length of the project and the need to stay within a strict time frame. When writing a book, the author must keep to deadlines and persevere or the book will never be completed.

REFERENCES

Al-Ubaydli, M., Whitehurst, K., Koshy, K., Gundogan, B., & Agha, R. (2017). How to publish a book. *Internal Journal of Surgery Oncology*, 2(6), e26. doi:10.1097/ij9.0000000000000026

Nicoll, L. H. (2013). Writing a book chapter. *Nurse Author & Editor*, 23(3). Retrieved from http://naepub.com/writing-basics/2013-23-3-2

Oermann, M. H. (2013). Writing a book: What you need to know. *Nurse Author & Editor*, 23(1). Retrieved from http://naepub.com/writing-basics/2013-23-1-7

Oermann, M. H., De Gagne, J. C., & Phillips, B. C. (2018). *Teaching in nursing and role of the educator: The complete guide to best practice in teaching, evaluation, and curriculum development* (2nd ed.). New York, NY: Springer Publishing.

Springer Publishing. (n.d.). Resources for authors. Retrieved from http://www.springerpub.com/authors

Watwood, C. L. (2016). Mapping the literature of pediatric nursing: Update and implications for library services. *Journal of the Medical Library Association*, 104, 278–283. doi:10.3163/1536-5050.104.4.005

IV

THE WRITING PROCESS

11

WRITING PROCESS

At this point in the process of writing, the author has identified the type of manuscript, the purpose of the paper, potential journals, and the audience for the topic. The author has obtained author guidelines from the target journal, has conducted or updated the literature review, has completed other preparations for writing, and is now ready to begin writing the manuscript.

Writing for publication involves an iterative process of forward momentum, pause, and circling back over previous ground. The forward motion of engagement in writing is the creative and energized time when thoughts and words are flowing onto the page or computer screen. But good writing also includes a time of retreat, when the author takes a step back from the newly created article before re-engaging to review, revise, refine, and enhance the material. Both kinds of involvement with one's written work are important to produce the article that will meet the author's goals.

The writing process is time consuming. Novice writers report that the most important strategy for success is to break the process into small structured tasks with frequent deadlines and reminders from colleagues with writing expertise (von Isenburg, Lee, & Oermann, 2017). This chapter reviews the many such steps in completing a manuscript appropriate for journal submission.

This chapter focuses first on preliminary questions to ask before starting to write and on organizing the content into an outline. Next, it describes how to write the first draft of the manuscript. Finally, this chapter describes the steps in revising the content and organization of the paper and then revising the writing structure and style. Some principles are provided for improving how the paper is written, although the chapter does not address all aspects of prose structure and style that are important in writing for publication.

PREPARING TO WRITE

Writing for publication requires careful planning, organization, and personal strategies to keep on target until the paper is completed. It cannot be done haphazardly. With an outline, even if brief, and materials assembled, the author can move quickly into writing the first draft. The author should plan on revising the first draft a number of times until satisfied with the final copy.

Before beginning the outline, the author completes other preparations to facilitate the writing process and eliminate unnecessary distractions. These preparations include reviewing the author guidelines for the journal to clarify the format and other requirements; gathering materials about the project, innovation, or practices described in the manuscript; and assembling analyses of data and other information about the research project. These preliminary activities are important to allow authors to focus on their writing once they begin rather than on time-consuming, and sometimes distracting, tasks such as finding evidence needed to support ideas, locating statistical analyses of data, and checking references. The goal is to assemble all materials prior to writing the first draft.

The accumulated literature review should be available so that references can be checked during the writing phase. No writer, even an experienced one, can rely on memory to cite a reference in a manuscript. Even in high-quality journals authors make too many errors in their reference lists. This can be avoided by carefully checking each reference when preparing the manuscript.

This phase of writing is not the time to learn a new word processing or reference management program or how to develop tables, and so forth. When the author begins to write, all other necessary activities of this nature should have been done so the author is able to concentrate on preparing the first draft.

Review Purpose and Audience

Before writing the first draft, the author should spend time planning how to approach the topic. Reviewing the purpose of the manuscript is the first step in this planning. It is often helpful to record the purpose on a note card that is visible as a way of keeping the manuscript focused on this main point. The author should be able to track the main point from the beginning of the manuscript to the end.

The author should then think about the intended readers. What is their level of knowledge and expertise? Why is the article important to them? The intended readers, combined with the purpose of the manuscript, guide the author in writing the first draft. If the primary audience is nurses in the same specialty field or a related one, authors are essentially writing for their peers and therefore are able to use technical and highly specialized language in the writing. Examples from nursing practice and case studies that focus on nursing care would be easily understood by readers and therefore appropriate for inclusion in the manuscript.

The primary audience of other journals, though, may be readers from disciplines beyond nursing. *The Joint Commission Journal on Quality Improvement* (The Joint Commission, 2017) is a journal that provides information on developing, adapting, and implementing quality and safety improvement practices in healthcare organizations. When writing for this journal, authors would avoid using terms and examples unique to nursing and instead would write for understanding by any professional involved in measuring and improving performance.

Review Writing Style of Journal

In writing the manuscript, the author needs to use a writing style consistent with the journal. Journal editors will not send a manuscript for peer review if it does not conform to the conventional writing style of the journal. Journal readers will find it easiest to absorb the information in the article if the author has used a form of writing that readers expect. Before beginning the process of writing, it is helpful to read paragraphs from several articles published in the journal to become familiar with its conventional style.

Formal Writing Style

There are different ways of categorizing writing style. One way is to classify styles of writing as formal or informal. A formal style is expected in scientific and scholarly journals. Authors using a formal style may refer to themselves in the third person, as "the researchers" or "the authors." Many sentences may be constructed in the passive voice. An example of a clearly written introductory paragraph in the formal writing style follows:

> Patients at the end of life often suffer from urinary difficulties, including incontinence and retention (Twycross, 2003; Glare et al., 2011). Strategies for managing these problems can be controversial. Although indwelling urinary catheters may relieve problems of retention and complications associated with intractable incontinence such as skin integrity (Grey et al., 2012), insertion may itself cause distress to a dying patient. An expert opinion paper by Kyle (2010) identified situations in which catheterization at the end of life is acceptable, and these indications were adopted as guidance by the Royal College of Nursing (RCN) (2012) in its advice to nurses on catheter use at the end of life. Despite this, a recent review (Farrington et al., 2013) found minimal research to indicate how incontinence should be managed at the end of life. (Farrington, Fader, Richardson, Prieto, & Bush, 2014, p. S4)

Informal Writing Style

An informal writing style may use more active voice sentences. Typically, with a more informal style, personal pronouns such as "I" and "we" are used as subjects of sentences.

Similarly, informal writing style often uses the personal pronoun "you" to engage the reader in the topic and personalize the information. In the following example of an informal writing style, the personal pronoun "you" is used:

> *You* can help the patient break down his overall stress into separate concerns that can be addressed one at a time. *You* can also refer the patient to the nurse practitioner if needed.

Develop an Outline

An outline is an overview of a manuscript's content and its organization. Outlines enable the author to specify content areas to include in the manuscript and decide how to organize these topics logically so the information is clear to readers. If the journal prescribes a basic structure for the type of article being drafted, the author can use the headings of that structure to frame the outline.

Some authors prefer not to develop an outline, but even experienced authors may drift in their writing and find near the end of a manuscript that certain content areas were omitted or that the organization was unclear. It is easier and quicker to revise an outline than an entire paper, so the time devoted to outlining is worth it in the long run.

The author should view the outline as a working document; the outline is not a final product but instead is a tool to aid writing. Some authors find it helpful before writing the draft to review the outline a few days after its initial development to assess if changes are needed and to add details to the content.

Advantages of Outlines

The American Psychological Association (APA, 2010) identified advantages of outlining before starting to write the first draft. An outline:

- Supports the logic of the research
- Distinguishes primary and secondary ideas
- Disciplines the writing such that tangents are avoided
- Illuminates gaps in logic
- Facilitates optimal headings and subheadings

Types of Outlines

Outlines may be formal or informal. A formal outline uses a standard format such as Roman numerals or decimals. Authors can prepare an outline themselves with Roman numerals or decimals, or can use the outline mode in the word-processing program. For instance, Microsoft Word's outline view automatically formats the outline and assigns numbers. When changes are made in the level of the outline, the content is automatically renumbered. For some authors, though, it is easier to develop an outline themselves rather than use word-processing software for this purpose.

Outlines can also take the form of tree diagrams, mapping, or other graphics (Gallaudet University, 2017). Authors may try several formats to stimulate thinking and idea generation. There is no right or wrong type of outline. The best outline is the one that fits the material, encompasses a comprehensive scope for the manuscript, and constrains the authors from wandering away from its focus.

Outlines can grow and develop from many sources. Some authors jot notes as they read through the background literature and following conversations with colleagues; others keep diaries or record their thoughts digitally.

These notes can then be transferred to sticky notes or note cards for development or reorganization into an outline. Outlines for an article may be generated from interim material used for other purposes. Presentations, procedure guides, lecture notes, learning resource packets, and other material prepared for uses other than writing an article can lend themselves naturally to an outline format.

How much detail to include in the outline depends on the author and what style best facilitates writing the manuscript. There is no single correct way to develop an outline. Every author should develop a style of outlining that best meets the need. For some authors, developing a detailed and formal outline is essential to stay on target and not have to think about how to structure the content. For these people, outlining saves valuable time later when writing the first draft. For others, a brief list of topics to be covered in order in the manuscript is sufficient to guide writing. Regardless of the format, it can be valuable to use the same type of outlining for each writing project.

Examples of outlines are shown in Exhibits 11.1 and 11.2. Exhibit 11.1 shows an outline and subsequent text developed from that outline. Exhibit 11.2 is a sample outline for a research manuscript.

EXHIBIT 11.1

Sample Formal Outline and Article

OUTLINE FOR ARTICLE ON BREAST CANCER SURVIVORS' USE OF EXPRESSIVE WRITING

A. Introduction
    a. Epidemiology of breast cancer
        I. Incidence, prevalence, and survival rate
        II. Survivor distress and its duration
        III. Barriers to interventions among survivors
    b. Emotional expression as intervention
        I. Use as coping strategy
        II. Findings in college populations
    c. Meta-analysis
        I. Inconsistent findings of improved psychological and physical health
        II. Limited findings on illness groups, dose, durability, mechanism, and generalizability
    d. Intervention components
    e. Theoretical model (with figure)
    f. Hypotheses: QOL over time following expressive writing regarding breast cancer/trauma vs. neutral topic
B. Methods
C. Results
D. Discussion

(continued)

EXHIBIT 11.1

Sample Formal Outline and Article (*continued*)

ARTICLE: "EXPRESSIVE WRITING IN EARLY BREAST CANCER SURVIVORS"

Breast cancer leads in the incidence of and deaths from cancer in women worldwide, including developed and developing countries, accounting for 23% of the cancer cases in women (Jemal et al., 2011). . . . A diagnosis of breast cancer can lead to physical, cognitive, and affective distress (Cimprich, 1999; Knobf, 2007), with the risk of distress extending well beyond the time of diagnosis (Spiegel et al., 1989; Hoskins, 1997; Ganz et al., 2004; Schmid-Buchi et al., 2011). . . . There are multiple barriers to providing psychosocial care, however, and the IOM report gave an astoundingly low rate of only 10% to 30% of women with breast cancer who receive any formal psychosocial care (Thiewes et al., 2004). . . .

Emotional expression has been studied for many years and has demonstrated success in helping women deal with the diagnosis of breast cancer (Spiegel et al., 1989; Servaes et al., 1999; IOM, 2004; Low et al., 2006, 2010), thus providing the root intervention of many support groups, online support mechanisms, and other structured interventions. . . .

Over 200 studies have been performed since James Pennebaker began studying expressive writing in college students in the mid-1980s. . . . Findings indicated predominantly that the experimental group (i.e., writing group) had reductions in symptoms, either physical or psychosocial.

Several meta-analyses have also been performed (Frisina et al., 2004; Frattaroli, 2006; Harris, 2006; Mogk et al., 2006), finding that expressive writing is associated with improvements in psychological health and in physical health; however, the reported effect size from the meta-analyses remains small, 0.07 to 0.21, and the results do not always follow predictions. There also remain many questions. . . .

Studies related to cancer usually require participants to write about their illness experience. . . . The results have included a decrease in physical symptoms, a decrease in medical care use, and an increase in perceived support.

Emotional inhibition, cognitive adaptation, and exposure/emotional processing have all been theorized to explain the multiple physiological and psychosocial results seen in expressive writing studies (Sloan et al., 2008). . . .

The research hypotheses were that . . .

Source: From Craft, M. A., Davis, G. C., & Paulson, R. M. (2013). Expressive writing in early breast cancer survivors. *Journal of Advanced Nursing, 69*(2), 305–315. doi:10.1111/j.1365-2648.2012.06008.x. Reprinted by permission of John Wiley & Sons.

EXHIBIT 11.2

Outline for Research Manuscript

Introduction
Extensive research on defining and measuring healthcare quality
Limited attention to consumers' perspectives of quality care

(*continued*)

EXHIBIT 11.2

Outline for Research Manuscript (*continued*)

Purposes
  Identify importance to consumers of indicators of quality healthcare and nursing care
  Examine relationships of health status and demographic variables to consumer views

Methods
  Exploratory design
  239 consumers, convenience sample
  How selected (waiting rooms of clinics and neighborhoods)
  Instruments
    Quality Healthcare Questionnaire
    SF-36

Results
  Indicators of quality healthcare most important to consumers (Table 1)
  Indicators of quality nursing care most important to consumers (Table 1)
  Differences based on race/ethnicity, income, and educational level (Table 2)
  Correlations of indicator ratings and health status (Table 3)

Discussion
  Consistency of findings with other studies
  Important implications for teaching patients in clinics
  Limitations of design and sampling
  Next steps in research agenda

Techniques for Outlining

Before beginning the outline, the author should review quickly the materials gathered, making a list of relevant topics and notes on how the material might be grouped into topics and in what order. This gives the author a general sense of how the content will be organized.

If unsure how to organize the content, the author might record key content areas on separate index cards. This can be done as the author is reviewing the materials in preparation for beginning the manuscript. Each index card should have a major content area listed on it; these content areas represent the main topics to be covered in the manuscript. The author can then arrange the cards in a logical order, rearranging as needed until comfortable with the organization. Subtopics can be recorded with the relevant content area and then organized logically. This technique allows the author to easily change the outline until it represents the best order in the author's judgment.

Some authors may prefer to outline their ideas in a picture or map. A concept map is a graphic or pictorial arrangement of key concepts and their interrelationships. Concept maps facilitate and record the author's thinking that underlies the understanding of the topic (Daley, Morgan, & Black, 2016).

Mapping concepts visually helps authors connect key ideas and organize them logically.

The shape of the related concepts is entirely dependent on the author's understanding. After the ideas are written down, the author can order the ideas to guide their logical presentation in the article. The authors can use different shapes (circles, triangles, squares) connected or combined by different types of lines to depict different types of information and their interrelationship. The logical order of the information can flow from left to right or top to bottom. The author's ideas may lend themselves to a scene, for example, an iceberg or forest, where elements of the picture are labeled. The important idea is for authors to get as much of the content of their ideas as possible onto paper to gain perspective on its best organizational structure.

When the outline is complete, it should clearly show the main topic or content area. Identifying the main idea prominently helps keep the writing focused on the purpose of the manuscript. This is especially important when writing the first draft because the main point should be highlighted early in the introduction to the paper.

WRITING THE FIRST DRAFT

Each author develops a *way* of writing—what works best for him or her. With a well-thought-out outline and materials available that might be needed during the writing, the author is ready to begin the draft. The draft can rarely be written all at one time. Instead, the author should find the best time for writing and work on the draft over the next few weeks. The author should be careful not to extend the time for writing the draft for too long a period. When this happens, it is difficult to keep track of ideas and remain motivated about the writing project.

In preparing the first draft, the author should write as quickly as possible to get the ideas on paper. This forward momentum can instill confidence and a feeling of productivity. There will be time in the future to be concerned about grammar, spelling, punctuation, and writing style. These will be revised later. The author may not feel ready to write, but it is important to begin (Halcomb, 2017). The goal with the first draft is to get the ideas on paper, using the outline for organizing them.

With the outline or concept map, the author should be able to start at the beginning of the manuscript with the main idea and write through each section to the end. Content can be reordered if needed by modifying the outline. Some authors, though, do not write each section of the manuscript in order. With experience, authors develop their own styles of writing and techniques for completing writing projects.

Drafting a Title and Abstract

A first draft of the title and abstract should accompany the first draft of the manuscript. The author may use these elements along with the outline to keep the draft focused as it is being written, or may craft a title and abstract once the first draft is complete. Since the title conveys the purpose of the paper and the abstract includes the main ideas in each section of it, writing these first may help the author clarify the main points to be conveyed in the paper. As the first draft is revised and refined, it is likely that the title and abstract will also undergo some change.

Managing Reference Citations in the First Draft

The references used in the body of the first draft should conform to the format requirements of the target journal. Most journals use either name-year or citation sequence system.

In the name-year system, such as with the APA (APA, 2010) reference format, the author's name and date of publication are cited in the paper. References are then organized alphabetically on the reference list. For example, a paper by Craft et al. (2013) used the name-year format in the introduction, as follows:

> Studies have shown that the distress of breast cancer survivors may persist from 2 to 5 years or longer (Mols et al., 2005; Schmid-Buchi et al., 2011).

In the citation-sequence system, references in the reference list are numbered in the order they first appear in the text instead of by the author and date. If the previous example had appeared in a journal requiring citation-sequence references, it would appear as

> Studies have shown that the distress of breast cancer survivors may persist from 2 to 5 years or longer.[1,2]

In the reference list at the end of the paper, number "1" refers to the reference Twycross published in 2003, and number "2" to Glare et al.'s paper published in 2011. Only the number, though, is listed in the text of the paper.

Even if the target journal uses the citation-sequence system, the author's last name and date of the publication should be recorded in the drafts of the manuscript. The references can be numbered later. If numbers are assigned prior to the final copy, they will need to be changed every time content is shifted and a reference is added or deleted. To make it easier to correct the reference format with the final manuscript, the author can insert a symbol before each citation in the text and can use the "find" function in the word-processing program. With this function, the author can move quickly through the document to find the references and then replace them with a number.

If using a bibliographic management program, references are marked in the text and then converted to the proper reference format later. The author should learn how to use this software before writing the first draft.

Even though this is the first draft, authors should be careful about how they cite references to avoid errors. Sometimes in an effort to quickly write the first draft and get ideas expressed, authors make notations about references as a way of remembering to include them in the manuscript but later forget to check them for accuracy.

Producing the Draft

The medium for preparing the first draft depends on author preference. Most authors compose the draft directly on the computer, although some people may prefer to write on paper first, then type it into an electronic file or have someone else type it. Regardless of the process used, each draft should be numbered and dated. This allows the author to refer back to earlier drafts. One easy way to number and date the drafts is by inserting this information in a header or footer; this is shown in Exhibit 11.3. Another way is to label the electronic file name with this information.

If writing alone and working from the beginning section to the end, pages can be numbered sequentially. However, some authors write sections in a different order from how they will eventually appear; in these instances, a system should be devised for numbering pages within each section. Otherwise, the author may be faced with a situation in which pages were printed off from the computer for review, but it is unclear as to their order. If there are coauthors who are submitting drafts of sections to the primary author, a system should be devised for noting the name of the contributor, numbering and dating the draft, and numbering the pages of the contributed section.

Line Numbering and Exhibiting Revisions of Drafts

When writing in a group, and exchanging sections of the manuscript for critique, it is helpful to number the lines. The lines can be numbered automatically by

EXHIBIT 11.3

Labeling Drafts

[Teaching Portfolio, 1st draft, 1/12/18]

Documenting the quality of teaching in the classroom, in clinical practice, and in the learning and simulation laboratories through student evaluations of teaching alone negates other sources of information about the teacher and the context within which the teaching has occurred. Teaching portfolios provide a solution to this issue because they allow faculty to compile materials that more fully represent the scope and quality of their instruction and supervision of students.

[Teaching Portfolio, 2nd draft, 3/5/18]

Teaching portfolios are being used more widely for documenting teaching effectiveness in nursing education programs. Promotion, tenure, reappointment, and merit decisions are based on an assessment of the quality of teaching, research, service, and clinical practice depending on the mission and purposes of the nursing program. Teaching portfolios allow faculty to compile materials that more fully represent the scope and quality of their instruction and supervision of students.

the word-processing program, which enables coauthors to communicate more easily where changes are needed. For example:

247 Studies have shown that the distress of breast
248 cancer survivors may persist from 2 to 5 years or
249 longer (Mols et al., 2005; Schmid-Buchi et al.,
250 2011). An Institute of Medicine (IOM) report on
252 psychosocial care in breast cancer stressed the . . .

With line numbering, an author can indicate easily to colleagues or reviewers where to direct their attention.

Other word-processing functions that can be used to show revisions of drafts are through annotations, inserting comments, and marking the revisions with different colors while editing. Manuscripts can then be sent electronically to coauthors, indicating the queries and suggesting revisions in the draft with one of these techniques.

PREPARING TO REVISE

After writing the first draft, an author may structure a period of retreat from writing. A writing break allows the author to rest, relax, and rejuvenate her energy for the next steps in the creative process. Another reason to retreat from active writing is to seek the comments and views of others. In this pre-submission phase when the article is emerging, the perspectives of other like-minded colleagues serve as proxies for the eventual readers of the article. Chapter 3 discusses in more detail the structure and processes of writing in a group context. A retreat from active writing allows the author to prepare for active writing in the revision stage.

Getting Feedback From Others

If the break from writing comes after the author completes the entire first draft of the manuscript, it can be sent to coauthors to read. Circulating the article to coauthors should be delayed until after the author has revised the draft for content and organization. Colleagues who are experts in the content or the method described in the manuscript can also serve as reviewers of the content and organization of the paper. Feedback from collaborators, experts, and readers who represent a constituency for the final draft is an essential ingredient for the writing process (Chichester & Wool, 2017).

As the author approaches the phase of writing when feedback from others is appropriate, the author may experience resistance to proceeding. If an author is working with other colleagues for whom publication is a high priority, group sessions for critiquing first drafts may be helpful. In one such group, the authors projected their manuscripts on a screen and read them out loud to each other in order to identify unclear or problematic reasoning. A collegial and constructive climate for such group feedback is critical (Oman, Mancuso, Ceballos, Makic, & Fink, 2016). In another working group of novice writers, pairing group members with a master-writer from the faculty or health services library has also proven to be a useful strategy for gaining internal feedback (von Isenburg et al., 2017).

Review by Coauthors

When to send the draft to coauthors is a decision of the first author or whoever is responsible for organizing the preparation of the manuscript. Usually, coauthors are asked to critique a second or subsequent draft of the manuscript rather than the first draft. The first draft may not contain the essential content, and the lead author may find in revising the draft that a reorganization of the content is warranted. However, it is best for coauthors to read an early draft after the content has been revised for accuracy and structure by the lead author. Coauthors have a variety of strengths and expertise such that comments from each may be focused on separate parts of the emerging article.

Drafts should be numbered, dated, and labeled with the coauthor's name as a means of tracking revisions of the manuscript. If contributors are reading drafts of individual sections of the paper, this should be noted. As the lead author receives suggestions for revisions, these can be made in subsequent drafts. All versions of the manuscript should be kept by the lead author or individual organizing preparation of the paper in case authors need to refer later to them. The "reviewing toolbar" of word-processing programs is useful for tracking changes and comments by coauthors in a digital format.

The final version of the paper must be read and approved by each coauthor to meet the requirements for authorship as described in earlier chapters. A record of which coauthors have drafted or provided critical revisions of each draft is crucial for required documentation affirming that authorship criteria have been met during the writing process.

Anticipating the Revision Phase

During the period of rest from writing, the author may think of new ideas or possible improvements for the first draft. To provide a record of any thoughts related to the topic or written draft, the author should keep notepads or tape recorders handy for recording them. It is not important to evaluate the usefulness of these thoughts during this time. If they are stored securely for retrieval during the revision phase, the author is free to allow the mind and body to take a needed break from the active writing process.

REVISING THE FIRST DRAFT

With the essential elements of the article arranged on the page into a preliminary logical order and with a period of retreat from the article, the author is ready to begin revising the first draft. The author should begin to revise based on the list of priorities developed at the end of the first phase of writing and any notes taken during the period of retreat. Some of the priorities may have changed, and ideas jotted down may be dismissed. However, these early changes allow the author to gain momentum for revising the draft.

Authors will revise the content, organization, grammar and punctuation, and writing style of the first draft. Some authors may revise content and organization first, until they are satisfied that all elements are in their logical place, and then focus on elements of style and accuracy. Other authors will choose to proceed from first paragraph to last paragraph, revising all elements as they go. Still others will work from the "inside outward," focusing first on the original material in the center of the article and then moving to "set up" that material well in the introduction and background section and "wrap up" the contributed material with the final section of the article. However, the following elements must be addressed before a final draft is complete.

Number of Drafts

There is no set number on how many drafts to write until satisfied with the finished product. Some authors need to revise their drafts more than others. In the first few drafts, authors should continue to focus on expressing the content clearly and thoroughly. Only when satisfied with the content should the author begin to revise grammar, punctuation, spelling, and writing style. The author should avoid trying to write a finished manuscript as a first draft and instead should focus on including the essential content. The key in writing the first and early drafts is to get the content on paper and organize it effectively. During the revising phase, the author engages in an iterative and interactive cycle of changes. Each article will emerge from its own pattern, and the author will develop increasingly comfortable patterns of writing, resting, seeking advice, incorporating the advice of others and authorial evaluations, resting, and so forth.

There comes a time, however, when the author needs to stop modifying the content, or the drafting phase will never end. "Perfection is the ideal, but an obstacle to done" (Williams, 2009, p. 5).

Revising for Content and Organization

In revising the content and its organization, the authors become their own peer reviewers and editors. It is important to allow oneself to be receptive to criticism of one's own work; the author should view the draft as a "work in progress" that needs to be revised rather than as a finished product. Change is a key ingredient for growth and development, as an author and as a professional. If convinced of the perfection of a draft of the article, the author may be unwilling to make changes that are essential to improve it. Authors must always keep in mind that the ultimate goal of the article is to communicate to the readers, whose needs guide all changes and improvements.

The principles described earlier for preparing each section of the manuscript may be used as a framework for revising the first and later drafts in terms of content and organization. Exhibit 11.4 provides a list of questions the author can use to revise the paper.

EXHIBIT 11.4

Revising Content and Organization: Questions to Ask

Title
- Does the title communicate the purpose of the manuscript?
- Is the title informative?
- Is it accurate?
- Is the title too long? If so, what words can be omitted?

Abstract
- Does the abstract summarize the most important content in the paper?
- Does the abstract of a research manuscript describe the background, purpose, methods, results, and conclusions of the study, within the length allowed?

Text
- Is the purpose of the paper clear and introduced early in the discussion?
- Does the introduction explain why the content is important to readers and how it will improve their knowledge or skill?
- Can the main concepts expressed in the purpose be traced from the introduction to the end of the text?
- Is important literature reviewed and synthesized?
- Is the literature review relevant for the goals of the paper and journal?
- Is the original contribution of the paper fully described?
- Is the literature current?
- Is any content missing?
- Is there any content that is repetitive in the text?
- What content can be omitted from the paper?
- Is the content accurate?
- Is the content sequenced clearly and logically?
- Is it clear how the content may be used in the nurse's own work and setting?

References
- Are all references essential?
- Have any important references been omitted?
- Are the references consistent with the citations in the paper?

Tables and Figures
- Do tables and figures display specific data that supplement and support the text?

(continued)

EXHIBIT 11.4

Revising Content and Organization: Questions to Ask (continued)

- Are they consistent with the text?
- Is each table and figure essential?

Headings and Subheadings
- Are the headings and subheadings effective in organizing the content of the manuscript?
- Are they substantive, informing readers of the content that follows?
- Do they provide transition from one topic to the next?
- Are the correct levels of headings and subheadings used to reflect the importance of the content area?
- Are there at least two headings or subheadings grouped sequentially at each level employed in the paper?

Additional Questions for Research Manuscripts
- Are the purposes of the study, research questions, and/or hypotheses stated clearly for readers?
- Are the gaps in knowledge and limitations of prior studies emphasized to provide support for the current study?
- Does the methods section adequately describe the study design, subjects, measures, procedures, and data analysis?
- Does the results section present the findings of the study, addressing the original purposes of the research?
- Are the main findings presented first?
- Are the findings presented without discussion, which is provided in the subsequent section of the paper?
- Are the results described accurately and precisely?
- Are statistics reported correctly, using conventional format?
- Does the discussion section interpret the results and explain what the findings mean in terms of the purpose of the study and how they advance previous studies?
- Are inconsistencies with prior research addressed?
- Are implications of the study discussed?

Review Title

If the author developed a working title, this can be reviewed first. The title should capture the purpose of the manuscript and, for research manuscripts, should indicate the objective of the study, which may have shifted in focus over multiple drafts. When writing the title:

- Be concise (avoid long titles)
- Use key words from the article (this helps with searching)

- Use specific terms
- Check word order
- Do not use abbreviations, acronyms, or jargon (Oermann & Leonardelli, 2013; University of California Irvine, 2017)

Regardless of when the title is prepared, following the final revision of the article, the author should critique the title to determine if revisions are needed in it.

Review Abstract

In reviewing the abstract, the author examines if it adequately summarizes the purpose of the current draft and indicates the most important content within the length allowed by the journal. For research manuscripts, the abstract should describe the key elements of the body of the article as ultimately developed (Price, 2015).

Review Text

After critiquing the title and abstract, the author is then ready to review the text. First, the author should reread the body of the article to determine if content is missing. It is helpful to read the draft as a whole without interruption. Sometimes, identifying missing elements requires the fresh eyes of a coauthor or colleague. It may be that the outline was missing a section of content or, in writing the paper, the author failed to elaborate sufficiently about a particular topic related to the central idea. The author may have made claims about the background issues that omit evidence from the literature. These gaps should be filled by appropriate references. Or, the author may have stated that there is one or more objectives for the article but neglected to describe the background for each of the concepts or population groups noted in the objectives. It is helpful to identify all of the nouns in the research questions or hypotheses or in each of the objectives to make certain that each has been addressed thoroughly in the article.

Second, the text should be reviewed to eliminate repetitive content and to assess if any content can be omitted, considering the purpose of the paper. In writing the first draft, authors often repeat ideas in different sections of the manuscript and frequently include more content than essential. Repetition should be avoided and information not immediately relevant to the topic should be deleted. It is better to prepare a shorter manuscript that is focused than a longer one with content not essential to the goals of the paper. It may be that entire sections or paragraphs of the manuscript may be eliminated; in these instances, the author should save the deleted content in a separate file in case it is needed later.

Because the author has devoted much time and effort to writing the first draft, it is sometimes difficult to delete content. The author, however, should be willing to make these changes to improve the manuscript and avoid having the material become distracting to the editor or peer reviewers during the submission process.

Third, once the author has revised the content of the draft, the next step is to assess its organization or structure. Although an outline was used for writing the draft, the content in the outline may not have been structured clearly, or the author may have strayed from the outline in writing the draft. The author also may find that the broad organization of content is consistent with the outline and is clear, but the content within each section of the paper needs reorganization. For research papers using the IMRAD format, the broad content areas are predetermined, but how the content is organized within each of these sections should be evaluated.

Some authors find that making a "reverse outline" from the first draft can diagnose problems with the structure and organization of the article (Duke Writing Studio, 2017). This strategy involves taking the first draft as the starting point and listing on a fresh piece of paper the concept or premise that is addressed in *each* of the paragraphs of the article. By examining the actual structure and organization of the ideas in the paper in this way, the author is frequently able to see where ideas were introduced too late or out of logical order for the reader.

Fourth, the accuracy of the paper should be reviewed. For research papers, it is particularly important to check the accuracy of the data reported in the manuscript, statistical results, and conclusions reached from the findings. Each statement in the draft should be reread for accuracy and whether it is supported adequately by the discussion.

Fifth, the end of the manuscript should bring the ideas to a closing, summarizing the main points covered in the paper. The author should check that the manuscript does not end in midair without concluding remarks. New concepts should not be introduced at the end, and the author should be able to trace the development of the main points of the paper from the beginning through the end. A few sentences are usually sufficient to summarize the conclusions from the article and to prioritize the next steps based on its implications for practice, teaching, administration, and future research.

Review References

The author should remember that the literature review in a paper provides the background information for readers but is not intended to be an exhaustive review of every article on a topic. In reviewing the references, the author should ask whether they are essential to support the goals of the paper and consistent with the intended journal and readers. Unnecessary references should be omitted. When citing support for a statement, key references should be used rather than a long list of citations.

Review Tables and Figures

Consistent with eliminating unnecessary content and ensuring accuracy, the author should review each table and figure to determine if it is essential to the paper and if its content matches what is described in the text. Some tables may be omitted because they duplicate the content in the text. Sometimes, new tables should be developed to replace material that became unwieldy as the text was revised. Tables and figures should supplement the text, not duplicate it. This is a good time for the author to recheck numerical data in the table for accuracy and consistency with the information reported in the text.

Review Headings and Subheadings

Headings and subheadings emphasize for readers the content covered in each section of the manuscript. They give structure to the overall paper, provide transition from one topic to the next, inform readers of the content that follows, and suggest the importance of each subject area. By dividing the manuscript into sections, headings also make the paper more attractive visually (American Medical Association [AMA], 2007). The revision of the paper provides an opportunity for the author to add headings and subheadings to the manuscript if not done already or to review those written.

Headings and subheadings are often identified by using the outline developed for the manuscript, but these should conform to the best organizational structure for the final draft. Headings of the same "level" represent topics of equal importance (APA, 2010). For example, research papers following the IMRAD format include four predetermined level 1 headings that are of equal importance (Introduction, **Methods**, **Results**, and **Discussion**). The author may choose to insert subheadings within these general areas or may be required by convention to do so, as with the level 2 subheadings of Methods (Design, Sample, Intervention, Measures, and Analysis). For nonresearch papers, the author should select headings and subheadings to organize the content and indicate for readers the topics that follow. The target journal prescribes the levels of headings and their formatting, and the author is advised to review sample articles in the journal to determine the levels typically included in its publications.

There is no correct number of headings to use in an article. Because headings are meant to subdivide material into multiple parts, there should be at least two headings at each level used. If two or more are not needed, then no headings at that level should be used.

Headings and subheadings can be short sentences, phrases, single words, or questions. Headings should not contain a single abbreviation, an abbreviation with its first explanation, a citation to figures or tables, or references (AMA, 2007). Exhibits 5.8 and 5.10 presented two examples of effective use of headings in a Measures and a Results section, respectively. These headings improve readability and make the organization clearer for readers.

Guidelines for preparing the headings and subheadings are as follows:

1. Develop substantive headings that inform readers of the content in the section that follows.
2. Write headings and subheadings as short sentences, phrases, single words, or questions.

3. Do not use a heading for the introduction because the first part of the manuscript is assumed to be the introductory section (APA, 2010).
4. Avoid having only one subsection in a section, similar to principles for outlining (AMA, 2007).
5. Follow the style manual or author guidelines for how to level the headings, how to position them in the manuscript, and other details for typing them.
6. Abbreviations should not be used in headings even if expanded earlier in the manuscript. Instead, the author should write out the term or phrase.
7. Subheadings within a section should have parallel grammatical structure.

Revising for Style

Publication of the manuscript depends more on the substantive content than on writing style; however, poorly written papers may influence the critique by peer reviewers and the editor, and ultimately the acceptance decision. If similar papers are under review, the one that is well written will more than likely be accepted. Poor writing structure and style also may result in the manuscript requiring extensive revisions prior to acceptance for publication. It is important, therefore, that the author carefully edit the manuscript so it is well written.

Writers do not intend to write without clarity and grace. Some bad writing occurs because the author does not understand the topic and adds words to mask the knowledge deficiency (Williams, 2009). Some writing is grammatically accurate but sounds jerky because authors write slowly and painstakingly to avoid breaking supposed rules of writing. Some writing is awkward because it represents a first attempt to mimic the style of a new and unfamiliar genre such as scientific writing. Whatever the reason for poor writing style, authors can improve their writing with attention and practice.

The following section provides a framework for revising the style of any draft of an article. The author revises for style only after being satisfied that the necessary content is in place and organized appropriately in major sections of the article. In other words, the content of the draft should be complete and accurate. Revising for style should be accomplished by focusing first on paragraphs and then on sentences and words (Figure 11.1). This system enables the author to edit broad elements of the paper first, then more specific ones. Otherwise, changes may be made in words, phrases, and sentences that need to be modified again when the paragraph is edited.

The discussion that follows is not intended to be an exhaustive list of points to consider when editing the draft to improve the writing. The discussion highlights some of the aspects the author checks when editing the writing structure and style.

Check paragraphs ⟹ Check sentences ⟹ Check phrases ⟹ Check words

FIGURE 11.1 Scheme for revising writing structure and style.

In these revisions, the author should continue to keep earlier versions of the paper for referral later if needed. If the author is making her or his own revisions, the manuscript may be modified easily on the computer. Alternately, some authors prefer to print hard copies and revise the prose on the hard copy so as not to be distracted by word processing. If revisions are made first on the hard copy, the author might use proofreading marks to indicate changes.

Revising Paragraphs

One way to begin revising a first draft is to edit the paragraphs. In editing the paragraphs, the author should check the (a) coherence, (b) length, (c) structure, and (d) transitions between paragraphs.

Coherence

Coherent paragraphs share a common theme and include all aspects of that theme and none from different themes. The subjects of all of the sentences in the paragraph are related to each other (Williams, 2009). At least one of those sentences—usually the first or the last sentence—explains to the reader the paragraph's basic claim. Sentences in coherent paragraphs "add up, the way all the pieces in a puzzle add up to the picture on the box" (Williams, 2009, p. 60).

Length of Paragraphs

Long paragraphs often can be divided into two smaller ones by identifying breaks in the flow of ideas or how details might be grouped together into separate thematic paragraphs. For example, a lengthy paragraph on different addiction models might be divided into separate paragraphs, each describing one of the models. The initial paragraph in the sequence could specify the models discussed, listing them in the same order as explained in the paragraphs that follow. As a rule of thumb, paragraphs that extend beyond a single double-spaced page are too long and should be divided (APA, 2010).

Structure

In editing the paragraph structure, the author is concerned with the sequence of ideas. As noted earlier, the beginning sentence often explains the basic premise of the paragraph. The author should then confirm that there is a clear sequence of ideas developed from sentence to sentence through the paragraph. Authors can make their sentences flow more gracefully by selecting subjects for each sentence that are related conceptually. Later in this chapter, we discuss ways to construct sentences in which the subjects are thematically related.

Authors can also use *metadiscourse* to guide the reader through the unfolding ideas in a paragraph. Metadiscourse includes all of the elements of writing that point not to the content of the article but rather to the writing itself, the readers, or the authors (Williams, 2009). For example, when constructing a paragraph, the author can alert the reader that a series of subthemes will be presented in the writing by using terms noting seriation, for example, "first," "second," "finally," to guide the reader through the paragraph. In a paragraph that begins, "There are two major principles in evaluating a burn wound," the reader expects the paragraph to cover these two principles, with a sentence that begins "First . . ." followed eventually by a sentence that begins with "Second. . . ." These words do not concern the topic of the paragraph, which is the evaluation of burns. Rather, the words are used to inform the reader about how the writing of the paragraph is constructed, that is, metadiscourse.

Transitions Between Paragraphs

To develop ideas in the paper, paragraphs need to be linked to one another. When the reader completes one paragraph and begins the following one, there should be a sense of moving to a new idea or different points about the topic. The first sentence of the new paragraph introduces the next theme to be discussed in the article and often echoes the preceding paragraph. Readers should be able to track the main idea from the beginning of the paper to the end by following the content from one paragraph to the next. Readers should not be disappointed to find a paragraph with a new theme that follows illogically from the preceding paragraph's theme.

To edit the transitions between paragraphs, the author should read the last sentence of a paragraph and the first sentence of the next paragraph. The example in Exhibit 11.5 shows how paragraphs are connected so there is a transition between them and how ideas are developed by reading a sequence of paragraphs.

EXHIBIT 11.5

Sample Paragraphing With Transitions

Evaluation fulfills two major roles: formative and summative. Formative evaluation judges students' progress in meeting the objectives and developing competencies for practice. It occurs throughout the instructional process and provides feedback for determining where further learning is needed. Considering that formative evaluation is diagnostic, it typically is not graded. Teachers should remember that the purpose of formative evaluation is to determine where further learning is needed.

Summative evaluation, on the other hand, is end-of-instruction evaluation designed to determine what the student has learned in the classroom, an online course, or clinical practice. Summative evaluation judges the quality of the student's achievement in the course, not the progress of the learner in meeting the objectives.

Source: Adapted from Oermann, M. H., & Gaberson, K. B. (2017). *Evaluation and testing in nursing education* (5th ed.). New York, NY: Springer Publishing.

Revising Sentences

Once the paragraphs in each section of the article are thematically coherent and flow logically from one to the next, the author focuses on improving each sentence within a paragraph. The following are several recommended strategies for constructing sentences that readers will find easy to understand.

Cohesion

Even when all of the sentences in a paragraph are focused on a single theme, sentences may need revision to ensure that they link together as pairs, that is, to ensure cohesion. Williams (2009) makes two recommendations for constructing sentences that link together as puzzle pieces. First, authors should "begin sentences with information familiar to your readers" (p. 59), using a keyword from the previous sentence or a word logically related to the topic of the previous sentence. Second, authors should "end sentences with information readers cannot predict" (p. 59), allowing readers to read each sentence from the familiar to the new, from easy to hard. Readers find material easy when the new sentence uses a word or two from the previous sentence.

In an example where linking sentences are used effectively, an article on benefits and barriers to advancing nurse education (Sarver, Cichra, & Kline, 2015) discussed trends in qualifications of nurses hired by Magnet® hospitals, as follows.

> Magnet hospitals typically employ greater numbers of BSN-prepared nurses (American Association of Colleges of Nursing, 2012) and currently require that all nurse managers and nurse leaders hold degrees at the BSN level or higher. For hospitals applying for Magnet designation, plans must be in place to achieve the IOM recommendation (2011) of 80 percent BSN preparation by 2020.

Notice that early in sentence 2, the word "Magnet" echoed the subject of the preceding sentence; then sentence 2 moved from the familiar topic of Magnet hospitals to the new information concerning the IOM recommendation (p. 153).

Characters and Action

Put the main character and its action up front. "Begin your sentences with elements that are relatively short: a short introductory phrase and clause, followed by a short concrete subject, followed by a verb expressing a specific action" (Williams, 2009, p. 69). The early short phrase or clause frames the subject for the reader, who wants to know quickly the subject of the sentence and what the subject did to what or whom. These basic elements can be followed for several lines of additional details about the topic. In Exhibit 11.5, the first sentence is short and direct: "Evaluation fulfills two major roles: formative and summative." The two types of evaluation are the active agents of action, that is, they judge. The remainder of the two paragraphs elaborates about what (progress, feedback, learning), where (classroom, clinical), when (throughout, end of instruction), and who (students, teachers).

Active Versus Passive Voice

Write as many sentences as possible in the active voice, which is preferred by editors for brevity and clarity (APA, 2010). The active voice states who or what the person is doing; the passive voice suggests that the subject is being acted upon. The active voice keeps readers' interest better than the passive voice (Williams, 2009). Here is an example of passive and active voices:

> **Passive voice:** The clinical guidelines were developed by the interdisciplinary team.

> **Active voice:** The interdisciplinary team developed the clinical guidelines.

Although the active voice is preferred, the passive voice may be more appropriate if the author does not know or the reader does not need to know who is responsible for the action.

Use of the First Person as Subject

Use first-person pronouns sparingly to indicate actions that are unique to the writers (Williams, 2009). In the introduction to the article, the authors might state: "In this paper we will explain (or address, present, review). . . ." In the concluding sections, the authors might summarize as: "In this paper, we have developed (or argued). . . ." This is a second type of metadiscourse that helps the reader understand the content and follow its logic by using words that refer to the authors rather than to the content of the manuscript.

When referring to actions of a research team that includes others besides the writers, authors should use the third person plural and avoid the first person plural. For example, state that the "Researchers recruited diabetic patients . . ." or "Interviewers implemented screening procedures . . ." rather than saying, "We recruited . . ." or "We implemented. . . ."

Length of Sentences

Authors naturally vary the length of their sentences, and most fall between 15 and 30 words. Short sentences suggest urgency or certainty (Williams, 2009). Long sentences require particular attention to assure balance and rhythm.

Balanced Sentences

Construct sentences so that they are internally balanced using coordinating words, punctuation, transitional words, or parallel word forms. Coordinating words such as *and, or, nor, but,* and *yet* contribute to internal balance between parts of a sentence. Punctuation, such as semicolons, between two or more related independent phrases indicate that these are generally balanced in importance. When transitional words are used, such as *although* or *since,* the sentence communicates to the reader the continuity of thought across a balanced sentence structure (APA, 2010). Parallel construction of verbs and nouns throughout the sentence also balances a sentence. Authors should check that parallel structure is used in sentences that contain a sequence of phrases or words.

In the following example, there is an unbalanced use of gerunds (ending in –ing) and infinitives (beginning with to . . .) as direct objects; these are revised to use gerunds throughout the sentence.

> **Original:** Benefits of simulations are learn*ing* how to use equipment, develop*ing* ability to perform a procedure, and *to practice* complex technological skills in a laboratory environment rather than with actual patients.

> **Revised for parallel structure**: Benefits of simulations are learn*ing* how to use equipment, develop*ing* ability to perform a procedure, and *practicing* complex technological skills in a laboratory environment rather than with actual patients.

Sentences That Compare Elements

To avoid ambiguous and illogical comparisons, identify both elements in the comparison and use parallel construction for each element.

> **Ambiguous:** "Previous research suggests that residents of public housing units are more disabled." (The reader is left wondering, more disabled than whom?)

> **Illogical:** "Previous research suggests that residents of public housing units were more disabled than single-family dwellings." (Dwellings are not disabled; people are disabled.)

> **Correct:** "Previous research suggests that residents of public housing units were more disabled than residents of single-family houses."

Mechanics of Sentence Construction

In this stage of revision, the author also ensures that each sentence is grammatically correct. One common problem with sentence mechanics is *subject–verb agreement.* The sentence's subject must match in number to the form of the sentence's verb(s). Subject–verb pairs must be consistently singular or plural. Two common problems occur when using intervening words or nouns of foreign origin. For example,

> The *number* (singular) of applicants to second-degree nursing programs *rises* (singular) during periods of unemployment.
> The *data* (plural) *show* (plural) a positive trend.

Another common problem is with *pronouns*. A pronoun must match in number and gender (masculine, feminine, neuter) the noun to which it refers earlier in the sentence. Pronouns used with present participles must be in the possessive form. Authors should check the antecedents of pronouns and, when using pronouns, make it clear to what word they are referring. For example:

> Jones and Smith reported that patients learned effectively with videotapes. *They* were satisfied with the quality of the instruction.

In the second sentence it is not clear to whom "they" refers—is it Jones and Smith who were satisfied with the quality of the instruction or the patients? Ambiguity often results when sentences begin with "it" and "this," requiring readers to refer to the prior sentence. Authors are advised to check each pronoun for clarity.

A third common problem is with *modifiers* and *adverbs*. Authors should place each modifying phrase and adverb as close as possible to the word it modifies in the sentence and be certain that the sentence contains the word that an existing modifier is intended to describe. They also should check for misplaced modifiers. Often, this problem can be avoided if the modifying word, phrase, or clause is placed close to the word it is modifying. In the first example, the modifier is misplaced; the patient has congestive heart failure, not the nurse.

> **Original:** The patient was transferred to the home health nurse with congestive heart failure.

> **Revision:** The patient *with congestive heart failure* was transferred to the home health nurse.

Lastly, authors need to check that the *punctuation* is correct. Style manuals such as the APA (2010) and AMA (2007) include extensive instructions regarding punctuation of sentences in scientific writing. Two of the most commonly misused elements in sentence construction are the comma and the semicolon.

The semicolon is used in only two circumstances. First, use a semicolon to separate two independent clauses (that could otherwise stand alone as separate sentences) but which are thematically related and are not joined by a conjunction such as *and* or *but*. Second, use a semicolon to separate a series of three or more elements, any of which already contain commas.

The comma is more common but has related uses. Its first usage is to separate two independent clauses that are joined by a conjunction. A second usage is to separate a series of three or more elements that do not already contain commas. A third usage is to separate from the main part of the sentence any nonessential or nonrestrictive clause (one whose omission would leave intact the meaning of that sentence [APA, 2010]). Other uses are to separate the year in a date, the year in a reference citation, and groups of three digits in most numbers. Commas should *not* be used to separate essential clauses (whose omission would change the meaning of the sentence) or between two parts of a compound predicate (which could not stand alone as separate sentences).

Revising Words

When revising sentences, the author likely made numerous changes in the words used to describe ideas and connect sentences. The focus of this last phase of revising the manuscript is to examine the words used in each sentence, to ensure that they convey the correct meaning and that the writing is clear, concise, and accurate. For some authors, reading the manuscript out loud helps identify where revisions are needed. Following are some recommended strategies for choosing words that readers will find easy to absorb.

Concision

Publishing is expensive, and the author should write as concisely as possible. Use of many words is not required to demonstrate a topic's importance. Authors should select only necessary and accurate words to express their ideas and eliminate all others.

Williams (2009) lists six types of words that should be deleted:

1. Words that mean little or nothing, for example, *really, certain, various*
2. Words that repeat the meaning of other words, for example, *each and every*
3. Words implied by other words, for example, *basic fundamentals, large in size*
4. Phrases that could be expressed in a word, for example, *if* rather than *in the event that*
5. Words in the affirmative that could replace a negative, *different* versus *not the same*
6. Useless adjectives and adverbs, for example, *abstract idea, tried as much as possible*

We applied these principles of concision to the following example.

Less concise: *In order to* evaluate neck masses, a thorough and complete examination of the head and neck region should be performed by the nurse practitioner *using a systematic process*.

"In order to" is an unnecessary phrase that can be omitted while still preserving the meaning of the sentence. Similarly, examinations are done systematically so the phrase "using a systematic process" is not needed. By eliminating unnecessary words in this sentence it reads:

> **More concise:** To evaluate neck masses, the nurse practitioner should perform an examination of the head and neck regions.

Precision

The value of journal space also underlies the need to choose the most precise and complete information available to inform the reader. Sizes and amounts can be described in more and less precise ways. In general, "approximations weaken statements" in the scientific literature (APA, 2010, p. 68).

> **Less precise:** There was a *large* increase in the number of patients admitted to home care with the initiation of case management.

"Large" in this sentence is vague; it would be better to present the actual increase in numbers of patients admitted to home care within a particular time period.

> **More precise:** Case management increased home care admissions by 35% over 1 year.

Words have precise meanings that communicate the same common understanding to all readers. Sometimes the meaning of simple words can confound the writer and confuse the reader as much as or more than long unfamiliar words. Authors should check their manuscripts for some of the most common imprecise word usages. For example:

- *Among* (for a group of three or more objects) versus *between* (for two objects): The work to be done was divided *among* the three nurse managers. The work to be done was divided *between* the nurse manager and the clinical coordinator.
- *Effect* (noun) versus *affect* (verb): The *effects* of the intervention were decreased pain and improved coping. Patients were *affected* positively by the intervention, reporting decreased pain and improved coping.
- *Normal* and *abnormal*; *positive* and *negative* (the findings and results of tests and examinations are normal, abnormal, positive, or negative, not the tests and examinations themselves):

> **Incorrect:** The physical examination given by the nurse practitioner was normal.

Correct: The *findings* from the physical examination given by the nurse practitioner were normal.

- *Which* (relative pronoun used to introduce a nonessential clause) versus *that* (relative pronoun used to introduce a necessary clause):
  The patient should have a complete assessment, *which* is described in this article, when admitted to the hospital.
  The author should check *that* the statistics are reported correctly.

Words to Avoid

There are a number of guidelines for word choice that will help readers engage with the text.

- Avoid abstract words. Authors may be tempted to use abstract words to make their writing seem more formal. This can be a mistake. Abstract words are often verbs that have been turned into nouns, called *nominalizations* (Williams, 2009). Examples of nominalized verbs are: investigation, expansion, intention, decision, and many others. Use of nominalizations obscures both the actor and action taken.

Instead of using abstract nominalized words as the subject or object of a sentence, authors should ask two questions: (a) What is the underlying action verb? and (b) Who is doing the action? Next, the author should construct a new sentence in which the actor serves as the subject and the previous nominalized verb serves as a true verb. Clearer and more concrete words (and sentences) emerge from this strategy. For example:

Abstract: A review of falls investigations in nursing homes was completed.

Concrete: We reviewed how investigators have studied falls in nursing homes.

Abstract: Understanding how nutrition problems impact overall health and mortality in late life has been limited by a lack of population-based samples and longitudinal designs.

Concrete: Researchers usually study late life nutrition using convenience samples and cross-sectional studies, which limits understanding of its impact on health and mortality.

- Avoid jargon, colloquialisms, and abbreviated terms, such as "temp" and "lab." Jargon represents technical shorthand that is immediately understood by a limited group of people and, as such, will be exclusive of and grating to larger communities of discourse (APA, 2010). Jargon and other shorthand terminology can be used in the drafts of the paper as a way of capturing the ideas for the manuscript, but they need to be rewritten during the revision.

Original: The nurse *prepped* the patient for surgery after checking lab values.

Revised: The nurse *prepared* the patient for surgery after checking *laboratory* values.

- Avoid words that imply a bias for or against any group of persons. Historically, such groups have been distinguished by gender, sexual orientation, racial and ethnic identity, disability, and age (APA, 2010). The following guidelines may assist authors in revising specific words to avoid bias:
  1. Be as specific as possible about relevant characteristics. Instead of *elders*, refer to *persons 65 to 83 years of age.*
  2. Avoid labels and impersonal terminology. Instead of *depressives* or *diabetics*, refer to *people with depressive disorder* or *patients with diabetes.*
  3. Acknowledge participation by using action verbs. Instead of "The survey was administered to students," state that "Students completed the survey" (APA, 2010, p. 73).
  4. Use the plural form of nouns and verbs. For example:

     Original: The nurse begins health teaching when she completes the initial assessment of learning needs.

     Revised: Nurses begin health teaching when *they* complete the initial assessment of learning needs.

     Original: The patient should have an opportunity to choose *his* own treatment.

     Revised: Patients should have the opportunity to choose *their* own treatments.

  5. Select nonspecific forms of words to avoid assumption of an unknown characteristic, for example, using *committee chair* or *chairperson* rather than *chairman.*

Mechanics of Word Choice

Rules and conventional uses of English grammar and scientific writing are myriad and complex. It is not possible to describe the universe of such conventions here. Three frequent stumbling blocks are particularly prevalent in formal writing.

- Check verb tense so it is consistent throughout the paper and the correct verb tense is used. The correct verb tense is needed so readers know when the action occurred. For instance, in the first statement listed here, the use of past tense indicates to the readers that the study was completed earlier and is presented for historical purposes.

In 2015 Jones completed the first study that evaluated the effects of using a smartphone for teaching patients in clinics.

If the study by Jones remains important, the author might revise the sentence using the present perfect tense and delete the date:

Jones has completed a study on evaluating the effects of using the computer for teaching patients in clinics.

In referring to current studies, present tense may be used:

Smith reports that computers are effective for teaching patients in clinics.

- Check for spelling errors. The spell-checking function in word-processing programs identifies misspelled words, although medical and specialized terms often need to be checked by the author. The author also should be alert to words that are spelled correctly but misused in the sentence, for instance, *principle* versus *principal*. Only careful reading by the author, not the word-processing program, will locate these errors.
- Check capitalization of proper nouns, names of organizations and institutions, and others. Exhibit 11.6 is a checklist for authors to use in revising their drafts for writing structure and style. As mentioned earlier in the chapter, this discussion is not exhaustive of principles to consider in improving writing but highlights some important ones for the author to follow.

EXHIBIT 11.6

Checklist for Revising Writing Structure and Style

Paragraphs
- Ideas sequenced clearly through manuscript as a whole and in each section
- Paragraphs focus on one topic and present details about it
- Clear sequence of ideas developed within and between paragraphs, using sequencing terms as needed
- Clear transitions between paragraphs
- First sentence of paragraph introduces subject and provides transition from preceding paragraph
- Paragraphs appropriate length

Sentences
- Sentences clearly written and convey intended meaning
- Characters and their actions are apparent in sentences
- Sentences appropriate length
- Variety in types of sentences and how they begin
- Clear transitions between sentences within paragraphs
- Subjects and verbs agree in each sentence

(continued)

EXHIBIT 11.6

Checklist for Revising Writing Structure and Style (*continued*)

- Comparisons specify all elements
- First person used sparingly
- Sentences are balanced by use of punctuation and coordinating, transitional, or parallel words

Words
- Words express intended meaning and are used correctly
- Clear antecedents for pronouns
- Information provided with maximum possible precision
- No misplaced modifiers
- Excessive and unnecessary words omitted
- Stereotypes, abstractions, nominalizations, jargon, and abbreviated terms avoided
- Active voice used

Throughout the Manuscript
- Correct grammar
- Correct punctuation
- Correct capitalization
- Correct spelling

Revising for Scientific Style

Publications in nursing and healthcare often include abbreviations, symbols, measures, and other labels for presenting specialized content. Similar to formats for references, journalistic style is particular and dictated by the editor and publishers. This information may be provided in the journal guidelines, but usually the author refers to a style manual such as the *AMA Manual of Style: A Guide for Authors and Editors* (AMA, 2007) or the *Publication Manual of the American Psychological Association* (APA, 2010). In the revision of the manuscript, the author verifies the proper use of abbreviations, nomenclature, units of measure, numbers and percentages, and statistics. Exhibit 11.7 summarizes these principles in the form of a checklist for the author to use.

Abbreviations

An abbreviation is a shortened form of a word, such as U.S. for United States. An acronym is a word formed from the initial letters of words in a phrase, such as CINAHL, which stands for Cumulative Index to Nursing and Allied Health Literature. An acronym is pronounced as a word. An initialism is a name formed from the initials of an organization, such as ANA for American Nurses Association (AMA, 2007). For the purposes of writing a manuscript, the author can think about these together, all representing a type of abbreviation in writing.

EXHIBIT 11.7

Checklist for Scientific Style

Abbreviations
- Expanded first time cited in text followed by initials in parentheses
- No abbreviations in title or abstract
- No author-invented abbreviations

Nomenclature
- Standard nomenclature used

Units of Measure
- The International System of Units (SI) used for measurements except for temperature, blood pressure, and time

Numbers and Percentages
- Figures used for numbers 10 and above
- Figures used for statistics, fractions, decimals, and percentages
- Words used for numbers below 10 except when grouped with numbers 10 and above in the same sentence
- Words used for common fractions
- Words used if sentence, title, or heading begins with number
- Percentage used when specific number not included

Statistics
- Statistical analysis and interpretations correct
- Data in text consistent with tables and figures
- Complete information reported with each statistic
- Accepted abbreviations and symbols used
- Statistics typed correctly

Most journals discourage abbreviations in manuscripts because abbreviations commonly used in one specialty in nursing may not be understood by readers with different clinical backgrounds and experiences. The exceptions are standard and approved abbreviations, such as those found in a style manual, and words that are repeated throughout a manuscript, for example, using CINAHL rather than Cumulative Index to Nursing and Allied Health Literature.

When abbreviations are used, the author writes out the words the first time the name or phrase to be abbreviated is cited in the manuscript, followed by the initials in parentheses. From that point on, the initials can be used alone. For instance:

> Length of stay (LOS) decreased from 4.0 to 2.5 days after implementation of the critical pathway. With improved medication management, LOS decreased by an additional 1.2 days.

Abbreviations, though, should not be used in the title or abstract (APA, 2010). The reader should understand words and phrases in the title and abstract without referring to the text. This is important, particularly in bibliographic databases that contain abstracts of articles; the abstract should be clear to individuals searching the database.

In the first draft, it is best to write out the words and avoid using abbreviations, then to add these during the revision. Otherwise, content might be reorganized, altering the first time the abbreviation is used in the manuscript. It also allows the author to keep a draft without abbreviations in case this information is needed later.

Nomenclature

For clinical papers, the author may need to refer to specific diseases, diagnostic tests, terminology, medications, and names for other entities. Nomenclature is the formulation of names to represent these entities. For example, the author might describe care of a patient with stage IV cancer, indicate that the patient had a grade 4 systolic murmur, report an Apgar score of 9 at 1 minute, and include the PO_2 value in a manuscript. Some symbols may be used without expanding them the first time cited in the paper, such as PO_2, while others should be written out the first time, such as positive end-expiratory pressure (PEEP). For medications, authors should use the nonproprietary (generic) name that is the official name of the drug (AMA, 2007). Authors are not expected to remember these rules and instead should write out the terms in the first draft, then in the revision refer to the style manual for how to correctly cite them in the paper.

Units of Measure

The International System of Units (SI) is considered the universal measurement standard, providing uniformity in expressing measurements (AMA, 2007). It is a refinement of the metric system. Non-SI units used in papers are measurements for temperature, blood pressure, and time. The requirements for metric style are well established, so authors should be careful to check the style manual to be consistent with it.

Numbers and Percentages

There are a number of style requirements when reporting numbers and percentages. A few are summarized here, but again the author is advised to check a style manual.

1. In general, use figures for numbers 10 and above, for example, 30 years old, 10 cm wide, 15% of the group, and 207 participants.
2. Use words for numbers less than 10; for example, subjects completed five instruments.
3. However, for numbers below 10 that are grouped with numbers 10 and above in the same sentence or paragraph, use figures. For example:

In 4 of the 27 patients, acute pain was reported.
The children ranged in age from 2 to 11 years.

4. Use figures for statistics, fractions, decimals, and percentages, for example, $P = .04$, 5½ days, 0.25, and less than 8%.
5. Use words for common fractions, for example, one fourth.
6. If a sentence, title, or heading begins with a number, use words to represent the number, for example, Twenty-four of the patients were discharged within 5 days of admission. Percent means by the hundred; the word *percent* and symbol % are used with a specific number (AMA, 2007). Percentage is used when a number is not included. For example:

Eighty percent of the nurses had high levels of job satisfaction.
Pain was reported by 25% of the patients.
Of the 120 patients, 62 (51.7%) had improved scores on the posttest.
Anxiety was reported by a small percentage of the nursing students.

Statistics

Reporting statistics in research papers was described in Chapter 6. In the revision of the paper, the author should check carefully that the statistical analysis is correct, the data in the text are consistent with the tables and figures, and complete information is included when reporting the statistics. What constitutes complete information depends on the statistic reported, and the author should consult a style manual or statistics book for direction.

In reporting statistics, accepted abbreviations and symbols must be used. Common ones are listed in Appendix A. Many statistical abbreviations, such as SD for standard deviation, are not expanded the first time cited in the text. Others, though, such as ANOVA, may be written out at the first mention in the text with the abbreviation in parentheses, depending on the style manual. The author should follow the guidelines specified in the style manual.

In checking the statistics, the author should do the following:

1. Review the original statistical analysis to confirm that the statistics reported in the manuscript and interpretations are correct.
2. Compare the data and statistics reported in the text with the tables and figures.
3. Refer to the style manual or statistics book to ensure that complete information is presented with each statistic reported, the appropriate abbreviations and symbols are used, and they are typed properly.
4. Use the statistical term, not the symbol, when referring to a statistic in the narrative. For example, instead of "The M score was 125," the text should read, "The mean score was 125."
5. Use an uppercase and italicized N for the number of subjects in the total sample, for example, $N = 206$. A lowercase n, also in italics, represents the number of subjects in a portion of the total sample, for example, "Group 1 included managers ($n = 32$) and staff ($n = 16$)."

SUMMARY

Before beginning the first draft, the author completes preparations to facilitate the writing process and eliminate unnecessary distractions. These preparations include reviewing the author guidelines for the journal to clarify the format and other requirements; gathering materials about the project, innovation, or practices described in the manuscript; assembling analyses of data and other information about the research project. The goal is to assemble all materials before writing the first draft.

After reviewing the purpose of the manuscript and intended audience, the author writes an outline, which is a general plan of the content to be included in the manuscript and its organization. Outlines may be formal, such as one developed using Roman numerals, or informal, such as topics listed in order.

Using the outline, the author writes the first draft. The important principle here is to get the ideas on paper. This is not the time to be concerned about grammar, spelling, punctuation, and writing style—these are revised later. The goal with the first draft is to present the content following the format of the outline and in a logical order.

Between the first draft and subsequent revisions, authors plan a period of retreat from writing. In anticipation of retreating, the author rereads the first draft, jots down any priorities for revision that come to mind, and schedules a firm time to begin the revision. Then, it is important to take a complete break from the manuscript, away from the desk, doing something physically active. If a first draft is circulated to colleagues or coauthors, the author should alert them to the stage of writing that has been achieved and what would be a helpful contribution from them. Any thoughts that occur to the author during the retreat period could be jotted on a notepad for later consideration.

The initial revisions of the draft focus on the content and how it is organized, not on grammar, punctuation, spelling, and writing style. There is no set number of revisions to make until satisfied with the content, although writing at least three drafts is likely.

If the author developed a working title, this can be reviewed first. In reviewing the abstract, the author examines if it adequately summarizes the purpose of the paper, indicating the most important content within the length allowed by the journal. For research manuscripts, the abstract should describe the study purpose and background, methods, findings, and conclusions.

In reviewing the main body of the paper, the author begins by reading the introductory section. The key is to assess if the introduction explains the content covered in the paper and its importance to readers. After critiquing the introduction, the author then is ready to review the rest of the text. The author should reread the draft to determine if content is missing, if content can be omitted, and if there is repetitive content; to assess the organization or structure of the paper; and to determine the accuracy of the content. Unnecessary references should be deleted at this stage, and each table and figure should be reviewed to determine if it is essential to the paper.

Headings and subheadings emphasize the content covered in each section of the manuscript. They indicate the organization of the manuscript, provide transition from one topic to the next, inform readers of the content that follows, and suggest the importance of each subject area. In the revision stage, the author has the opportunity to add headings and subheadings to the manuscript.

After the first draft is revised, the author continues revising the drafts until satisfied with the content and its organization. Usually, coauthors are asked to critique a second or subsequent draft of the manuscript rather than the first draft. The final version of the paper must be read and approved by each coauthor to meet the requirements for authorship.

Publication of the manuscript depends more on the substantive content than on writing style, but poorly written papers may influence the critique by peer reviewers and the editor and, ultimately, the acceptance decision. Therefore, the author must carefully edit the manuscript so that it is well written. The author can begin by editing paragraphs and then move to revising sentences, phrases, and words. This system enables the author to edit broad elements of the paper first, and then move to specifics. In the revision of the manuscript, the author verifies the proper use of abbreviations, nomenclature, units of measure, numbers and percentages, and statistics.

This chapter discusses some of the aspects of writing for the author to check when editing the writing structure and style. It also emphasizes the importance of authors being cautious about giving proper credit to their sources.

REFERENCES

American Medical Association. (2007). *AMA manual of style: A guide for authors and editors* (10th ed.). New York, NY: Oxford University Press.

American Psychological Association. (2010). *Publication manual of the American Psychological Association* (6th ed.). Washington, DC: Author.

Chichester, M., & Wool, J. (2017). Before journal submission, build your own peer review board. *Nursing for Women's Health*, 21(2), 137–141. doi:10.1016/j.nwh.2017.02.004

Craft, M. A., Davis, G. C., & Paulson, R. M. (2013). Expressive writing in early breast cancer survivors. *Journal of Advanced Nursing*, 69(2), 305–315. doi:10.1111/j.1365-2648.2012.06008.x

Daley, B. J., Morgan, S., & Black, S. B. (2016). Concept maps in nursing education: A historical literature review and research directions. *Journal of Nursing Education*, 55(11), 631–639. doi:10.3928/01484834-20161011-05

Duke Writing Studio. (2017). Reverse outlining. Retrieved from https://twp.duke.edu/sites/twp.duke.edu/files/file-attachments/reverse-outline.original%281%29.pdf

Farrington, N., Fader, M., Richardson, A., Prieto, J., & Bush, H. (2014). Indwelling urinary catheter use at the end of life: A retrospective audit. British Journal of Nursing 23(Sup9), S4–S10. doi:10.12968/bjon.2014.23.Sup9.S4

Gallaudet University. (2017). Mapping. Retrieved from http://www.gallaudet.edu/tutorial-and-instructional-programs/english-center/reading---english-as-second-language/reading-and-mapping-strategies/mapping

Halcomb, L. (2017). Break down the barriers to writing and simply start now. *Nurse Researcher*, 25(2), 5. doi:10.7748/nr.25.2.5.s1

Oermann, M. H., & Gaberson, K. B. (2017). *Evaluation and testing in nursing education* (5th ed.). New York, NY: Springer Publishing.

Oermann, M. H., & Leonardelli, A. (2013). Make the title count. *Nurse Author & Editor, 23*(3). Retrieved from http://www.nurseauthoreditor.com/article.asp?id=230

Oman, K. S., Mancuso, M. P., Ceballos, K., Makic, M. F., & Fink, R. M. (2016). Mentoring clinical nurses to write for publication: Strategies for success. *American Journal of Nursing, 116*(5), 48–55. doi:10.1097/01.NAJ.0000482966.46919.0

Price, B. (2015). Writing up research for publication. *Nursing Standard, 29,* 52–59.

Sarver, W., Cichra, N., & Kline, M. (2015). Perceived benefits, motivators, and barriers to advancing nurse education: Removing barriers to improve success. *Nursing Education Perspectives, 36,* 153–156. doi:10.5480/14-1407

The Joint Commission. (2017). *The Joint Commission Journal on Quality and Patient Safety.* Retrieved from http://www.jointcommissionjournal.com/content/aims

University of California Irvine. (2017). *Writing a scientific paper: TITLES.* Retrieved from https://guides.lib.uci.edu/c.php?g=334338&p=2249904

von Isenburg, M., Lee, L. S., & Oermann, M. H. (2017). Writing together to get AHEAD: An interprofessional boot camp to support scholarly writing in the health professions. *Journal of the Medical Library Association, 105*(2), 167–172. doi:10.5195/jmla.2017.222

Williams, J. M. (2009). *Style: The basics of clarity and grace* (3rd ed.). New York, NY: Pearson Longman.

REFERENCES

Most papers written for publication in nursing include references. The references in the manuscript document the literature reviewed by the author in preparation of the paper and provide support for the ideas in it. Chapter 4 discussed how to conduct and write a literature review for a manuscript. It described purposes of a literature review, bibliographic databases useful for literature reviews in nursing, selecting databases to use, search strategies, analyzing and synthesizing the literature, and writing the literature review. The outcome of Chapter 4 was to develop skill in conducting literature reviews for writing papers in nursing.

In this chapter, the focus is on citing the references in the manuscript and preparing the reference list. Journals have different reference formats, and the author needs to prepare the references according to the journal guidelines. Examples are provided of how to cite references in the text and on the reference list using the name-year format and citation-sequence format. The author will need to consult a style manual for more information about preparing different types of references using each of these formats. The examples provided in this chapter are based on the reference styles in use at the time this book was written; however, these reference styles are updated every few years, and authors should check the current edition of the style manual.

REFERENCE STYLES

Journals differ in the styles they use for citations and references. Two of the reference styles used widely in nursing and healthcare journals are the name-year format and citation-sequence format. The name-year format, such as found in this book, uses the author surname and year of publication. The American Psychological Association (APA) publication style uses this format: the citations in the text are the author(s)' last name(s) and publication year in parentheses, and the references on the list at the end of the paper are in alphabetical order. A study of author guidelines of nursing journals indicated that most journals ($n = 142$, 67.9%) use the APA style (Nicoll et al., 2018).

The other reference style is the citation-sequence format. With this format, the citations (in the text) are numbered sequentially, either in superscripts, brackets, or parentheses. The references on the list at the end are placed in numerical order. The American Medical Association (AMA) uses this format (AMA, 2007). This is the second most common reference style in nursing journals ($n = 55$, 26.3%) (Nicoll et al., 2018). The International Committee of Medical Journal Editors (ICMJE) recommends the National Library of Medicine style for references, which is used in MEDLINE/PubMed (ICMJE, 2017). This reference style is similar to the AMA. The National Library of Medicine, though, does not provide guidelines about how to cite documents in the text (U.S. National Library of Medicine, 2017). When submitting a manuscript to a journal, authors should follow whatever reference style is specified for preparing the manuscript.

Citations are how the work is documented in the text. The citation informs the readers that the statement or idea in the text was developed by the author(s) cited. In some reference styles, such as APA, the citations are documented by author surname and year of publication, allowing readers to find the complete reference on the alphabetized list at the end of the manuscript. Other formats, such as AMA, call for the citations to be noted by a number that corresponds to a publication on the reference list.

The reference list, at the end of the manuscript, provides the documentation of the publications reviewed by the author in preparation of the paper and the means for readers to retrieve those publications for their own work. A reference list cites the resources actually used in preparing the manuscript, whereas a bibliography includes other publications and information related to the content of the paper. The bibliography provides additional readings about the topic not cited in the manuscript. Most journals require reference lists, not bibliographies, although the author might prepare a bibliography for other types of writing projects.

References are placed at the end of the paper following the text and before the tables and figures. All references cited in the text must be on the reference list, and there can be no publications on the reference list that were not cited in the text. The author is responsible for verifying this.

Because one of the purposes of the references is to allow others to retrieve them, information about each publication must be complete and accurate. Although there are numerous variations of reference formats, references to journals contain

- Author(s) surname and initials
- Year of publication
- Title of article (and subtitle)
- Name of journal
- Volume number
- Issue number if journal is paginated by issue
- Inclusive page numbers

For many reference styles, such as APA, the issue number is not included if pages are numbered consecutively across issues; however, other styles, such as AMA, require the issue number for all references to journals (AMA, 2007).

References to books contain

- Author(s) surname and initials
- Year of copyright
- Book title (and subtitle)
- Volume number and title if more than one volume
- Edition number (other than first edition)
- Place of publication
- Name of publisher

When referring to a chapter in a book, the reference also includes the

- Chapter author(s) surname and initials
- Chapter title
- Inclusive page numbers of the chapter

There are specific formats for preparing references to articles in journals, books, book chapters, technical reports, proceedings of meetings and conferences, theses and doctoral dissertations, unpublished materials, online references, audiovisual media, and other sources of information. The author guidelines either provide examples of how to prepare each type of reference or indicate the reference style to be used for manuscript preparation. In addition, some journals may limit the number of references to include, which would be specified in the author guidelines.

Authors cannot assume that the reference style they used for writing papers in their nursing programs or with which they are familiar is the same one used by the journal for submission of the manuscript. If the manuscript is rejected and then sent to a different journal, the author is responsible for revising the citations and references to be consistent with that journal's style.

Name-Year Format: Citations

In the name-year format, citations in the text include the surname of the author(s) and year of publication in parentheses. The author's name and publication date are placed next to the statement being referenced:

Smith (2018) found a significant relationship between student stress in the clinical setting and performance.

A significant relationship was found between student stress in the clinical setting and performance (Smith, 2018).

Once the reference is cited in a paragraph, subsequent references in that same paragraph do not have to include the date of publication. For example:

Smith (2018) found a significant relationship between student stress in the clinical setting and performance. The higher the level of stress, the lower the performance ratings. Smith also found differences in student stress across clinical courses in the nursing program.

For publications by multiple authors, different principles are followed for citing author names in the text. When the publication has two authors, both names are included each time the reference is cited in the text:

Jones and Mayflower (2018) found a significant relationship between student stress in the clinical setting and performance.

A significant relationship was found between student stress in the clinical setting and performance (Jones & Mayflower, 2018).

When there are three to five authors, the names of all the authors are included the first time the reference occurs in the text, but for subsequent citations only the name of the first author is included followed by "et al." and the year published (APA, 2010). For example:

Doe, Jones, Kaelig, Brown, and Dowd (2018) reported that . . . [first citation in text]

Doe et al. (2018) reported that . . . [subsequent citations].

For references with six or more authors, only the surname of the first author is cited followed by "et al." (APA, 2010). In using "et al." (which means "and others"), only the surname of the first author is included, without a comma after the name and with a period after "al."

If the citation refers to a specific part of the original work, such as a quotation or statement on a particular page, then the page number also is included in the citation. An example follows.

Patients described their conditions as living with a "time bomb with no possible way out" (Brown, 2018, p. 24).

Name-Year Format: References

In the name-year format, the references are listed at the end of the manuscript in alphabetical order based on the surname of the first author. The year of publication, in parentheses, follows the last author name cited with the reference. When there is more than one reference by the same person(s), they are arranged by year of publication with the earliest listed first (APA, 2010). An example follows:

Basco, S., Gumbel, A. C., & Davies, R. (2017).

Brown, M. J. (2018).

Doe, L. H., Jones, J. Y., Kaelig, M. P., Brown, M. J., & Dowd, B. B. (2018).

Jones, T. B., & Mayflower, J. K. (2018).

Mathews, A. M. (2018).

Mathews, A. M., & Coleman, T. Z. (2015).

Smith, J. B. (2014).

Smith, J. B. (2018).

If there is more than one reference by an author, or by the same two or more authors in identical order, published in the same year, these would be arranged alphabetically by title (APA, 2010, p. 182). Lowercase letters are placed after the year of publication to differentiate the citations. For example:

Smith, J. B., & Thompson, M. (2016a). Behavioral . . .

Smith, J. B., & Thompson, M. (2016b). Stress . . .

The APA *Publication Manual* provides detailed information about preparing references using the name-year format. Some journals use a variation of this format by listing the references in alphabetical order and then numbering them. These numbers are used for the citations in the text rather than the name and year of publication. Exhibit 12.1 presents sample references prepared according to the two commonly used reference styles in nursing journals. As noted earlier, these reference examples are based on the style manuals currently in use at the time this book was written. Readers need to check if the reference styles have been updated since the publication of this book and use the current sources.

EXHIBIT 12.1

Different References Styles With Examples of References to Journal Article and Book

American Psychological Association (APA) Style

Read, C. Y., Shindul-Rothschild, J., Flanagan, J., & Stamp, K. D. (2018). Factors associated with removal of urinary catheters after surgery. *Journal of Nursing Care Quality, 33*, 29–37. doi:10.1097/ncq.0000000000000287

Oermann, M. H., & Gaberson, K. B. (2017). *Evaluation and testing in nursing education* (5th ed.). New York, NY: Springer Publishing.

American Medical Association (AMA) Style

Read CY, Shindul-Rothschild J, Flanagan J, Stamp KD. Factors associated with removal of urinary catheters after surgery. *J Nurs Care Qual.* 2018;33(1):29–37.

Oermann MH, Gaberson KB. *Evaluation and Testing in Nursing Education.* 5th ed. New York, NY: Springer Publishing; 2017.

Citation-Sequence Format: Citations

To improve uniformity across journals, the ICMJE developed the *Recommendations for the Conduct, Reporting, Editing, and Publication of Scholarly Work in Medical Journals*, which uses a citation-sequence style (ICMJE, 2017). These recommendations, which can be accessed from the ICMJE website at www.icmje.org/, provide valuable guidelines for authors not only in citing references but also on ethical principles in the conduct and reporting of research and other aspects of writing for publication. Sample references using this style can be found at the U.S. National Library of Medicine (U.S. NLM) website (www.nlm.nih.gov/bsd/uniform_requirements.html). The reference format in the *Recommendations* of the ICMJE has been adapted by the NLM (U.S. NLM, 2017). The *AMA Manual of Style* uses a citation-sequence format.

In the citation-sequence format, citations are numbered consecutively in the order in which they are first mentioned in the text. The same number is used each time the citation is included in the paper. In the *AMA Manual of Style*, the citations in the text, tables, figures, and legends are indicated using Arabic numerals in superscripts. The superscript numeral is placed outside periods and commas and inside colons and semicolons (AMA, 2007, p. 43). When more than two references are cited in a series, a hyphen is used to join the first and last number of the series. Two examples follow:

Recently, these guidelines have been implemented in the emergency department and outpatient clinic.[1-4]

The teacher can prepare different types of objective test items for the course[7]: true–false, multiple choice. . . .

One advantage of using the citation-sequence format is that the numbered citations do not interrupt the text and flow of ideas as sometimes occurs with the name-year format. A long list of references cited in a sentence may interfere with the ease of reading it and may affect remembering the preceding idea; at a minimum, it can be distracting.

Citation-Sequence Format: References

In the citation-sequence format, references at the end of the manuscript are numbered consecutively in the order in which they are first cited in the text (AMA, 2007; ICMJE, 2017). Journal titles (names) are abbreviated, and the year of publication follows the title, which differs from APA. Authors cannot shorten the titles themselves; the names of the journals need to be abbreviated according to the NLM style as used in MEDLINE/PubMed. The list of journal title abbreviations can be accessed through PubMed (www.ncbi.nlm.nih.gov/pubmed) by using the link "Journals in NCBI Databases" (right side of screen). That link brings the reader to the NLM catalog (www.ncbi.nlm.nih.gov/nlmcatalog/journals) with information about journals in the database including the abbreviated titles. The abbreviated journal title also is used with each citation in PubMed.

Authors should use reference management software for preparing their manuscripts. There are many types available, including some that are open source. This software saves information about the publication during a search, automatically renumbers citations as changes are made in the paper, and reformats the reference based on different styles. If the author is not using reference management software in preparing the draft, citations in the text should be indicated by the author's name and publication date rather than numbered. Otherwise, as revisions are made in the draft and references are reordered, these numbers will change. The citations can then be numbered in the final version of the paper.

The references for the following citation are prepared using the *AMA Manual of Style*. Because there are many variations to the citation-sequence format, the author needs to follow the journal guidelines.

Recommendations for integrating patient and worker safety initiatives include building worker safety as a core value of the organization, identifying opportunities to link patient and worker safety activities across departments and programs, understanding and measuring performance on safety-related issues, and maintaining successful patient and worker safety improvement initiatives.[1,2]

References

1. Riehle A, Braun BI, Hafiz H. Improving patient and worker safety: exploring opportunities for synergy. *J Nurs Care Qual*. 2013;28(2):99–102.
2. The Joint Commission. *Improving Patient and Worker Safety: Opportunities for Synergy, Collaboration and Innovation*. Oakbrook Terrace, IL: The Joint Commission; 2012. http://www.jointcommission.org/assets/1/18/TJCImprovingPatientAndWorkerSafety-Monograph.pdf. Accessed June 26, 2013.

ELECTRONIC REFERENCE FORMATS

The proliferation of electronic information resources continues, and authors need to follow the style manual for citing these references. Internet resources are prone to being moved and deleted, resulting in URLs in the reference lists that can no longer be accessed (APA, 2010). In a study of 2,822 articles in medical journals, the number of citations to websites increased since January 2006, but accessibility to the URLs decreased with time (Habibzadeh, 2013). Authors should be cautious about using websites as primary sources of information for manuscripts except for documents from reputable sources.

Because of these problems with electronic information sources, publishers assign a digital object identifier (DOI) to journal articles and other bibliographic materials. A DOI is used to permanently identify an object or entity and provide a link to it on the Internet (doi, 2017). While URLs may change, the DOI is a persistent link to the digital content. More information about the DOI system can be found at www.doi.org/index.html. The DOI system is implemented through agencies such as Crossref, which provides citation linking services for publishers (Crossref, 2018).

The sixth edition of the APA *Publication Manual* includes the DOI with references to journal articles if one was assigned. For example:

Read, C. Y., Shindul-Rothschild, J., Flanagan, J., & Stamp, K. D. (2018). Factors associated with removal of urinary catheters after surgery. *Journal of Nursing Care Quality, 33*, 29–37. doi:10.1097/ncq.0000000000000287

The DOI is generally located on the first page of the article, including papers published ahead of print and in the published version. The DOI is also listed on the article's database page in MEDLINE/PubMed, CINAHL, and other bibliographic databases.

In general, citations for web documents and other electronic resources follow a format similar to that for print, with additional information about the location of the site (URL). For example, the citation for a document found at the Agency for Healthcare Research and Quality website using APA style is:

Agency for Healthcare Research and Quality. (2017). *Patient safety organization programs*. Retrieved from https://www.ahrq.gov/cpi/about/otherwebsites/pso.ahrq.gov/index.html

In citing an entire website, rather than a specific document on it, it is usually sufficient to give the address of the site in the text without including a reference. For example, "The American Heart Association provides valuable information on how to maintain a healthy life style, cardiac diseases, and early warning signs of heart attack and stroke. This information can be found at http://www.heart.org." In this situation, the resource would not need to be included on the reference list.

The author should be aware of the type of information required for electronic references to ensure that information is recorded when the materials are accessed. In a search, the author can copy the URL and other information from the web page that will be needed for the reference or can print the page. Because of the rapid changes on the web, the author is cautioned to check the reference prior to submitting the paper to the journal and again when reviewing the page proofs to validate the URL and other information. To ensure that electronic resources, of which there are many types, are cited correctly, authors should follow the style manual used by the journal or the author guidelines.

REFERENCE MANAGEMENT SOFTWARE

Reference management software, such as EndNote, RefWorks, and Zotero (which is a free, open-source tool), among others, allows authors to search online bibliographic databases, store records, organize references in a database, and create reference lists automatically. It also enables the author to format manuscripts complete with citations and references for hundreds of reference styles. If the author decides later to submit the manuscript to another publication, which uses a different reference style, the software automatically reformats the citations and references. This avoids retyping them. If using this software, the author needs to select the style that is required by the journal, making preparation of the citations and references easier.

VERIFYING REFERENCES

Being careful to prepare accurate references cannot be overemphasized. Errors that can occur with reference lists are (a) mistakes in the information provided in the reference, (b) errors in matching the citation with the correct reference, (c) not including all of the information needed with the reference, and (d) incorrect reference style. Authors can avoid many of these problems by using reference management software. However, even with this software, errors can occur, and it is the author's responsibility to ensure the references are complete and accurate, and in the correct format (Chinn, 2016; Kratochvil, 2017; Nicoll et al., 2018).

The author should verify the accuracy of each reference against the original document, paying particular attention to the spelling of authors' names, initials, order of names, title of the document and publication it is in, and publication data. Book titles should be taken from the title page rather than the cover.

In reviewing the paper, the author should check that each citation is placed properly in the text and that the name or number corresponds to the correct reference at the end of the manuscript. In the name-year format, the spelling of authors' names and the year of publication cited in the text should be identical to the reference list, and references should be alphabetized correctly. In the citation-sequence format, the author should check that the citation number in the text matches the correct reference on the list at the end of the paper. Once

EXHIBIT 12.2

Checklist for Verifying References

VERIFY THE FOLLOWING BEFORE SUBMITTING A MANUSCRIPT

Spelling of authors' names and year of publication in text with spelling and year in reference list
Number of citation in text with correct reference on reference list
Spelling of authors' names and accuracy of initials on reference list
Order of authors' names listed in reference and if all names included
Date of publication
Accuracy of title of document (e.g., title of article, chapter, report)
Accuracy of title of publication in which document appears (e.g., journal title, book title)
Abbreviation of journal title if relevant (using MEDLINE/PubMed Journals Database)
Accuracy of volume number, issue number (if included with reference style), page numbers
Capitalization
Order of references

the information is verified, then the author can check that all of the data are included in the reference, depending on the style, and that the reference format is correct. Exhibit 12.2 provides a checklist for verifying the references.

SUMMARY

Journals differ in the styles they use for citations and references. Citations are how the work is documented in the text. The citation informs the readers that the statement or idea in the text was developed by the author(s) cited. A reference list includes the resources actually used in preparing the manuscript, whereas a bibliography provides additional readings about the topic not cited in the manuscript. Most journals require reference lists, not bibliographies.

Two of the reference styles used widely in nursing and healthcare journals are the name-year format and citation-sequence format. In the name-year format, citations in the text include the author name and year of publication in parentheses. References are listed at the end of the manuscript in alphabetical order based on the surname of the first author.

In the citation-sequence format, citations in the text are placed in Arabic numerals (in superscript for AMA style) and numbered consecutively. References are listed and numbered at the end of the manuscript in the order they are first cited in the text. There are many adaptations of these formats by journals; authors need to follow carefully the journal guidelines or style manual adopted by the publication.

Authors make errors in their references that can be avoided by verifying the reference with the original document and matching the citations in the text with the reference list. Reference management software prevents many of these errors. With this software, authors can select the reference style required by the journal; the citations and references are then prepared according to this style. However, even with this software, errors can occur, and it is up to the author to check the references to ensure they are accurate and in the correct format.

REFERENCES

American Medical Association. (2007). *AMA manual of style: A guide for authors and editors* (10th ed.). New York, NY: Oxford Press.

American Psychological Association. (2010). *Publication manual of the American Psychological Association* (6th ed.). Washington, DC: Author.

Chinn, P. L. (2016). Paperpile and Google Docs. *Nurse Author & Editor*, 26(4), 4. Retrieved from http://naepub.com/wp-content/uploads/2016/11/NAE-2016-26-4-4-Chinn.pdf

Crossref. (2018). Crossref DOI display. https://www.crossref.org/display-guidelines/

doi®. (2017). Factsheet: Key facts on Digital Object Identifier system. Retrieved from https://www.doi.org/factsheets/DOIKeyFacts.html

Habibzadeh, P. (2013). Decay of references to Web sites in articles published in general medical journals: Mainstream vs small journals. *Applied Clinical Informatics*, 4, 455–464. doi:10.4338/aci-2013-07-ra-0055

International Committee of Medical Journal Editors. (2017). Recommendations for the conduct, reporting, editing, and publication of scholarly work in medical journals. Retrieved from http://www.icmje.org/recommendations

Kratochvil, J. (2017). Comparison of the accuracy of bibliographical references generated for medical citation styles by EndNote, Mendeley, RefWorks and Zotero. *Journal of Academic Librarianship, 43*(1), 57Y66. doi:10.1016/j.acalib.2016.09.001

Nicoll, L. H., Oermann, M. H., Chinn, P. L., Conklin, J. L., Amarasekara, S., & McCarty, M. (2018). Guidance provided to authors on citing and formatting references in nursing journals. *Journal for Nurses in Professional Development, 34,* 54–59. doi: 10.1097/NND.0000000000000430

U.S. National Library of Medicine. (2017). *Samples of formatted references for authors of journal articles.* Retrieved from https://www.nlm.nih.gov/bsd/uniform_requirements.html

TABLES AND FIGURES

Tables are essential when the author needs to report detailed information and numeric values. It is often clearer and more efficient to develop a table than to present the information in the text. Figures, such as graphs and charts, are valuable for demonstrating trends and patterns. For some manuscripts the author may even include an illustration of a new procedure or equipment, or a photograph. Not every manuscript, though, needs tables and figures; whether to include them is a decision made during the drafting phase of writing the paper. This chapter provides guidelines for deciding when to prepare tables and figures and how to develop them.

NUMBER OF TABLES AND FIGURES

In writing the draft, the author needs to know the maximum number of tables and figures allowed. With this information the author can avoid developing too many tables and figures for the length of the manuscript and specifications of the journal. It is helpful to prepare a draft of each table and figure as the manuscript is being written to confirm that the essential data are presented. The author can format these at a later point when the manuscript is revised.

Many journals limit the number of tables and figures to about three, because of the space they require in the publication. This information should be included in the author guidelines of the journal. If the number is not specified, the author can review current issues of the journal for the typical number of tables and figures per article.

Tables and figures taken from journals and other copyrighted materials cannot be reproduced in a manuscript without written permission from the copyright holder, for example, the publisher of the journal or book where the original document was found. Permission to reuse published material can be obtained from the Copyright Clearance Center (www.copyright.com). For journal articles, a link to the Copyright Clearance Center via RightsLink is often provided at the journal website. To learn how this process works, as an example, the reader can go to the *Nurse Educator* website (journals.lww .com/nurseeducatoronline/pages/default.aspx), select an article, and on the next screen with the article title and abstract, click the link "Get Content & Permissions" on the right side of the web page. This link goes to the Copyright Clearance Center to request permission to reuse content from the article in another publication. In addition to obtaining this permission, authors need to add a credit line at the bottom of the table or figure that indicates the original developer and copyright holder and that the material was "reprinted with permission." Authors need to consider if it is worth the space in the manuscript to reproduce tables and figures that readers can find elsewhere; instead, authors can refer readers to the original publication.

TABLES

Tables are an effective way of presenting detailed and complex information succinctly and clearly. Tables should be used when the author wants to report exact values, present a large amount of information, display different quantitative values simultaneously, and show relationships among data. For research articles, tables are valuable for presenting the findings of the study with statistical results. In a table, the author can compare groups and show how differences across the groups were analyzed with accompanying results.

The purpose of tables is to present detailed information that supplements the text and supports statements made in it without duplicating it. The text and table should not contain the same data (Cook, 2016). In the text, the author can discuss main findings from the table and highlight key points for readers to look for in the table. As an example, using the data from Exhibit 13.1, a statement in the text might be as follows:

> Of the 150 registered nurses, the majority (122, 81.3%) were in classifications II and III (Table 1).

Additional information about the number of nurses in each classification is available in the table, which avoids duplicating the text.

While tables support the text, they should be clear enough to "stand alone." Sufficient information should be included in the table for readers to understand it without referring to the explanation in the text. The author should reread each table when the draft of the manuscript is completed to ensure that the tabled material is integrated into the text yet is clear enough to be understood without reference to the text.

The data in tables should be accurate and consistent with the information reported in the text. To check this, the author can place each table next to the page(s) in the text where it is referenced and compare them for accuracy and consistency.

Types of Tables

There are two types of tables authors can include in a manuscript: a traditional table and tabulation. Boxes or textual tables can be developed for nontabular material to supplement the text. These are discussed later in the chapter.

Table

A table contains information arranged in columns and rows. It is used to present quantitative data, statistical results, and detailed information. Most of the examples in this chapter are tables. Each table has a title, headings to explain the columns and rows, and lines that visually organize the data for the reader. Examples are provided in Exhibits 13.1 and 13.2.

EXHIBIT 13.1

Presenting Information in Table and as Text: Text Preferred

As table:

Table 1 *Classifications of Registered Nurses*

Classification	n (%)
I	28 (18.7)
II	56 (37.3)
III	66 (44.0)

As text:

Of the 150 registered nurses, 28 (18.7%) were in classification I, 56 (37.3%) were in classification II, and the remaining nurses ($n = 66$, 44.0%) were in classification III.

EXHIBIT 13.2

Presenting Information in Table and as Text: Table Preferred

As table:

Table 1 *Differences in Importance Ratings Between Men and Women*

Importance Ratings	Men M (SD)	Women M (SD)	t
Able to ask nurse questions	4.13 (.83)	4.12 (.85)	0.07
Having nurse teach me about illness and treatments	4.58 (.81)	4.51 (.89)	0.61
Having nurse teach me self-care after discharge	4.56 (.89)	3.91 (.98)	2.51*

*$p = .006$.

As text:

There was no difference in the importance of being able to call a registered nurse (RN) with questions after the visit to the nurse-managed clinic between

(continued)

EXHIBIT 13.2

Presenting Information in Table and as Text: Table Preferred (continued)

men (M = 4.13, SD = .83) and women (M = 4.12, SD = .85), $t(120)$ = 0.07, P = .47. Teaching by the RN about the illness and treatments also was equally important to men (M = 4.58, SD = .81) and women (M = 4.51, SD = .89), $t(120)$ = 0.61, P = .27. However, having an RN teach patients about self-care at home was significantly more important to men (M = 4.56, SD = .89) than to women (M = 3.91, SD = .98), $t(120)$ = 2.51, P = .006.

Tabulation

A tabulation is a short, informal table in the text that sets the content off from the text (American Medical Association [AMA], 2007). Tabulations usually contain only one or two columns that are not placed within a formal table structure and instead are developed as part of the text (Exhibit 13.3).

Use of Tables

In planning the manuscript, the author determines what information should be reported and then decides if this information is best communicated in a table or in the text. There are two general principles for using tables in a manuscript.

EXHIBIT 13.3

In-Text Tabulation

Nursing faculty reported the use of multiple strategies for assessing student performance in the clinical setting. As expected, the predominant method in all schools of nursing was observing students as they care for patients. The strategies used by educators in baccalaureate nursing programs were:

Observation of performance by faculty	114 (93%)
Written assignments	100 (82%)
Skills testing	79 (65%)
Contributions to clinical conferences	90 (74%)
Self-assessment	70 (57%)
Simulations	56 (46%)

In associate degree programs, some differences were found in assessment methods in clinical courses. In those programs, faculty ... [text continues]

First, tables should not be used when the information can be reported in the text. Sometimes authors develop tables with information that could be presented easily in the text. When that is the case, tables should not be used. Readers may have difficulty following the data presented in a large number of tables and may lose track of the message (American Psychological Association [APA], 2010). Too many tables "break up" the text, and tables and figures are expensive to produce in a publication. For these reasons, tables should be used judiciously by authors.

An example of this principle can be seen in Exhibit 13.1. The information in the exhibit is presented in the form of a table and as text. As can be seen in this example, the information can be conveyed easily and concisely in the text; for this reason, a table should not be developed.

Second, tables should be used when the author needs to report a large amount of data and exact numbers. Tables are an efficient way of presenting detailed information in a small amount of space and facilitating the comparison of information. In Exhibit 13.2, data are presented in two ways, as a table and in the text. In contrast to the previous example, these data are best reported in the form of a table. They are too detailed for readers to follow in the text, limiting the ability to draw comparisons between the groups. Another example is Table 13.1. The correlations reported in this table are too extensive to include in the text, and the table provides a means for presenting all of the correlations, significant and not significant, in one place.

TABLE 13.1 SAMPLE TABLE

Table 1
Correlations of Patient Satisfaction Scores With Health Status

SF-36	Medical Care	Patient Teaching	Provider Competence	Type of Provider	Nurse–Patient Provider Interaction	Convenience of Appointments
Physical Functioning	.10	.42**	.23*	.11	−.24*	−.48**
Role Limitations (Physical)	−.22*	−.36**	−.04	.10	−.23*	−.24*
Pain	.08	−.09	−.03	.04	−.03	−.32**
Vitality	.12	−.06	−.04	.11	−.12	−.18*
Social Functioning	.09	−.06	−.03	−.02	−.14*	−.12
Role Limitations (Emotional)	.06	−.26*	.01	.04	.02	−.32**
Mental Health	.12	−.18*	.02	.01	−.26*	−.09
General Health	.25	−.47**	.23	.34**	−.12	−.46**

$^*p < .05; ^{**}p < .01.$

Guidelines for Constructing Tables

The content in tables should be arranged logically and presented clearly so that readers can understand it and locate specific data easily. In drafting the manuscript, the author plans what information will be reported in the text and in tables. The next decision is how best to organize the information so it is clear to readers. The content is usually organized into columns (vertical) and rows (horizontal). Most tables are read first from left to right (horizontally), then from top to bottom (vertically; AMA, 2007, p. 84). In deciding how to place data in a table, the author should keep this in mind: The key information should be placed horizontally on the table. For example, if the table is intended to compare groups or make before-and-after comparisons, it should be constructed for readers to review the data horizontally across the table. In Exhibit 13.2, readers can compare scores for men and women on each of the three importance items by reading the scores horizontally across the table.

Tables contain five major parts: title, column headings, row headings, body of the table, and notes (Figure 13.1). This chapter provides general guidelines on how to construct tables, and the author is directed to a style manual such as the APA *Publication Manual* (APA, 2010) and *AMA Manual of Style* (AMA, 2007) for more details.

Title

Every table needs a title. The title should be short, descriptive of the content in the table, and written as a phrase rather than as a sentence. The word "table"

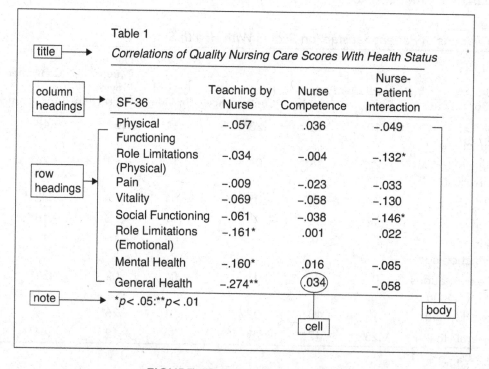

FIGURE 13.1 Parts of a table.

and its number are part of the title. In some style manuals such as the *AMA Manual of Style*, the entire title is placed on one line (Example 1), whereas in other styles such as the APA *Publication Manual*, two lines are used and the title is italicized (Example 2):

Example 1: Table 1. Classifications of Registered Nurses
Example 2: Table 1
     Classifications of Registered Nurses

The first letter of each major word should be capitalized but not articles, short prepositions, nor conjunctions such as "and" and "but." With APA (2010), all words of four letters or more are capitalized (p. 101).

Column Headings

A table provides a means of organizing information and presenting it logically, and the headings inform the reader of how the information is organized. The main categories of information should be in a separate column (AMA, 2007). Each column should have a brief heading that identifies the type of information reported in it. This includes the left-hand column of the table, referred to as the *stub column*. For research papers, this column usually contains the independent variables. When numerical data are reported in a column, the heading should include the unit of measure, which should be consistent for all of the information in that column. Only one category of information should be reported in a column.

If groups of columns relate to one another, they can be labeled with a heading, and a line can be placed over the column headings included under it. For example:

	Education				
Measure	ADN	BSN	MSN	DNP	PhD

Row Headings

The left-most column of a table contains the row headings that describe the content included in the rows of the table. Similar to column headings, these should be brief statements that adequately label the row and all of the items in that row. If groups of rows are related, a heading can be included and subheadings used to clarify this in the table. This can be seen in Table 13.2 in which race/ethnicity, highest education, and marital status are used as headings to group the information reported in the rows that follow.

Body of Table

The body of the table is also referred to as the *field* (AMA, 2007). The body is the content of the table—its numerical values or words and phrases—organized

TABLE 13.2 SAMPLE TABLE WITH SUBHEADINGS TO GROUP INFORMATION IN ROWS

Table 1

Background of Patients Receiving Home Care

Variable	n (%)
Race/ethnicity	
Caucasian	67 (56.8)
African American	46 (39.0)
Hispanic	3 (2.5)
Asian	2 (1.6)
Highest education	
<12th grade	40 (34.8)
High school graduate	64 (55.6)
College graduate	11 (9.6)
Marital status	
Married	72 (61.0)
Divorced/separated	19 (16.1)
Widowed	9 (7.6)
Single	18 (15.3)

in columns (vertical) and rows (horizontal). The intersection of a column and row, a *cell*, is where the specific numbers and text are placed. If the cell is empty because the information is not applicable, the cell can be left blank. If the cell is empty because data are missing, however, the author should insert a dash and include a note if further explanation is necessary.

Numerical values are usually placed in the columns; this facilitates totaling the scores and percentages. The author should verify that totals and percentages reflect the numbers and percents given in the table. When a discrepancy exists, such as the percents not equaling 100 because of rounding, an explanation can be included in a note with the table if needed. Column data should align vertically, for example, by decimal points, so the numbers are not misinterpreted. This can be seen in the sample tables in this chapter.

Information in the rows of a table should be aligned horizontally to facilitate reading from left to right across the table. If the lines of text do not fit in the space allotted and run over into the next line, the numbers or words in the cells are placed on the first or top line. For example, in Table 13.1, because the text "Physical Functioning" and "Role Limitations (Physical)" runs over into the next line, the numeric values within the table cells are positioned on the first or top line.

When reporting the results of statistical analyses, the author should check in the reference style manual or statistics book the information that should be contained in the table. There are accepted conventions to follow when reporting statistics in a manuscript; for example, for a *t*-test, authors should include the *t* value, the degrees of freedom, the value, and an effect size estimate such as Cohen's d (Stephens, 2015). Statistical abbreviations, such as M (mean) and standard deviation (SD), may be used in tables without an explanation in a note. Some statistics are reported with upper-case letters and others with lower-case letters, and some are in italics (Stephens, 2015). A list of statistical abbreviations is provided in Appendix A. Other examples of how to report statistics are often included in the reference style manual.

In the text and tables, the exact probability values should be reported to two or three decimal places rather than using $P < .05$ or $P < .01$ (AMA, 2007, p. 96; APA, 2010, p. 139). These values should be reported to two digits to the right of the decimal point; if those digits are zeros, then the three digits should be used, for example, $P = .003$. When the P values are less than .001, then $P < .001$ should be used in both the text and table (AMA, 2007; APA, 2010).

Notes

Notes placed at the bottom of the table provide additional details about the table in general or a specific column, row, or cell. They also are used to explain abbreviations in the table and define the symbols; for example, asterisks to indicate the P values. Notes make the table understandable for readers.

Style manuals differ in how notes are designated. The APA *Publication Manual* (2010) refers to a note that pertains to the entire table as a "general note." These are labeled as *Note* (in italics and followed by a period) and are placed at the bottom of the table. For example:

Note: S = student; RN = registered nurse.

Notes for columns, rows, and the specific entries in the cells are designated by superscript lowercase letters (a, b, c) placed after the item and then explained at the bottom of the table. These superscripts are ordered from left to right and top to bottom, beginning at the top left point in the table (APA, 2010, p. 138). An example is

[a]n = 125. [b]n = 129. [c]Control variables were age, gender, and smoking history.

The third type of note, a probability note, explains the symbols used in the table to represent the P values. The exact probability values should be reported unless it makes the table difficult to prepare and read, such as with a correlation matrix. In those instances, P values are designated by asterisks, such as *$P < .05$ and **$P < .01$, or by superscript lowercase letters. Sample notes are seen in Table 13.3.

AMA style designates footnotes (rather than notes) for both tables and figures with superscript lowercase letters (AMA, 2007). The style indicated in the author guidelines dictates how tables and their component parts are prepared in a manuscript.

TABLE 13.3 TABLE WITH NOTES

Table 1

Differences in Role Stress Based on Highest Degree of New Graduate

Role Stress scores[d]	ADN[a]		BSN[b]		Master's[c]			
	M	SD	M	SD	M	SD	F	p
Overload	2.89	.69	3.36	.72	3.93	.70	5.96	.004
Conflict with physicians	2.88	.96	3.36	.89	3.54	.78	3.28	.04
Lack of support from manager	2.65	.71	3.23	.78	3.34	.83	3.86	.05
Personal impact	2.57	.48	2.93	.61	3.14	.43	3.69	.02

Note: New graduates completed tool within first 6 months of practice.
[a]$n = 46$; [b]$n = 52$; [c]$n = 6$. [d]New Graduates' Role Stress Assessment.

Relationship of Table and Text

Every table must be referred to in the text, and the author should inform readers what to look for in the table. Tables are numbered consecutively, using Arabic numerals, in the order they are first mentioned in the text. This number is then used in the text to refer the reader to the table. Two examples follow:

As seen in Table 1, there were differences in the importance of teaching by the nurse to men and women.
Men and women differed in the importance they placed on teaching by the nurse (Table 1).

When the article is published, tables are placed close to where they are first referenced as determined by the publisher. As such, in the manuscript authors should not write "the table on page 7" because it may not be in that position or place when published.

Formatting Tables

Tables are double-spaced throughout, including the title and headings. Because journals differ in how they format tables, the author should follow the style manual or use a standard format such as found in this book. Generally, horizontal lines (rules) are placed between the table title and column headings, which are used to separate the column headings from the body of the table, and placed at the bottom of the table to separate it from the notes. Lines also are used to group similar columns together, as shown earlier in the chapter. If any additional formatting is needed for a particular journal, this will be done by the publisher.

Authors can construct tables using the "Table" feature of Microsoft Word. Tables developed with this feature, however, are enclosed in boxes and include additional lines between rows and columns. Authors will need to modify this to meet the style requirements, as discussed earlier. In some situations, authors may attempt to use scans of tables that were developed using other formats, but generally these will not be clear enough for publication. Smaller type should not be used because the submitted table (and figure) will be reduced in size when published, making smaller type difficult to read. The author guidelines of the journal will specify requirements for producing tables and figures, and authors should adhere to them. If unfamiliar with developing tables, the author should practice how to develop them before beginning to type the manuscript to avoid being distracted during the writing phase.

Each table is placed on a separate page. When tables extend beyond one page, they are continued on the next page and labeled with the table number and title, followed by the word "continued" (AMA, 2007). For wide tables, the author might orient them horizontally (landscape) rather than vertically (portrait), consider preparing two tables, or shift the columns with their headings to the rows, and the rows and headings to the columns if appropriate. Exhibit 13.4 provides a checklist for authors to ensure their tables reflect principles for their development.

EXHIBIT 13.4

Checklist for Reviewing Tables

- Is the table essential to the paper, or can the information be conveyed in the text?
- Does the table stand alone—is the information in the table sufficient for readers to understand it without referring to the explanation in the text?
- Does the title communicate the content in the table and is it short?
- Does every column and row have a heading, and do the headings reflect the information in them?
- Is the content in the table arranged logically and presented clearly for readers to understand it?
- Is the table designed for readers to easily locate specific data?
- Are the data in the table accurate and consistent with the information reported in the text?
- If the table has totals and percentages, are they correct based on the numbers given in the table?
- Are abbreviations and symbols in the table explained in the notes?
- Are the notes listed in this order: general, specific, then probability (APA, 2010)?
- Are the lines in the table done correctly, for example, horizontal lines between the title and column headings, to separate the column headings from the body of the table, and at the bottom?
- Are p values identified correctly?

(continued)

EXHIBIT 13.2

Checklist for Reviewing Tables (*continued*)

- Are exact probability values reported and asterisks used only when needed?
- If part or all of a copyrighted table is reproduced, is there a note in the caption giving credit to the copyright owner?
- Was written permission obtained to reproduce the table in the manuscript, and was a copy of the permission submitted to the journal with the manuscript?
- Is each table numbered (consecutively) and referenced in the text?
- If there are multiple tables in the paper, are they consistent in format, font type and size, and other aspects of the presentation?

Nontabular Material

Word or textual tables can be used to highlight key points, summarize information, and provide additional details to support the text. These are used to set the material off from the text, emphasizing it to readers. Word tables display words, phrases, and sentences, usually in lists. Similar to tables that present numerical data, word tables convey information that helps readers understand the content but is too detailed to be included in the text. For example, a word table may be developed for a paper on care of the burn patient that lists potential patient problems, data to collect in an assessment with related laboratory tests, and interventions for each problem. Boxes, sidebars, and similar types of exhibits (that have one column only) may be used in place of a word table. Word tables, similar to ones that report quantitative data, should not be developed if the information can be presented clearly and concisely in the text. Table 13.4 is an example of a word table that could be included in a publication.

FIGURES

Figures include graphs, charts, diagrams, photographs, and other illustrations. They can be used to illustrate the findings of a study; display trends in the data; make comparisons; and show equipment, procedures, and other objects described in the text. For research papers, figures have the advantage of

TABLE 13.4 SAMPLE WORD TABLE

Table 1
Phases of Nursing Process

Phase	Definition
Assessment	Recognizing problems and collecting data
Diagnosis	Analyzing data and identifying nursing diagnoses
Plan	Setting priorities, developing goals, selecting interventions
Implementation	Carrying out nursing interventions
Evaluation	Evaluating outcomes of care

allowing readers to visualize trends and patterns in the data more easily than when written in the narrative.

Figures should be used only when essential to facilitate understanding of the content in the paper. They should add value to the paper, displaying the results and other information more clearly than can be done by the text alone. Figures are useful for illustrating trends in data over time and showing the relationships between variables. However, if those same outcomes can be described adequately in the text, figures should not be developed. Journal editors are allotted a certain number of pages for each issue of the journal, and tables and figures take space to produce.

Types of Figures

There are various types of figures that can be prepared by the author:

- *Graphs*: Graphs show the relationship of two variables, for example, hospital length of stay to number of days on a ventilator. Graphs displaying quantitative data are valuable to indicate changes and patterns in the data. These include line graphs, survival plots, scatterplots, histograms and frequency polygons, bar graphs, pie charts, and dot or point graphs (AMA, 2007).
- *Diagrams*: Diagrams depict the sequence of a process, such as a flowchart to show the steps in a process or how subjects moved through a study. A flow diagram to report the progress of participants through a randomized controlled trial, from the Consolidated Standards of Reporting Trials (CONSORT) Statement, is included in Figure 13.2. Authors can download a template of this diagram from the CONSORT website to use in their own manuscripts (CONSORT, 2017). Diagrams also include charts such as organizational charts and algorithms.
- *Maps*: Maps show relationships and trends that involve locations and distance (AMA, 2007). For instance, they may be used to display the prevalence of health problems in particular communities.
- *Photographs*: Photographic images of patients and objects are usually submitted as separate digital files, and need to have the appropriate level of resolution (APA, 2010). Photographs of patients require the patients' written informed consent. Identifying information about the patient should not be published with the photograph unless the information is essential, and the patient gives written informed consent for publishing it (International Committee of Medical Journal Editors [ICMJE], 2017). The ICMJE also states that patient consent should be written and archived with the journal, the author, or both, depending on local standards. The author is advised to consult with the journal office and his or her own legal department when considering using photographs of patients in a manuscript. When copied from another source, in addition to obtaining permission for use of the photograph, the author should request an original version; copies of photographs and other illustrations or figures are often blurry.

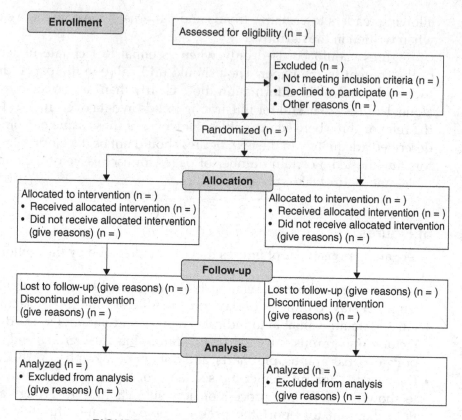

FIGURE 13.2 CONSORT 2010 flow diagram.

CONSORT, Consolidated Standards of Reporting Trials.

Source: From CONSORT. (2017). The CONSORT 2010 flow diagram. Retrieved from http://www.consort-statement.org/consort-statement/flow-diagram. The CONSORT Statement is distributed under the terms of the Creative Commons Attribution CC BY 2.0, which permits use, distribution, and reproduction in any medium, provided the original work is properly cited.

Guidelines for Developing Figures

How to develop each of the figures described earlier is beyond the scope of this book, and the author can obtain this information in a style manual. A few general guidelines, though, follow.

- Use letters, symbols, numbers, lines, and other objects that are large enough to allow figures to be read once reduced in size to fit the journal page. Figures are usually smaller when published, and this should be taken into consideration when they are constructed. The final printed figures must be easy to read and clear.
- Use standard symbols, such as open and closed circles, triangles, and squares, that are defined in the legend or caption of the figure.
- If shadings are used, they should be sufficiently different and limited to two or three types in one bar graph. The ideal option is to use no shading and black bars (APA, 2010, p. 161).
- Label each axis as to what it is measuring and the units in which it is measured.

- Number figures consecutively, for example, Figure 1, Figure 2, and so forth, and include a title immediately following the number. This is not part of the figure.
- Prepare a legend or caption for each figure that is placed below the figure. The legend provides information for understanding the figure and all the symbols in it without referring to the text. This is illustrated in Figure 13.3.
- Submit the originals of all figures with the manuscript. Most figures will be reproduced as submitted, and for this reason it is important to be careful that the original is without flaws.
- Follow the author guidelines or style manual as to how to prepare the figures. Figures developed for presentations with PowerPoint, for example, are likely to need revision because the type will be too large for use in a manuscript. APA (2010) style indicates that lettering should be no larger than 14 points.

Exhibit 13.5 provides a checklist for authors to ensure that their figures reflect principles for their development.

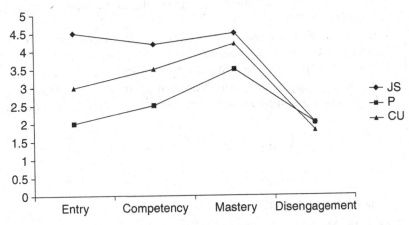

Figure 1. Scores are for new graduates' job satisfaction (JS), productivity (P), and commitment to the unit (CU) by stages.

FIGURE 13.3 Sample figure.

EXHIBIT 13.5

Checklist for Reviewing Figures

- Is the figure essential to the paper, or can the information be conveyed in the text?
- Does the figure stand alone—is the information in the figure sufficient for readers to understand it without referring to the explanation in the text?
- Does the title communicate the content in the figure and is it short?
- Is the information shown in the figure accurate and consistent with what is reported in the text?

(continued)

EXHIBIT 13.5

Checklist for Reviewing Tables (*continued*)

- Is the figure easy to read and understand?
- Is it free of unnecessary details?
- Are standard symbols used, and all parts of the figure labeled clearly?
- Are letters, symbols, numbers, lines, and other objects large enough to be read once reduced in size to fit the journal page?
- Is there a caption with each figure, which is placed below it?
- Does the caption provide information for understanding the figure and all the symbols in it without referring to the text?
- If there is more than one figure, is the same scale used for their preparation? (APA, 2010)
- Are the figures in a file format consistent with the author guidelines and publisher specifications?
- Are the figures at a sufficiently high resolution to allow for accurate reproduction? (APA, 2010)
- If a copyrighted figure is reproduced, is there a note in the caption giving credit to the copyright owner?
- Was written permission obtained to reproduce the figure in the manuscript, and was a copy of the permission sent to the journal editor?
- Is each figure numbered (consecutively) and referenced in the text?

Relationship of Figure and Text

Similar to tables, figures are numbered consecutively, using Arabic numerals, in the order they are first mentioned in the text. Every figure is referred to in the text by its number, for example:

> Changes in infant mortality over the time period of the evaluation project are shown in Figure 1.

When the article is published, figures are placed close to where they are first referenced in the text. Similar to tables, authors should not indicate the placement of the figure because it may not be in that position when published. As far as placement in the manuscript, tables and figures follow the references, with tables first, then figures. As one last reminder: Tables and figures should only be used when essential, and it is the author's responsibility to know the maximum number allowed with a manuscript.

SUMMARY

Tables are an effective way of presenting detailed and complex information succinctly and clearly. Tables should be used when the author wants to report exact values, present a large amount of detailed information, display different quantitative values simultaneously, and show relationships among data. Tables should not be used, however, when the information can be reported instead in the text.

There are two types of tables authors can include in a manuscript: the traditional table with information arranged in columns and rows; and a tabulation, a short, informal table developed as part of the text. Word tables, boxes, and similar types of exhibits also can be developed; these are valuable for emphasizing important information from the text and highlighting key concepts.

Tables contain five major parts: title, column headings, row headings, body of the table, and notes. The title should be short, descriptive of the content in the table, and written as a phrase rather than as a sentence. The body or content of the table is usually organized into columns (vertical) and rows (horizontal). The intersection of a column and row, a cell, is where the specific numbers and text are placed.

A table provides a means of organizing information and presenting it logically, and the headings inform the reader of how the information is organized. Each column has a brief heading that identifies the type of information reported in it. Only one category of information is reported in a column. The leftmost column of a table contains the row headings that describe the content included in the rows of the table. Notes provide additional details about the table in general or a specific column, row, or cell in the table.

Every table should be referred to in the text, and the author should inform readers what to look for in the table. Tables are numbered consecutively, using Arabic numerals, in the order they are first mentioned in the text. Each table is placed on a separate page following the references.

Figures include graphs, diagrams, maps, and photographs. They can be used to illustrate the findings of a study, display trends in the data, make comparisons, and show equipment, procedures, and other objects described in the text. Figures are usually reduced when published, so the letters, symbols, numbers, lines, and other objects should be large enough that they can be seen once reduced to fit the journal page. The legend or caption for the figure is placed below it and includes details about the figure. Most figures will be reproduced as submitted, and the author should take care that the original is without flaws. Similar to tables, figures are numbered consecutively, using Arabic numerals, in the order they are first mentioned in the text. Every figure is referred to in the text by its number. Tables and figures should only be used when essential, and it is the author's responsibility to know the maximum number allowed with a manuscript.

REFERENCES

American Medical Association. (2007). *AMA manual of style: A guide for authors and editors* (10th ed.). New York, NY: Oxford University Press.

American Psychological Association. (2010). *Publication manual of the American Psychological Association* (6th ed.). Washington, DC: Author.

CONSORT. (2017). The CONSORT 2010 flow diagram. Retrieved from http://www.consort-statement.org/consort-statement/flow-diagram

Cook, D. A. (2016). Twelve tips for getting your manuscript published. *Medical Teacher, 38*(1), 41–50. doi:10.3109/0142159X.2015.1074989

International Committee of Medical Journal Editors. (2017). *Recommendations for the conduct, reporting, editing, and publication of scholarly work in medical journals.* Retrieved from http://www.icmje.org/icmje-recommendations.pdf

Stephens, R. (2015). Editorial: Reporting statistical analyses in peer review journal articles. *Health Information & Libraries Journal, 32,* 81–83. doi:10.1111/hir.12106

V

FINAL PAPER THROUGH PUBLICATION

FINAL PAPER AND SUBMISSION TO JOURNAL

At this point in the writing process, the author has completed the revisions of the content and format of the paper; has prepared the references, tables, and figures; and is ready to submit the paper to the journal. Prior to submission, there are some final responsibilities of the author to ensure that the manuscript is consistent with the journal requirements and contains all the required parts for submission. The manuscript is then ready to send to the journal for review.

This chapter describes the steps in preparing all elements of the final paper to submit to the journal and details associated with this submission. Examples of these elements are provided in the chapter, and a checklist is included for authors to ensure that all items are submitted with the manuscript to avoid delays in its review.

PREPARATION OF FINAL PAPER

Chapter 11 provided guidelines for revising the content and format of the paper so it is ready for submission. Because journals differ in their requirements, the author needs to complete one final check of the manuscript to ensure it is consistent with these requirements. This final check begins by reviewing the guidelines for preparing manuscripts described in the author information page. The author reads these while preparing the manuscript, but this final review confirms that the paper has all essential parts and meets these requirements. Some journals provide a presubmission checklist that summarizes the requirements. Most manuscripts are submitted electronically, and the author needs to register at the journal website. This registration can be done at any point during the process but needs to be completed for the author to upload the manuscript to submit it. Instructions at the journal website describe the electronic submission process, and the software prompts the author to upload the manuscript and other documents, such as the copyright transfer agreement, required by the journal.

This chapter begins by describing all of the required elements for submission of a scientific manuscript. Exhibit 14.1 provides a checklist for authors to use to ensure that all of the essential elements are addressed. The chapter concludes with considerations for using a website to submit a manuscript to the journal.

EXHIBIT 14.1

Checklist of Elements for All Submissions

- Manuscript title
- Authors and author information
- Designated corresponding author
- Running title (if journal requires)
- Funding support
- Acknowledgments
- Abstract
- Keywords
- Text with appropriate headings, subheadings, citations, and reference list
- Tables (each table in separate file)
- Figures (each figure in separate file)
- Disclosures
- Preferred and nonpreferred reviewers (if requested by journal)
- Permissions
- Cover letter
- Copyright forms

ELEMENTS OF A FINAL SUBMISSION

Title Page

Every manuscript needs a title page, which is the first page of the paper. Journals differ in their requirements of elements on the title page. Journals that use American Psychological Association (APA) formatting require five elements: title, running title, all authors, their organizational affiliations, and an author note (APA, 2010). Journals that use American Medical Association (AMA) style do not require a running title but rather compose running heads during the production process after acceptance (AMA, 2007).

For refereed journals, manuscripts are reviewed anonymously. Reviewers must receive title pages that include only the title(s) and omit elements that could identify the authors or their affiliations. If one or more title pages are required by the journal, authors should read the journal's author guidelines carefully to learn what elements are required on each version of the title page and prepare them accordingly.

When information about the manuscript is entered separately into the fields at the journal website, each is coded and assembled into requisite versions of the title page, depending on the stage of submission. For example, full and running titles are entered separately and placed automatically on title pages that will go to reviewers. Title pages that are sent to copy editors after acceptance include some combination of the following elements: the title of the paper; authors' names, credentials, positions, and institutions in which employed or with which affiliated; corresponding author and contact information; grant support or other type of support; disclosure of financial or other benefits and conflicts of interest; keywords; and a running head. Prior to submission online, authors should gather all materials that will be needed when submitting the manuscript.

Title

As discussed in Chapter 11, the title may have undergone multiple changes as the manuscript emerged. In the presubmission phase, the author has the opportunity to refine the title to capture the essence of the article. The author should craft a final title to capture the attention of the target audience.

Author Information

The author should confirm all of their contact information with each of the coauthors. This includes the full name with middle initials, correct academic degrees and certifications, institutional affiliations, physical addresses, telephone numbers, and email address(es). It is advisable to include a work and an alternate email address, such as a personal email, when registering at the journal website. This facilitates contact with the editorial office in case the author changes employment during the manuscript review and production periods. Correspondence about the manuscript is done electronically, and authors need to ensure that the editorial office has a current email address.

The authors should decide before submission who will serve in various submission-related capacities. The first author and all coauthors should be listed in order in the appropriate fields. One of these should be designated as the "corresponding author." The corresponding author is the one who will have the responsibility for being available to the editorial office during the review process. Typically only one author can be identified as corresponding author. Some journals also require information from the "submitting agent," who may or may not be an author on the manuscript. For example, a staff assistant may submit the manuscript but not be either the first author or a coauthor.

Running Title

Some journals include a running title, which is a short version of the title, usually 50 characters or fewer, to be used on each page of the published paper. In the final printed copy, this short title is printed at the top (running head) or bottom of the page (running foot) to assist the reader to find the desired article. Journals differ regarding their requirement for authors to compose a running title. This is typically specified in the journal's information for authors.

Funding Support

If the author received a grant or another type of support for the project reported in the paper, this should be noted. Some funding agencies and organizations require that authors use specific language when acknowledging their support. This information is usually available on award letters or on the website of the agency. If there is any doubt about the correct acknowledgment, authors should contact the agency directly for information. If the journal does not provide a separate field to enter funding information, the authors should use the field for Acknowledgments to include this information.

Acknowledgments

The journal website for submitting manuscripts usually includes a field for the acknowledgments. If not, the author can include this information on the title page or at the end of the text prior to the references. The acknowledgments allow the author to give credit to people who made contributions to the manuscript but do not meet the criteria for authorship. These contributions can be in many forms: consultation on the content of the paper, statistical assistance, editing of the paper, and financial support, as described in Chapter 3. Authors need written permission to publish the names of people listed in the acknowledgments section. Often journals provide a permission form that can be used for this purpose. Exhibit 14.2 is an example of a title page.

EXHIBIT 14.2

Sample Title Page

Evaluation of Educational Program for Patients With Congestive Heart Failure

Mary Smith, MSN, RN
Clinical Nurse II

John Peterson, DNP, APRN-BC
Nurse Practitioner

Jane Doe, MSN, RN
Nurse Manager

Robert Jones, PhD
Statistician

Grace Memorial Hospital
Reading, PA

Funding provided by Grace Memorial Hospital, Grant #2014-37.

The authors declare no conflict of interest.

Correspondence to:
Mary Smith, MSN
[mailing address, phone number,
and email addresses]

Abstract Page

The next page of the paper is the abstract page. How to write the abstract was described earlier in the book. In reviewing the abstract page, the author should confirm that the information is consistent with the text. The author should also check again that the length of the abstract is within the limits of the journal.

At the journal submission website, the abstract is usually uploaded into a separate field and not included with the text of the manuscript. Some journals, however, include the abstract and keywords at the beginning of the manuscript. The format will be specified in the author guidelines. The heading "Abstract" can be centered at the top of the abstract page. The abstract should be double-spaced, consistent with the rest of the paper.

Keywords

Most journals require authors to designate a short list of keywords (usually three to 10) that represent the most important topics of their article and that readers will use to search online databases for articles of interest (AMA, 2007). Keywords are usually listed at the end of the abstract in published manuscripts.

Several of the major databases use their own controlled vocabulary indexing system to assign keywords to published articles. MEDLINE uses the MeSH vocabulary; the Cumulative Index to Nursing and Allied Health Literature uses the Nursing and Allied Health Subject Headings (AMA, 2007). If authors are requested to submit their own keywords, they should use these databases to select terms. When keywords are consistent between the printed article and the indexing system, readers can more easily find individual and related articles on the topic.

Text

The next part of the paper is the text. Although this should be in final form, and not require any further revisions of content or writing style and format, the author should check the leveling of the headings and subheadings for consistency throughout the manuscript, the citations, and the consistency between the text and any tables and figures.

Headings and Subheadings

Guidelines for determining the level of headings and where to position them in the text are determined by style manuals, publishers, or journals. The *AMA Manual of Style* (2007) defers to publishers and journals with regard to headings. The *Publication Manual of the American Psychological Association* (APA, 2010) describes how to use five levels of headings in a paper, although for most manuscripts only two to three levels are needed. The format and placement of the heading depend on its level. For instance, when levels 1 and 2 of headings are used, the first one is centered, bolded, and uses uppercase and lowercase; the second-level heading is also bolded and uses uppercase and lowercase but is placed at the left margin. The text begins on the following line (APA, 2010).

At the final presubmission check, there are two important issues regarding headings. The first issue is to have consistency in how the headings and subheadings are typed throughout the manuscript, regardless of what format is used. It may be helpful to write the headings and subheadings, and their leveling, on a separate sheet of paper and confirm that this is how the content should be organized and divided into sections. The second issue is to use headings strategically to link the manuscript into a coherent whole and help the reader keep track of what the author is describing.

Citations

Although the need for accuracy in preparing citations and references has been discussed throughout this book, the author should check the citations in the text one final time. Citations should be consistent with the style used by the journal, all citations should be included, and they should match the references in the reference list.

Consistency of Text With Tables and Figures

The need for consistency between the text and related tables and figures has been emphasized in Chapters 5, 11, and 13. The author should check that the data in the text are consistent with the tables and figures and that each one has been cited accurately in the text. The tables and figures also should be numbered correctly.

References

The reference list follows the text and is prepared according to either a citation-sequence system, in which references are listed in the order they are first cited in the text, or name-year format, in which they are alphabetized. The author should have verified already the accuracy of the references against the original documents; if this was not done previously, it is an important step in preparing the final copy for submission. The author also checks that each reference on the list is cited at the correct place in the text, the reference format is consistent with the journal requirements and style manual, and each reference includes complete information.

For manuscripts cited in the text that are "in press," the author can include these on the reference list and insert them in the appropriate space as "In press."

Papers under review should not be included as background information or listed in the reference list. Other unpublished papers should be noted according to the style manual required by the journal.

Tables

Each table should begin on a new page, numbered consecutively in the order to which it is referred in the text. Tables are not placed within the text unless the author guidelines state specifically to place them there. The author checks that the tables are cited in the text at the correct place and that the information in the table supports the text. The author also should review the titles of the tables and verify that they are formatted consistently with the style used by the journal or general principles provided in this book. The author should have identified earlier how many tables and figures are allowed with each manuscript; if not, this limit should be confirmed before submitting the manuscript. Tables follow the reference list when uploading the parts of the manuscript during the submission process.

Figures

Figures follow the tables, with each figure beginning on a new page similar to the tables. Figures are numbered consecutively in the order they are cited in the text, and they should be uploaded in that same order. Figure captions provide an explanation of the figure and are placed below the figure; the caption serves as the title (APA, 2010, p. 158).

Disclosures

Online submissions may have separate fields for disclosing pertinent information related to responsible author practices. Such checklists or statements may be related to the following actions: complied with author guidelines, blinded the manuscript, did not previously publish the article or simultaneously submit it to another journal, or other concerns that will impede the prompt processing and review of the manuscript. It is important that the submitting author pay special attention to these disclosures. Careless or incorrect information in these fields can come back to haunt the group of authors, at best by delaying review or publication and at worst by requiring retraction of an article.

If there were any financial or contractual associations between the authors and others that might bias a study or how the findings are interpreted, this should be disclosed to the editor (AMA, 2007). A statement may be included in the cover letter, but in addition authors typically complete and sign a separate form for disclosing any conflicts of interest. When submitting a manuscript that involves the use of a product, it is important for the author to disclose if there was a financial association between the author and the commercial company that makes the product featured in the manuscript.

In addition to financial interest, authors need to disclose any other type of involvement that might represent a potential conflict of interest, such as being a paid consultant on a project evaluated in the manuscript, owning stock in the company that manufactures the product described in the paper, and receiving an honorarium for participating in the evaluation of the product, to name a few. For example, a statement such as this might be included on the title page:

> Ms. Smith is a consultant for Software Incorporated that produced the software evaluated in this paper.

If there are no conflicts of interest to disclose, this statement can be used on the title page: "The authors declare no conflict of interest."

OTHER ELEMENTS OF ONLINE SUBMISSIONS

Journals must often triage incoming submissions to the appropriate persons across multiple layers of editors and reviewers. In order to sort and track different types of manuscripts to the appropriate associate or review editor, journal submission websites may request additional information from the authors about their manuscript at the time of submission. Types of information may include whether the manuscript reports original research, the type of data analysis (qualitative, quantitative, or mixed methods), or subject characteristics (diagnostic focus, setting, age group, or other). The author will probably be familiar enough with the content to provide the requested information but should confer as needed with coauthors.

Some journals request submitting authors to provide the names of reviewers who would have the requisite expertise to serve as invited reviewers, as well as any persons whom the authors prefer not be invited to review their manuscript. Authors may suggest other authors whose work has been important to the development of their ideas, but authors should not inquire directly of any suggested reviewers whether they would be willing to serve as a reviewer of the manuscript, as this information would compromise the blinded peer-review process.

Authors might list as nonpreferred reviewers any colleagues at other universities or organizations who have served in an advisory capacity on the material in the article but who were not coauthors. This information also supports the blinded peer-review process. The editors are free to disregard both preferred and nonpreferred reviewers at the time of reviewer selection.

If relevant, the author should have available any permissions needed. These may include permissions to reprint information in the manuscript, letters granting permission to publish the acknowledgments and to cite the names of institutions in the manuscript, and permissions to publish photographs and other illustrations.

FORMATTING THE FINAL MANUSCRIPT

The manuscript must be formatted according to the specifications in the journal's information for authors. Papers are double-spaced throughout, including the title page and abstract and continuing through the last page of the manuscript. This includes double-spacing the references, tables, and figure captions. The references themselves are double-spaced, not only the lines between each reference on the list.

There are some other important guidelines for preparing the paper of which the author should be aware. If the paper is too long, do not attempt to include more lines per page by using narrow margins. The journal guidelines may specify the size of the margins, but if unsure about them, refer to the style manual or use 1-inch margins on all sides. Paragraphs should be indented, and spaces should not be left between each paragraph unless the author guidelines specifically ask for this format. Pages should be left-justified (aligning the text at the left margin), not double-justified (where the text is aligned at both the right and left margins). When double-justified, there may be large spaces between words and symbols in a line.

Pages are numbered consecutively, considering the title page as the first page. Some journals specify the placement of page numbers, but if not indicated in the author guidelines, pages can be numbered in the right-hand corner of each page either at the top or bottom.

SUBMISSION OF MANUSCRIPT TO JOURNAL

The paper is now ready to submit to the journal. Submission to the journal requires writing a cover letter to accompany the manuscript, obtaining signatures on the transfer of copyright form, and creating an author account on the journal website.

Cover Letter

The cover letter accompanies the manuscript and provides the editor with information about the paper and corresponding author (Exhibit 14.3). The cover letter should include these relevant elements:

- Title of the paper
- Length of manuscript (pages or word count) and number of tables and figures
- Statement that the paper is original and has not been published already
- Confirmation that all authors have read and approved the final version

- Information about previous presentations, for example, at a scientific meeting
- Information about closely related manuscripts submitted to other journals, in press, or published
- Explanation of conflicts of interest
- Full name, affiliation, and complete contact information of the corresponding author

EXHIBIT 14.3

Sample Cover Letter

[Date]

Dr. Ann Brown
Editor, *Nursing Journal*
1234 Main Street
Anytown, Anystate 56789

Dear Dr. Brown:

Attached please find our manuscript, "Evaluation of Educational Program for Patients With Congestive Heart Failure," for your review for possible publication in *Nursing Journal*. The manuscript includes 4,978 words, two tables, and one figure.

The manuscript is based on a symposium paper delivered on November 4, 2017, at the ninth National Council of Nurses Education Summit meeting in Indianapolis, IN. A companion paper describing the development of the educational program is "in press" in the *Education Evaluation Journal*. That manuscript describes the pilot data ($n = 32$) from one hospital that informed the content of the program described in the current paper; however, the current paper is based on follow-up data and describes the process and outcome evaluations of the program in three hospitals ($n = 291$). Please let me know if you would like us to forward to you a copy of the companion manuscript. Neither the enclosed manuscript nor any part of its content has been submitted to, accepted for, or published by another journal.

The undersigned have no financial interests in any element of the study, which was approved by the institutional review boards of Our Town University and each of the three hospitals.

The study is based on a conceptual model copyrighted to Wiley Interscience. We attach a copy of the permission granted by that publisher to reprint the model herein.

Mary Smith will serve as the corresponding author on this paper. The four authors contributed significantly to and have read and approved the current version.

(continued)

EXHIBIT 14.3

Sample Cover Letter (*continued*)

Thank you for your consideration.

Sincerely,
Mary Smith
Mary Smith
Our Town University
1 River Road
Reading, PA 19709
313.888.8888 (voice)
mary.smith@otu.edu

John Peterson
John Peterson

Jane Doe
Jane Doe

Robert Jones
Robert Jones

Some journals have departments that publish different types of articles. The cover letter can state if the paper was written for a particular department.

Because of issues with duplicate publications, discussed in the beginning of this book, authors should include a statement in the cover letter indicating that the paper is original and has not been published already, in its entirety or in part. A sample statement that can be used is: "Neither the entire paper nor any part of its content has been published or has been accepted by another journal. The manuscript is submitted only to this journal." Inclusion of this statement in the cover letter can be seen in Exhibit 14.3.

If the manuscript being submitted is based on the same dataset or has similar content as previously published or submitted papers, the author should indicate exactly how the manuscript differs from these other publications. Journals also may ask the author to submit these articles with the manuscript. If the manuscript is based on a conference presentation, the author should indicate such to the editor.

The cover letter should specify the full name and affiliation of the corresponding author. Contact information should be consistent with that listed on the title page or elsewhere in the online submission website.

Copyright Forms

For some journals, the author submits the signed transfer of copyright form with the submission; for others, this is only completed when the paper is accepted for publication. If the copyright transfer is needed for submission, this will be noted on the author guidelines and will be available at the website of the journal. For many journals, each coauthor completes and signs his or her own copyright transfer agreement, but for others the corresponding author signs for all the authors as a group. For journals that require the copyright transfer when the paper is submitted, typically the copyright questions are web based and are answered by the author(s) as part of the manuscript submission, or a separate electronic form needs to be uploaded with the manuscript for the author to complete the submission process.

Creating an Author Account for Web-Based Submissions

The first time that authors log onto a journal website, they will be instructed on how to initiate an account dedicated to their submission. If the author is already a reviewer of manuscripts for that journal, an account may already be available for manuscript submissions.

The same author account is used to process manuscripts being submitted, to track the progress of submitted manuscripts through the editorial process, and to respond to invitations to revise and resubmit an article. For a new manuscript being submitted, the author is prompted through sequential steps to provide each element needed and respond to specific queries relevant to the submission. The final screen provides the opportunity to check all of the inputted elements and displays any missing elements, which can then be uploaded. Once the author is satisfied with all uploaded elements, the author clicks a link that "submits" the manuscript to the editorial office. The author account will confirm the receipt of the manuscript, and the corresponding author will receive an email confirmation. Chapter 15 describes the editorial processing of a manuscript.

SUMMARY

The author needs to complete one final check of the manuscript to ensure that it is consistent with the requirements of the journal specified in the information for authors page. This final review confirms that the paper has all essential parts and meets these requirements.

The author should check the title page, abstract page, and text. Although the manuscript should be in final form, and not require any further revisions of content or writing style and format, the author should check the (a) leveling of the headings and subheadings and if typed consistently throughout the manuscript, (b) citations, and (c) consistency between the text and any tables and figures. The author should complete one last check of the references.

Each table and figure is placed on a separate page and numbered consecutively in the order referred to in the text. The author checks that the tables and figures are numbered consistently with their placement in the text.

The manuscript should be prepared according to the journal specifications. Most manuscripts are submitted online at the journal's website. Submission to the journal requires writing a cover letter to accompany the manuscript, obtaining signatures on the transfer of copyright form if required for submission, and uploading the files. The author now awaits the results of the review of the paper.

REFERENCES

American Medical Association. (2007). *AMA manual of style: A guide for authors and editors* (10th ed.). New York, NY: Oxford University.

American Psychological Association. (2010). *Publication manual of the American Psychological Association* (6th ed.). Washington, DC: Author.

EDITORIAL REVIEW PROCESS

Chapter 14 presented the final steps in preparing a paper for submission to a journal. This same process is used in writing a grant, a report for an organization, and other types of papers. When the paper is completed, another person or group will more than likely read and critique it, whether for publication, funding, or some other purpose. The process of writing drafts and revising them for content and format was emphasized in earlier chapters, so the final paper contains the essential content, is organized clearly, and is well written. The cycle of writing a draft and revising it, combined with attention to other details described earlier, results in a paper that should be competitive with others that are also being reviewed.

This chapter presents the editorial review process from the point at which the paper is received in the journal office through the final editorial decision. The roles and responsibilities of the editor, editorial board, and peer reviewers are discussed, and examples are provided of criteria used by reviewers when asked to critique a manuscript for publication. Peer review is not without issues, and some of these are examined in the chapter.

Manuscripts submitted to a journal may be accepted without revision or accepted provisionally pending revision, may be returned to the author for a major revision and resubmission, or may be rejected. Each of these editorial decisions has implications for the author and how the author responds to the editor.

WHO IS INVOLVED?

When the manuscript is completed, and all materials assembled, the manuscript and supplementary document are forwarded to the editorial office of the journal to begin the review process. The editorial office might include a large number of staff in a dedicated office for journals widely circulated and published frequently or an editor and limited, if any, support staff working online from their home offices. Journals differ in the resources needed to process manuscripts and, once accepted, to prepare them for production. For example, health-related newspapers and journals published monthly will need more editorial staff to handle the number of manuscripts to be processed in comparison with a specialty nursing journal published quarterly that receives and processes fewer manuscripts. The number of people involved in the editorial process and their roles, therefore, will differ based on the needs of the journal.

Editor

The editor of a nursing journal is an expert in the nursing specialty or content area covered by the journal. Depending on the focus of the journal, editors may have expertise in clinical practice, administration, management, education, research, and other areas. Few nursing editors are prepared as such, and most are selected for the position because of their knowledge of the topics covered by the journal.

In addition to content expertise, editors usually have additional knowledge and skills related to the types of articles published in the journal. For example, editors of journals that publish research have an understanding of statistics and research methods and often have conducted research themselves. Clinical journals that focus on a particular nursing role, such as publications for nurse practitioners, are generally edited by someone functioning in that role or with an understanding of it.

To maintain their expertise, editors spend much of their time keeping current by reading the professional literature; by attending professional meetings; through their own research, writing, and work; and by maintaining contact with experts in the field. This also serves as a way of soliciting manuscripts for the journal.

Some editors of journals began initially as assistant or associate editors, then moved into the editor's position. Most, however, served on editorial or advisory boards of journals, were manuscript reviewers, and have experience themselves writing articles, books, and other types of publications.

One or more editors are appointed by the owners of a journal. Although the owner is responsible for all important business decisions about the journal, the editor is accorded full authority over journal content (International Committee of Medical Journal Editors [ICMJE], 2017). Editors work with their owner–publishers under contractual arrangements that state the duties, responsibilities, and terms of both parties.

Functions of the Editor

Editors may work full time in their role or function as part-time editors who hold other positions in nursing. Part-time editors receive an honorarium from the publisher for serving in that role. The publisher of the journal is the individual or group that produces, distributes, and markets the journal. Editors report to the publisher of the journal through different types of organizational arrangements.

The editor is accountable to the readers for quality manuscripts that promote the development of the field. The editor also is accountable to the editorial board and reviewers for carrying out the editorial process and arriving at decisions consistent with their recommendations and advice. Since editors report to the publisher, they are responsible for meeting the publisher's expectations associated with editing the journal.

Responsibilities of the Editor

The editor's first responsibility is to readers: to inform and educate them by providing high-quality scholarly papers that were fairly selected (American Medical Association [AMA], 2007). In service of this first responsibility, the editor's overall responsibilities are for the editorial content and quality of the journal; direction of staff and consultation with board members; development and maintenance of procedures; and creation and enforcement policies that focus efforts to achieve the journal's mission effectively, efficiently, expeditiously, and ethically (AMA, 2007, p. 260). In addition and in service to these responsibilities, editors provide regular editorials and consult with the publisher on indexing the journal and website development (Kapoor, 2016).

To fulfill these responsibilities, the editor functions to

- Solicit high-quality manuscripts
- Work with authors to develop their ideas into manuscripts that are suitable for publication
- Assess the quality of manuscripts submitted to the journal honestly and impartially
- Select reviewers to critique papers
- Decide on manuscripts to publish based on recommendations from the reviewers
- Address appeals of decisions and conflicts of interest
- Maintain confidentiality concerning all submitted manuscripts
- Edit manuscripts
- Decide on the papers to include in each issue
- Complete other tasks to prepare the manuscripts for publication
- Exhibit courtesy, tact, and empathy with authors and reviewers (AMA, 2007)

With most journals, the editor is responsible for deciding whether to accept or reject a manuscript. With refereed journals, peer reviewers critique the submitted manuscript and advise the editor on the acceptance decision, but the editor makes the final decision. For tenure and promotion considerations, refereed publications carry more weight because they include this peer-review process, thereby providing an external review of the quality of the work and its contribution to nursing. There are other journals though that are not peer reviewed, and the editors read and critique the manuscripts in-house and make the acceptance decisions. These are considered nonrefereed journals.

Editors work with authors, editorial board members, peer reviewers, the production editor, and other personnel associated with publishing the journal.

Many editors subscribe to the *Code of Conduct and Best Practice Guidelines for Journal Editors* (Committee on Publication Ethics, 2018), which details the high standards to which editors aim when interacting with their many constituencies. Because the editor interfaces with the production editor, there is an opportunity to maintain the quality of the content of the manuscript as it moves through production.

The editor also establishes the editorial policies for the journal and develops the author guidelines for submitting manuscripts. These policies and guidelines are generally prepared with input from the editorial board and peer reviewers. If the journal is an official publication of a professional organization, the editor works closely with the officers and board of the organization so there is consistency between the goals of the journal and those of the organization.

In some journals, the editor writes an editorial or solicits other people to write it. When associated with a nursing organization, the editorials often reflect the positions of that organization.

For journals with columns and departments, the editor has a role in soliciting manuscripts for them or working with the assistant or associate editor who has this responsibility. The editor and the assistant or associate editor review these papers and suggest revisions to the authors rather than sending them to peer reviewers for critique.

Managing Editor

In addition to the editor, some journals also have a managing editor. The managing editor is the staff member responsible for the administrative details associated with processing the manuscripts from submission through publication. The managing editor sends the manuscripts to reviewers, tracks the status of reviews, and oversees the processing of the manuscripts once accepted for publication to ensure their consistency with style requirements (J. D. Baker, 2014).

Editorial Board

Editors do not make decisions in isolation about the journals they edit. They consult with an editorial board, which is a group of individuals with expertise in the content covered by the journal and who contribute that expertise in advising the editor about strategic plans for the journal as well as in reviewing the quality, accuracy, and currency of manuscripts submitted to the journal. The editor makes the decisions as to who will serve on the editorial or advisory board to the journal.

The editorial board members may represent the board in community outreach; give the editor advice on policies, content, and direction of the journal; provide feedback from journal constituencies; review and write manuscripts; and assist with editorial decisions (AMA, 2007). Board members are listed on the journal website and in the masthead. Editorial boards meet at least annually and confer by conference call as needed.

Peer Reviewers

Peer reviewers are experts in the topic of the manuscript; they are considered "peers" of the author because they have similar expertise, allowing them to critique the paper. Depending on the journal and type of manuscript, peer reviewers may have published on the topic, may be practicing in the same specialization as the focus of the manuscript, or may have research or statistical expertise needed for the review. The principle is that peer reviewers have expertise to critique the manuscript and make recommendations to the editor. Peer reviewers are sometimes called *external reviewers* or *referees*.

The panel of peer reviewers of a journal is usually larger than the editorial board because expertise is needed for a wide range of topics. The editor chooses peer reviewers based on their expertise. The editor also may ask ad hoc reviewers—people who do not serve on the review panel but have specialized knowledge—to read a particular manuscript. With some journals, the editorial board also serves as the review panel, with the board members reviewing manuscripts in their areas of specialization.

Peer review is a privilege. Peer reviewers have an obligation both to conduct their review within the domain dictated by the particular journal and also to adopt a professional approach to the review (Gallagher, 2013). Such an approach includes providing constructive and noncaustic feedback to authors (J. D. Baker, 2014). The domain of a review includes whether the manuscript topic will be of interest to the journal's usual readers and whether its quality will contribute to their scholarly endeavors. It is not within the purview of the reviewer to agree or disagree with the findings or conclusions. A professional approach to reviewing a manuscript includes identifying positive features of the work, treating the process collaboratively rather than as a test, providing as much detail as possible about literature that should be but was not considered, and to acknowledge one's own limitations of expertise when evaluating the work of others.

PEER REVIEW

Peer review is an extension of the scientific process whereby a journal submits the manuscripts it receives to outside review (ICMJE, 2017). The review policies and procedures used by journals to review manuscripts differ widely across journals. For this reason, general principles of peer review are described here, recognizing that each journal will have its own way of conducting peer reviews and its own criteria and format for doing so. Some journals publish statements in the information for authors page on their peer-review process and policies.

Peer review began in the 18th century when committees were set up by medical societies to evaluate papers sent to them for publication in their journals and has been integral to biomedical research since the mid-1940s (Csiszar, 2016). As medicine became more specialized and more journals developed, editors found they lacked the knowledge to review manuscripts out of their specialization and sought experts to give them opinions about the submitted papers. Specialization became a driving force in the acceptance of peer review (AMA, 2007). As more manuscripts became available, peer review also was seen as a way of accepting the best papers for the journal.

Blind Review Process

Many peer-reviewed journals use a process of blind review in which submitted manuscripts are sent to reviewers with the identity of the author and institution concealed (Kapoor, 2016). The editor or publishing company website conceals identifying information that might suggest the author and institutional affiliation. The principle behind sending a "blinded" copy, free of identifying information, is that there is less chance of bias when the reviewer does not know who wrote the article or the author's credentials. When the author also does not know the name of a reviewer, the process is called "double-blinded." However, blinding of authorship does not always work because in specialized areas the reviewers often know the research and projects of others (Tomkins, Zhang, & Heavlin, 2017).

Authors are usually blinded as to the identity of the reviewers. When reviews are returned to the author, the identities of the reviewers are masked so the author does not know who evaluated the paper. With this anonymity, reviewers are free to evaluate a paper honestly and without fear of repercussions from the author if they give a negative review. It is believed that these reviews are fairer. Unblinded reviews may also deplete the ranks of reviewers significantly due to potential reviewers' concerns about damage to collegial relationships or even retribution by disgruntled authors.

Unfortunately, some authors have had experience in receiving highly critical reviews without feedback that could be used to modify the manuscript. Unless the editorial decision is to accept the manuscript, reviews can be considered negative. Some novice authors, upon receiving a negative review, may abandon all future attempts to write for publication. We discuss later in this chapter how authors can prepare proactively for the results of the review process by developing strategies to address negative reviews.

Whether certain kinds of peer-review procedures actually improve the quality of scientific publications is debatable. Use of checklists and standardized guidelines for peer reviews are strongly recommended by editors as having a positive effect on overall quality of published manuscripts (DiDomenico, Baker, & Haines, 2017). Despite the complexity of such research, more studies are needed on the effects of editorial peer review on biomedical publications, including on the quality of nursing journals.

Purposes of Peer Review

Peer review supports the fundamental purpose of writing for publication in nursing. Reviewers evaluate the manuscript's value for informing practice and stimulating discovery, for archiving fundamental knowledge of the profession, for quality control, and for attribution to the appropriate developers of that knowledge (DiDomenico et al., 2017).

The review process assists the editor in establishing the manuscript's relevance to the journal, the value of its content to readers, and its timeliness, thereby providing a sound basis for the editor's decision. Peer reviewers give the editor and author their judgment and expert opinions about the manuscript. The editor uses the review as a basis for making the acceptance decision, and authors use the review for revising the paper.

With some journals, reviewers do not state their judgments on whether the paper should be published. For others, reviewers recommend to the editor if the manuscript should be accepted, revised, or rejected; the editor then makes the acceptance decision considering these recommendations.

Journals differ in the focus of the manuscript reviews by the nature of the articles they publish. Journals that publish clinical articles emphasize more of the practical implications of the paper and how readers might use the ideas. Reviewers for journals that publish research focus more on the adequacy of the research design, how the research was carried out, appropriateness of the statistical methods, and conclusions drawn from the evidence.

Although there are differences across journals, reviewers commonly evaluate whether the:

- Ideas and information in the paper are new and innovative
- Paper contributes to nursing and to the knowledge and skills of readers
- Content is important and warrants publication
- Content is relevant to readers of the journal
- Content is at the appropriate level for readers
- Content is applicable for the reader's practice
- Paper is well organized
- Ideas are expressed clearly and developed logically
- Research methods are adequate
- Evidence is sufficient to support conclusions drawn from the research
- Point of view that is advanced is balanced
- References are current (within the past 5 years) and relevant (AMA, 2007; American Psychological Association [APA], 2010)

Review Forms and Guidelines

Most journals conduct peer reviews online. Reviewers establish online accounts for reviewing in the same way that authors establish online accounts for submitting manuscripts, as described in Chapter 14. Once the reviewer accepts an invitation to review, the journal administrator makes available digital links to the manuscript, instructions, and the review forms.

Online reviewing entails some general responsibilities for reviewers. Reviewers should familiarize themselves with the journal's web page and review-related links, addressing any questions to the journal administrator or managing editor. Spam filters may interrupt the flow of some crucial information or communication and should be disabled. It is important for reviewers to monitor whatever email inbox they designated for journal communication so that no messages are missed. Reviewers should not hesitate to alert the journal staff or editors about any special needs or considerations related to their participation. If professional or personal circumstances will prevent them from accepting any invitations to review for a significant period of time, the software program can automatically be set to alert the editor not to interrupt the reviewer with unwanted messages during that time. The setting also avoids delaying the completed review process. If a reviewer recognizes an assigned manuscript as having been authored by a close colleague or student or otherwise suspects a conflict of interest, the reviewer should contact the journal immediately so that the manuscript can be reassigned.

Most journals use review forms or checklists that specify the criteria for judging the manuscript and provide space for reviewers to support their ratings with comments about the paper. An example of a rating form is shown in Exhibit 15.1.

Review forms vary in their format and wording. Most forms give the reviewer an opportunity to rate features of the paper as present or absent. For example (yes or no), "Does the abstract accurately reflect the text, are the references current, and so on?" Some forms ask the reviewer to compare the features of the submitted manuscript to other published papers in the field.

EXHIBIT 15.1

Sample Manuscript Review Form

Nurse Educator

Manuscript Review Questions (web based)

YES	NO	
Introduction:		
_____	_____	Is the purpose of the paper clear?
Content:		
_____	_____	Is it timely/relevant?
_____	_____	Is it logically and clearly developed?
_____	_____	Is it sophisticated enough for our readers?
_____	_____	Is it innovative?
_____	_____	Is it on cutting edge of knowledge on topic?
Methods (if applicable):		
_____	_____	Is the design appropriate?
_____	_____	Are the sample and sampling method adequate?
_____	_____	Was there institutional review board (IRB) approval (or is IRB indicated)?

(continued)

EXHIBIT 15.1

Sample Manuscript Review Form (*continued*)

		Are the instruments reliable and valid?
		Are statistical tests appropriate?
		Are data adequately and appropriately presented?
		Do conclusions/generalizations/implications go beyond what findings/data/theory support?

General:

		Are most references from the past 3 years?
		Are the references relevant?
		Is the content's application/utility made explicit to the reader's practice setting?
		If there is no cost-benefit analysis, does the content warrant its addition?
		Was the paper interesting to read?

Rate the overall quality of this manuscript on a scale of 1–5:

1 = excellent; 2 = good; 3 = acceptable; 4 = uncertain of acceptability; 5 = unacceptable.

Reviewer Blind Comments to Author:

_____

_____

Reviewer Confidential Comments to Editor:

_____

_____

For example, "Compared to published articles of similar content or methods, is the quality of the data presented (or the mechanics of the writing, etc.) in the top 10%, top 25%, top 50%, lower 50%, or lower 25%?" Following the specific ratings, the review form may ask for an overall assessment of the manuscript and a recommendation to the editor concerning the editorial decision. The editor takes such comments under consideration, but the final decision rests with the editor. Examples of overall assessment and recommendation schema are shown in Exhibit 15.2.

EXHIBIT 15.2

Example of Scales for Reviewer's Overall Rating and Recommendation to Editor

RATING OF THE MANUSCRIPT OVERALL

- Excellent—Presents an important new approach, new ideas, or new information.
- Good—Improves significantly on previous work of its type or contains new interesting information.
- Average—Good work, but contains little novelty and may be of limited interest to most readers.
- Routine—No errors, but likely to have narrow or little interest to journal's main readership.
- Flawed—Contains serious flaws in project design, data analysis, or presentation.

RECOMMENDATION OF ACTION TO EDITOR

- Accept subject to minor revision. No need for reevaluation by reviewer.
- Possibly accept with moderate revision. May need reevaluation by reviewer.
- Revise and resubmit. Major revision required, with reevaluation by reviewers.
- Reject. Not acceptable for publication by this journal.

Following the forced-choice ratings, the reviewer is invited to expand on the ratings in a narrative format. The additional comments are not required but are useful to both the editor and the author. The narrative customarily begins with a sentence or two that summarize the topic of the manuscript and one or more strengths or contributions. This is followed by an evaluation of each part of the manuscript that could be improved; the most helpful reviews are specific in these comments, suggestions, and questions. They encourage authors to refine and focus their manuscripts for the intended readership. Exhibit 15.3 presents questions that a reviewer may consider appropriate to discuss in a narrative evaluation when reviewing research and other types of manuscripts.

These reviews and narrative comments are given to the author for use in revising the paper. They also provide documentation for the editorial decision. With some journals, reviewers indicate the page and line of the manuscript in question or needing revision.

Peer reviewers should be provided with guidelines for an appropriate review, so that it is fair and unbiased. Journals take care that reviews are solicited consistently for each manuscript submitted, using the same process, criteria, and format. Reviewers are required to disclose to the editor any conflict of interest that would bias their judgment of the manuscript and disqualify them from the review process (ICMJE, 2017).

Editors, editorial board members, and peer reviewers treat manuscripts and reviews as privileged communication. The manuscript is not publicly

EXHIBIT 15.3

Topics Appropriate to Reviewer's Narrative Evaluation of Manuscript Sections

TITLE

- Does the title contain keywords that interested readers would logically use in an index search?
- Was the title too long, too general, inaccurate, nonprofessional, or boring?

ABSTRACT

- Was the abstract complete, that is, did it contain the objectives or research questions; study design, sample, and measures (if appropriate); key findings; and conclusion?
- Were there discrepancies between the abstract and the full manuscript?

KEYWORDS

- Did the keywords accurately reflect the content of the manuscript?

RATIONALE, BACKGROUND, AND OBJECTIVE(S)

- Rationale
  - o Did the introduction identify a significant problem?
  - o Was the chief aim of the article stated clearly and concisely?
- Background
  - o Were there gaps in the background literature described? Did the reviewer need more or different information about prior research?
  - o Was unnecessary background literature described?
  - o Was the background literature described logically, for example, from the more general to the more specific problem?
  - o Was the reviewer ultimately convinced of a significant gap in knowledge and the importance of filling it?
- Objective(s)
  - o Do the authors propose specific and concrete objectives or research hypotheses or questions?

SUBSTANTIVE *ORIGINAL* CONTRIBUTION

- For a data-based study
  - o Was the design of the study appropriate to the rationale?
  - o Were subjects chosen with clear inclusion and exclusion criteria and any groups clearly distinguished? Was the sample size large enough to draw useful conclusions? Were human or animal subjects protected?
  - o Were the assessment measures appropriate to the problem described in the Introduction?
  - o Was the data analysis strategy fully explained and did it fit the research questions?

(continued)

EXHIBIT 15.3

Topics Appropriate to Reviewer's Narrative Evaluation of Manuscript Sections (*continued*)

- Was enough information provided to support replication in another setting?
- Were results described completely and logically, in accordance with the tables?
- For nondata-based manuscripts
  - Did the newly proposed material follow logically from the background literature?
  - Were all elements and dimensions of the new material identified, defined, and explained?
  - Did you have enough information to apply the new material in another setting, if appropriate?

CONCLUSIONS AND IMPLICATIONS

- Were the conclusions justified or were they "over-interpreted," that is, did they claim more than flowed logically from the background and original material?
- Did the authors discuss similarities and differences between their work and the work of others, and possible reasons for differences?
- Did the authors discuss implications of their findings for patients, students, communities, human subjects, faculty, clinicians, and/or researchers?
- Did the authors discuss potential limitations to their conclusions and how future work might improve or extend their work?

REFERENCES

- Were the references more than 5 years old, or were classic articles on the topic missing?

TABLES AND FIGURES

- Were the tables and figures clear, complete, and effectively designed?
- Could tables and figures be improved to reduce bias when displaying results?

STYLE

- Did the authors use standard English prose style?
- Was the prose style direct and clear? If not, what are the specific examples of difficult sections?
- Did the authors avoid jargon, typographical, and grammatical errors?
- Was the manuscript compliant with required style guidelines, for example, headings, citations, references, tables, and so on?

discussed prior to publication, and reviewers are not allowed to copy the manuscript they receive, use the ideas in a paper for their own work, or share the ideas with others (ICMJE, 2017).

MANUSCRIPT REVIEW PROCESS

When the manuscript is submitted to the journal, it is given a number that is used throughout the review process to track the manuscript. This number is recorded in the author account on the journal website or in the email to the author acknowledging receipt of the manuscript, and should be used by the author in all subsequent correspondence with the editor.

The editor or managing editor establishes careful records so the manuscript can be tracked through the review process beginning from its receipt in the editorial office, through the review and revision stages, and into production. Records are digitalized into audit trails, based on the software used by the journal and including email correspondence.

Reasons Manuscripts Returned to Author

Not all manuscripts are sent out for review. If the manuscript is not relevant for the journal, the editor will likely return it to the author without its being reviewed. The editor usually will specify in the letter to the author why the manuscript is not suitable for the journal and its readers or other reasons for its return. The editor may suggest an alternative target journal for the topic. The author, however, can avoid this situation by carefully selecting journals for submission as discussed earlier in this book.

The second reason a manuscript may be returned to the author rather than its being reviewed is when it is incomplete or does not conform to the journal requirements. The manuscript may not be properly formatted, may not be written using standard English grammar and syntax, or the reference format may not be consistent with the journal guidelines. The importance of carefully preparing the manuscript and checking it before submission was described earlier. If authors do not follow these principles, the review of the manuscript may be delayed.

Steps in Review Process

After the editor determines the suitability of the manuscript for the journal, the review process begins. How many peer reviews are done depends on the journal, but generally at least two reviews are completed of each manuscript. For some papers an additional review might be included to assess a specific aspect of the paper, such as the statistical analysis used for a research study.

The editor decides who should review the manuscript. This decision is based on who has the expertise to evaluate the manuscript and make a judgment of its relevance for readers, importance, timeliness, and quality, among other criteria. For papers with highly specialized content, the editor may seek ad hoc reviewers, that is, people not on the review panel and who do not normally review for the journal. They may have the expertise, however, to judge a particular manuscript.

The results of the peer review are then sent (electronically) to the author with the editorial decision on whether the paper is accepted, should be revised and resubmitted, or is rejected. The editor also sends questions about the content, issues to be resolved, and suggestions for revision that were identified during the review process. The reviews provide data for the editor to use in making an acceptance decision and feedback for authors in revising the paper to strengthen it. In some instances the manuscript may be accepted without further revision, but usually authors revise their papers using the comments and suggestions from reviewers.

After revising the manuscript, the author submits it at the journal website. The editor may review the changes and make a final acceptance decision without another external review. If substantial changes were made in the manuscript or the author was directed to revise and resubmit it, the reviewers will critique the revised version and make recommendations to the editor. This revision process continues until the paper is accepted for publication.

Editorial Decisions

Not every paper sent to a journal will be accepted, nor should it be, to maintain the quality of the journal and meet reader needs. Rejection rates vary across journals. Some journals receive a large number of manuscripts, significantly more than could be published within a reasonable time frame, and therefore reject many of these papers. Other journals have fewer submissions and work with authors in revising their papers until acceptable for publication. Authors may ask the editor about the journal's rejection rates, as this information is proprietary and calculated by publishers.

Editors monitor the number of papers accepted for publication to avoid a backlog of papers accepted but not published. Journals are allotted by the publisher a predetermined number of pages for each issue. This is known as a "page budget." Because of the cost, only this contracted number of pages is allowed. As such, the editor plans which manuscripts to include in each issue, estimating the number to accept so the time between acceptance and publication is not unreasonable. A delay in publishing accepted papers hinders dissemination of new knowledge to readers, and when too much time elapses, papers may need to be updated. Some backlog though is needed to ensure that a sufficient number of papers is available for each issue and to allow for fluctuations in submissions without creating a delay in publication.

Criteria for Acceptance of Manuscripts

The criteria used by editors to decide whether or not to accept a manuscript vary by journal, but the AMA (2007) identified nine criteria for importance and quality that most editors use in making this decision.

Importance

1. Represents a nontrivial scientific advance
2. Has clinical relevance (for clinical specialty journals)
3. Presents original information
4. Will be interesting to reader

Quality

5. Design and methods are appropriate to the research questions or hypotheses
6. Research questions and methods are adequately described and rigorously conducted
7. Data analysis is appropriate
8. Conclusions are supported by the findings
9. Subjects are treated ethically (pp. 303–304)

The editor also considers the number of papers on the same or similar topics that have already been accepted. It is unlikely that the editor will accept too many articles on similar topics because of the need to publish new content for readers. If the author is notified that the paper is rejected, the backlog of papers may have been an influencing factor, and the rejection may have less to do with the paper's quality and relevance for readers than the backlog of manuscripts.

Types of Editorial Decisions

Editors generally make one of three decisions, based on their own review and suggestions from reviewers: (a) accept for publication, (b) revise minor or major issues and resubmit, or (c) reject (J. D. Baker, 2014).

Accept for Publication

Accept-for-publication decisions may involve an acceptance with no revisions or limited ones, or a tentative acceptance pending revision. An acceptance without revisions is rare. Even if the paper is accepted for publication because of its important and timely content, it is likely that the author will need to make some changes to strengthen it. The author should make these revisions, or provide a rationale for not making them, and return the paper as soon as possible to the editor. It may be that the editor has space to include the paper in an upcoming issue or, if not, the paper will have a better chance of earlier rather than later publication.

Other acceptances are provisional, with the final decision resting on whether the author revises the manuscript to reflect the changes suggested by the editor and reviewers. Changes might be needed in the content, for example, adding or deleting content, preparing or omitting a table, including a new section of content, and so forth, or the changes might be in the writing style and format. As with acceptance decisions, the author should revise the paper without delay.

Revise and Resubmit

A second type of editorial decision is to revise and resubmit the manuscript for another review. When authors are asked to revise and resubmit the manuscript, it suggests that the paper has merit and would be strengthened by a revision. Although a revision does not guarantee acceptance, there is interest by the editor and reviewers in the paper and its message. For this reason, the author should take the time to revise the paper as recommended. Once again, the author should not delay in resubmitting it (Albarran & Dowling, 2017).

Reject

The third editorial decision is a rejection. Perhaps the content was not new, and the author missed this in the literature review. The journal might have recently published a series of articles on the same or a similar topic or accepted a paper with the same theme. The content may be too specialized or not specialized enough for the readers of the journal, or may be of limited interest to readers. The organization of the paper and writing style may be unclear. These are among the World Health Organization's (2018) list of the top 10 reasons for manuscript rejection. An example of a rejection letter is shown in Exhibit 15.4.

Editors intend no personal offense when they reject a manuscript (AMA, 2007), and authors should not take a rejection personally. In an excellent set of essays, the Editorial Board of the *Western Journal of Nursing Research* argues that rejection of manuscripts and grant applications should be "normalized" as an integral part of the scientific process. They detail the practical steps that one can use to manage one's feelings upon receipt of a rejection letter, including

EXHIBIT 15.4

Sample of a Rejection Letter

Ref: JRN-D-18-00452
Manuscript Title: Clergy–Laity Support and Patients' Mood During Serious Illness
Journal of Research Nurses

Dear Dr. Turnbull,

Thank you for submitting your manuscript to the *Journal of Research Nurses*. We have now completed the review of your manuscript. Based on the comments and concerns of the external reviewers, we cannot accept your manuscript for publication. As you will see, our reviewers felt that, while the paper addressed an issue that is clearly of importance, the manuscript topic will not likely meet the needs of our readership. Taken together, the reviewers' comments resulted in a priority score for your manuscript that did not reach the bar for acceptance. The manuscript may be a better fit with a palliative care or religion and health journal. We hope that you find the three reviews to be helpful in improving this paper, should you decide to send the paper elsewhere.

We hope this decision will not discourage you from submitting other work to us in the future. Thank you for letting us consider your work.

With best wishes,
Dr. Mary Jones
Dr. Frank Barton
Senior Editors of *Journal of Research Nurses*

recommendations for how to reframe, share, cope with, and ultimately accept the experience as highly beneficial to one's professional development (Conn et al., 2016).

There are many reasons a manuscript may not be suitable for a publication, and the feedback from the editor and reviewers gives the author information about why the paper was rejected. Many well-written papers are rejected because the content and focus do not reflect the needs of the readers, and the paper would be better suited for a different journal and audience. When the reasons for rejection relate to the quality of the writing and development of the content, the author should get editorial assistance in revising the paper and should ask colleagues to critique the content.

Arguments given by reviewers against publication of a manuscript occur when its content is incomplete, insufficiently focused on the journal's target audience, written as a thesis or class paper (J. D. Baker, 2014), or when unethical, outdated, or nonreplicable methodologies were used (DiDomenico et al., 2017). Journal editors work diligently to ensure that reviewers are knowledgeable, constructive, and specific in their suggestions (J. D. Baker, 2014; DiDomenico et al., 2017; Kapoor, 2016).

The author should evaluate the comments made by the editor and reviewers, for these may provide a basis for revising the paper and submitting it to another journal. It may be that the second or third journal is a better fit for the content and writing style, or these journals may have fewer submissions and accept more papers than did the first journal to which the paper was sent. In revising the paper and submitting it to a different journal, remember to reformat it to fit the new journal's requirements, including the reference format, writing style, page limits, and so forth, so it appears to be written for that journal.

This revision and resubmission process can be continued until the manuscript is accepted or the author determines that no further revisions are possible. The author might even try a nonrefereed journal or newsletter as an option for publication.

MANUSCRIPT REVISION

Authors should understand the review process. Few papers are accepted without some revision. Generally, manuscripts need to be revised whether they are accepted for publication, tentatively accepted pending revision, or need a major revision prior to resubmission. If the paper is not rejected, the author should revise it using the feedback from the editor and reviewers and resubmit it to the journal within the deadline specified by the editor.

Authors should adhere to this deadline because some editors may accept the manuscript when returned. If the modifications were substantial, the editor may elect to send it back to one or more of the previous reviewers. If the criticisms made by the reviewers were resolved, an acceptance decision is more likely.

Except for unqualified acceptances and rejections, all other editorial decisions following peer review are returned to the authors with feedback in the form of comments or suggestions. The comments may request minor or major changes to the manuscript (J. D. Baker, 2014). Minor changes may involve typographical errors, gaps in referencing, or requests for elaboration of background material or findings. When an author receives requests of a more substantive nature, it is highly recommended to put the manuscript aside before trying to digest what may appear at first receipt to be a highly negative review (Albarran & Dowling, 2017; W. L. Baker, DiDomenico, & Haines, 2017; Cook, 2016). After a period, sharing such reviews with a trusted group of colleagues allows for debate about how to interpret reviewer responses, what may have prompted them, and how to revise the manuscript in response to the comments in a way that preserves the essence of the manuscript and the voice of its authors. Such colleagues will likely have stories of their own experiences with major or negative reviews, how they reacted and responded, and to what end, which can provide mutual support. The comments from reviewers are intended as constructive criticism, and usually their questions point out areas needing revision. The author can respond by revising the paper as suggested or can provide a rationale as to why those changes are not appropriate.

Not all revisions have to be made in the paper, but the author should justify why changes were not made rather than sending the paper back without the suggested revisions. The author should indicate which revisions would not strengthen the paper and provide a rationale. "Slavish compliance with all recommendations of all reviewers may result in a manuscript that is difficult to comprehend, which is not the intent of the review process" (APA, 2010, p. 228). Sometimes the proposed revisions would not strengthen the paper, but they also might give the author a clue as to areas of the paper that are not clearly written or have missing information. It may be that the writing is unclear or there is another flaw in the presentation that created the problem for the reviewer. W. L. Baker et al. (2017) provides helpful tips for how to word a response when the author declines to make a requested change.

Letter to Send With Revision

In revising the paper, the author should prepare a letter to accompany the revised version of the paper that explains each revision suggested and made in the paper as well as changes not made and why. The letter should indicate:

- Each change proposed by the editor and reviewers
- The specific revisions made in response to each of these proposed changes
- The location of the revisions (e.g., the exact page number, paragraph, and sentence (or line) where the revision is located)
- Changes proposed but not made in the manuscript, with a rationale for those decisions

Exhibit 15.5 provides an example of a cover letter to submit with a revised manuscript; Exhibit 15.6 presents two alternatives for summarizing the changes suggested by the editor and reviewers and those made in response by the author. Both formats include an example of how to respond to a reviewer's suggestion that was not made in the revised version of the paper. Authors should refer to each change suggested by reviewers using the reviewer's number, for instance, Reviewer #1, so it is clear to the editor who had suggested the revision.

Conflicting Reviewer Comments

There are times when reviewers might give conflicting advice to authors (Albarran & Dowling, 2017; W. L. Baker et al., 2017; Conn, 2015). One reviewer may suggest expanding a content area whereas another recommends eliminating it. As a result, the author is unsure how to revise the paper to improve it. The first step is to reread the comments to confirm that they are conflicting. It may be that both reviewers identified the same problem in the text or graphics, even though their suggestions for revision are quite different. If the author is asked to expand a content area by one reviewer and to delete it by the other, it may be that the paper is not clearly written in that section; the conflicting comments suggest some problem with that area of content. If neither of the reviewers suggested a change that would solve a specific concern, the author should develop another approach that could be used.

Decision Not to Revise

There are times, however, in which authors cannot modify the paper sufficiently to reflect the concerns of the editor and reviewers. In these situations,

EXHIBIT 15.5

Example of a Cover Letter Sent in Response to Reviewer Comments

Dear Dr. Smith,

Thank you for your invitation to revise and resubmit Manuscript #2018-0074 Medication Safety Initiative in Intensive Care. We found the comments and suggestions from you and the reviewers helpful to us in strengthening and focusing the paper. Please see the changes made to the manuscript in response to each comment.

We appreciate your time and attention and hope you will find the manuscript improved and appropriate for publication. Please do not hesitate to contact us with any other concerns or questions. We look forward to hearing from you at your earliest convenience.

Sincerely,
Jane Doe, MSN, RN

EXHIBIT 15.6

Examples of Alternative Formats for Displaying Revisions Made by the Authors in Response to Comments and Suggestions by Editors and Reviewers

Example #1:

Outcomes of Using Admission and Discharge Nurses in Acute Care Settings

Revisions Proposed (page numbers refer to original manuscript)	Revisions Made (page numbers refer to revised manuscript)
Editor:	
Change first heading of Abstract to "Issues and Purpose" and include statement of issue that prompted research.	Heading revised and statement added (p. 2, paragraph 1).
Discuss rationale for factor analysis considering sample size of 75.	Factor analysis was done in the original study with 120 admission and discharge nurses throughout the health care system. Paragraph on factor analysis revised to clarify this (p. 10, paragraph 2, sentence 1).
Reviewer #1:	
Add "qualitative portion" to description of questionnaire in abstract (p. 2).	Sentence revised (p. 2): "Nurses ($n = 75$) completed a modified satisfaction questionnaire *that collected both quantitative and qualitative data.*"
On pp. 3–4, include edits on text.	Included as suggested.
On p. 5, include statement as to why nurses were concerned about initiative.	Sentence included on p. 5, paragraph 1, sentence 2.
On p. 7, line 4, add "as compared to nurses on other units."	Added (see p. 7, line 11).
(page numbers refer to original manuscript)	(page numbers refer to revised manuscript)
On p. 8 (and on p. 9, paragraph 3, line 1; p. 11, paragraph 1, line 1), were stress and challenge measured as separate variables? How did instrument collect qualitative data (also questioned on p. 10, paragraph 3, line 1, and on p. 15, line 3)?	Stress and challenge measured by individual Likert scales; 6 open-ended questions collected qualitative data. Description of instrument revised (p. 8, paragraph 2).

(continued)

EXHIBIT 15.6

On p. 8, Procedure: Were instruments anonymous?	Instruments were anonymous; no identifying information was collected. Added on p. 8, paragraph 1, line 3. Also added to text as recommended (p. 9, paragraph 2, line 3).
Add table with data.	Table 1 added (p. 19).
On p. 10, paragraph 2, last sentence: How did these findings compare with other groups in the study?	Consistent with original study of new role for nurses; added (p. 10, last sentence).
On p. 12, paragraph 2, line 2: Move M and SD to follow "staff."	Moved (p. 12, paragraph 2, line 4).
Reviewer #2:	
In abstract and on p. 11, only report P (not r).	Prefer to include the actual correlations with the p values. Rationale from *AMA Manual of Style* (10th ed.): Correlations should be reported with coefficient followed by significance, for example, $r = 0.61$, $P < .001$ (p. 541).
On p. 3, paragraph 2, line 7: Change patient to patients.	Done
(page numbers refer to original manuscript)	(page numbers refer to revised manuscript)
On p. 4, line 5: Add n.	$n = 75$; added (p. 4, paragraph 1, line 3).
On p. 4, paragraph 1, delete last sentence.	Deleted
On pp. 4–5: Move paragraph 2 to p. 5 and sentences on Klehamer et al. study (p. 5, lines 4–6) to p. 4.	Revisions made as suggested, with minor editing.
On p. 5, paragraph 2, lines 4 and 5: Were the goals the same as patterns found in ethnographic data analysis?	Author of article uses "goals."

(continued)

EXHIBIT 15.6

Examples of Alternative Formats for Displaying Revisions Made by the Authors in Response to Comments and Suggestions by Editors and Reviewers (continued)

On p. 6, paragraph 1: Change "area" to "theme."	"Area" changed to "theme."
On p. 6, paragraph 2 and 3: Consider moving these two paragraphs to earlier section of literature with other quantitative studies.	The first set of studies reported in literature review (pp. 4–5) relate to experiences of nurses with other new models of care. Research on p. 6 is on studies about admission and discharge. For this reason, literature review was not reorganized.
On p. 7, line 1, change "Several studies" to "The studies noted here."	Done
Results: Add table	Table 1 added (p. 19).
On p. 13, delete last two sentences.	Sentences deleted.
On p. 15, add sentence written on text.	Sentence added and all other editing done as recommended (p. 15, last paragraph).

EXAMPLE #2:

Parents' Views of Quality Health Care

Editorial Suggestions:

1. Add a table on demographic data, comparing the two groups: Table added (see p. 16, Table 1).
2. Include a list of pertinent websites: Added (see pp. 18–19).

Reviewer 1 Comments/Suggestions:

1. Weakness of study is lack of information about consumers: Findings added in text (see pp. 6–7, lines 12–16). Table added that presents demographic data (see p. 16, Table 1).
2. Add information on consumers, such as age, educational level, marital status, views of nursing care of children, and so on: Ages of consumers (see p. 7, lines 2–7); educational level (see pp. 6–7, lines 12–13, and p. 16, Table 1); marital status (see p. 7, lines 8–10, and p. 16, Table 1). Other demographic data presented on p. 7, lines 10–12. Views of nursing care of children are part of the Results.

(continued)

EXHIBIT 15.6

Examples of Alternative Formats for Displaying Revisions Made by the Authors in Response to Comments and Suggestions by Editors and Reviewers (continued)

3. Indicators not specific to care of children but, nevertheless, are general enough to provide information on perception of quality; investigator should have completed a pilot study: Paragraph on this limitation was rewritten (see p. 11, lines 3–4). Pilot study was completed but did not reveal this limitation (see p. 6, paragraph 1).

Reviewer 2 Questions/Suggestions:

1. How were subjects identified and accessed? Sentence added on p. 5, paragraph 2, sentence 3.
2. Did the study go through IRB? Yes, sentence added on p. 5 (line 8).
3. In terms of the Quality Health Care Questionnaire (QHCQ), is most of the literature used to identify indicators (for instrument) included in reference list of manuscript? If so, add statement to this effect: No, the literature used to identify indicators for the QHCQ is much more extensive than that reported in manuscript. For this reason, statement was not added.
4. Indicators and factors used interchangeably in this section: Differences between the indicators and factors are explained on pp. 5–6 (lines 9–11). No revisions were made in this section.

the author might send it to another journal or rewrite the paper for a different type of publication: for example, modifying a research report for submission to a clinical journal with more of an emphasis on patient care rather than the research itself, describing how the instrument was developed and validated, and preparing an integrated literature review for a publication. At some point, the author may need to abandon the attempt to publish the work.

In other situations, the author may decide not to take the time to revise the manuscript substantially in order to address the editor's and reviewers' concerns. This decision should be made carefully by weighing the alternatives of revising the paper for a journal with some interest in it versus sending it to another journal where there may be minimal interest in its content. If the author decides not to revise and return the manuscript, the editor should be notified so records can be kept up to date.

Time Frame for Decision

If the editor decides not to review the manuscript, the author will be notified of this decision within a few weeks. If the manuscript is sent to peer reviewers, the length of time varies widely for the reviewers to critique a manuscript, for the editor to compile and summarize the reviews, and for an editorial decision to be made. Many journals ask peer reviewers to complete their critiques within 3 weeks, but not everyone is able to meet this deadline. Reviewers have competing demands, and it sometimes takes longer than anticipated.

The earliest the author would be notified about the decision on whether to publish the manuscript is approximately 8 weeks after it is submitted to the journal. Some editors make their editorial decisions more quickly than others, but generally it takes at least 8 weeks to complete the review process and notify the author of the publication decision. If the author has not heard by 12 weeks, the author should contact the editor to inquire about the status of the review.

Length of Time to Publication

Journals vary in their backlogs of accepted manuscripts waiting to be published. Some journals have a backlog of a year or 2 while others may publish the manuscript 6 months after the final version is accepted. Journals are increasingly publishing papers electronically before print, either the final version of the manuscript as it will appear in print or prior versions so readers can follow the revisions of the paper. These papers are identified in MEDLINE as "[Epub ahead of print]," and journal subscribers can often access them at the journal website at no cost. Other readers can obtain these electronic versions similarly to print publications.

Honorarium

Most scientific journals do not reimburse the author when a manuscript is accepted for publication. Unlike magazines for consumers, which generally pay authors for an accepted paper, most nursing and healthcare journals do not give an honorarium.

Some journals provide complimentary copies of the issue in which the article appears as well as a specified number of hardcopy reprints. Reprints can usually be downloaded from the journal's website to members of subscriber organizations such as libraries. Reprints can also be purchased following publication through the publisher website.

SUMMARY

The primary responsibilities of the editor are to solicit manuscripts, work with authors to develop their ideas into manuscripts that are suitable for publication, assess the quality of manuscripts submitted to the journal, decide on manuscripts to publish based on recommendations from the reviewers, edit manuscripts, and complete other tasks to prepare them for publication. Editors work with authors, editorial board members, manuscript reviewers, the production editor, and other personnel associated with publishing the journal.

In addition to these roles, some journals also have a managing editor who is a paid professional responsible for the administrative details associated with processing the manuscripts from submission through publication.

Journals rely on external or peer reviewers, sometimes called referees, to read and critically judge the manuscripts submitted to the journal. Peer reviewers are experts in the topic of the manuscript; they are considered "peers" of the author because they have similar expertise, allowing them to critique the paper. Peer reviewers give expert opinions about the manuscript and make recommendations to the editor concerning its acceptance.

Many peer-reviewed journals use a process of blind review in which submitted manuscripts are sent to reviewers with the identity of the author and institution concealed. The editor conceals identifying information that might identify the author and institution with which affiliated. The principle behind sending a "blinded" copy, free of identifying information, is that there is less chance of bias.

Reviewers also are unknown to the author. When reviews are returned to the author, the identities of the reviewers are masked so the author does not know who read the paper. With this anonymity, reviewers are free to evaluate a paper honestly and without fear of repercussions from the author if they give a negative review. It is believed that these reviews are fairer.

When the manuscript is submitted to the journal, it is given a number that is used throughout the review process to track the manuscript. Not all manuscripts are sent out for review. If the manuscript is not relevant for the journal, the editor will likely return the manuscript to the author without its being reviewed. The second reason a manuscript may be returned to the author rather than being reviewed is when it is incomplete or does not conform to the journal requirements.

After the editor determines the suitability of the manuscript for the journal, the review process begins. The editor decides who should review the manuscript based on who has the expertise to evaluate the manuscript. Usually at least two reviews are completed of each paper. The results of the peer review are then sent to the author with the editorial decision on whether the paper is accepted, should be revised and resubmitted, or is rejected. The reviews provide data for the editor to use in making an acceptance decision and feedback for authors in revising the paper to strengthen it.

The criteria used by editors to decide whether to accept a manuscript vary by journal, but there are some general criteria most editors use in making this decision: (a) relevance of the paper for the journal, (b) importance of the content, (c) if the content is new and innovative, (d) validity of evidence to support the conclusions of the paper, (e) usefulness to the journal considering other topics published in it, and (f) the number of papers on the same or similar topics that have already been accepted.

There are three main types of decisions that can be made by the editor based on his or her own review and suggestions from reviewers: (a) accept for publication, (b) revise and resubmit, and (c) reject. Accept-for-publication decisions may involve an acceptance with no revisions or limited ones, or a tentative acceptance pending revision. An acceptance without revisions is rare; even if the paper is accepted for publication, because of its important and timely content, it is likely that the author will need to make some changes to strengthen it. Other acceptances are provisional, with the final decision resting on whether the author revises the manuscript to reflect the changes suggested by the editor and reviewers.

The second type of decision is to revise and resubmit for another review. When authors are asked to revise and resubmit the manuscript, it suggests that the paper has merit and would be strengthened by a revision. The third editorial decision is a rejection.

A good review suggests changes that the author should consider. The author can respond by revising the paper as suggested or can provide a rationale as to why those changes are not appropriate. Not all suggestions have to be made in the paper, but the author should justify why changes were not made rather than sending back the paper without the suggested revisions. The author should prepare a letter to accompany the revised version of the paper that explains each revision suggested and made in the paper as well as changes not made and why.

When the manuscript is accepted for publication, the paper moves into the next phase. The author has some responsibilities here, such as answering queries and correcting page proofs, but the publisher completes most of the work performed at this stage.

REFERENCES

Albarran, J., & Dowling, S. (2017). Getting published: A practical guide—Part II. *British Journal of Cardiac Nursing, 12*, 274–279. doi:10.12968/bjca.2017.12.6.274

American Medical Association. (2007). *AMA manual of style: A guide for authors and editors* (10th ed.). New York, NY: Oxford University Press.

American Psychological Association. (2010). *Publication manual of the American Psychological Association* (6th ed.). Washington, DC: Author.

Baker, J. D. (2014). Artistry of peer review. *Association of periOperative Registered Nurses (AORN) Journal, 101*, 4–11. doi:10.1016/j.aorn.2014.10.020

Baker, W. L., DiDomenico, R. J., & Haines, S. T. (2017). Improving peer review: What authors can do. *American Journal of Health-System Pharmacy, 74*, 2076–2079. doi:10.2146/ajhp170187

Committee on Publication Ethics. (2018). About COPE. Retrieved from http://publicationethics .org/about

Conn, V. S. (2015). Close but not quite: How to get to the publication goal. *Western Journal of Nursing Research, 37*, 1379–1382. doi:10.1177/0193945914531697

Conn, V. S., Zerwic, J., Jefferson, U., Anderson, C. M., Killion, C. M., Smith, C. E., . . . Loya, L. (2016). Normalizing rejection. *Western Journal of Nursing Research, 38*, 137–154. doi:10.1177/0193945915589538

Cook, D. A. (2016). Twelve tips for getting your manuscript published. *Medical Teacher, 38*, 41–50. doi:10.3109/0142159X.2015.1074989

Csiszar, A. (2016). Peer review: Troubled from the start. *Nature, 532*, 306–308. doi:10.1038/532306a

DiDomenico, R. J., Baker, W. L., & Haines, S. T. (2017). Improving peer review: What reviewers can do. *American Journal of Health-System Pharmacy, 74*, 2080–2084. doi:10.2146/ajhp170190

Gallagher, A. (2013). The ethics of reviewing. *Nursing Ethics, 20,* 735–736. doi:10.1177/0969733013506646

International Committee of Medical Journal Editors. (2017). *Recommendations for the conduct, reporting, editing, and publication of scholarly work in medical journals.* Retrieved from http://www.icmje.org/urm_main.html

Kapoor, P. M. (2016). Editor's importunate role towards medical journalism in 2016—Way to go! *Annals of Cardiac Anaesthesia, 19,* 1–3. doi:10.4103/0971-9784.173012

Tomkins, A., Zhang, M., & Heavlin, W. D. (2017). Reviewer bias in single-versus double-blind peer review. *Proceedings of the National Academy of Science (PNAS), 114,* 12708–12713. doi:10.1073/pnas.1707323114

World Health Organization. (2018). Top 10 reasons for rejecting a manuscript. Retrieved from http://www.who.int/bulletin/contributors/rejection/en

PUBLISHING PROCESS

When the manuscript is accepted for publication, the paper moves into the publishing phase. The author has some responsibilities here, such as answering queries and correcting page proofs, but most of the work is done by the publisher of the journal or by the group or individual responsible for the publication. The manuscript is edited for clarity and consistency with the journal style and format; the copy editor more than likely will have questions about the manuscript for the author to answer. These questions, or queries, must be answered and the proofs must be reviewed, to confirm the accuracy of the content after editing and to check other details, in the time frame allowed.

This chapter describes the publishing process that begins with the acceptance of the paper and continues through its publication. In general, publishers engage in three key functions: editing, producing, and marketing the journal (Orchard, Jackson, & Bishop, 2016). Publishers have different ways of handling the manuscript editing phase and forms of the manuscript that they return to the author for proofing. The publishing process is described in this chapter, but the author should recognize that it may differ across journals. When the paper is published by an organization or individual, the process may vary from what is described in this chapter.

WHAT HAPPENS NEXT?

The time from acceptance of the paper to its publication varies with the journal, depending on that journal's backlog and other factors such as the relationship of the topic to others waiting to be published, the focus of a particular issue, and other editorial priorities. It could take a few months to a year or longer before the paper is published. When the editor decides on the issue in which the paper will appear, the author is notified of this and when to expect the proofs to review. The manuscript is edited first by a copy editor, who formats the manuscript to be consistent with the journal style, corrects grammatical errors, and edits the paper. The copy editor works for the publisher, not the author, and will not rewrite the manuscript; authors who need help with writing should get editorial assistance before they submit the paper to the journal.

The author receives proofs of the edited manuscript, which are in portable document format (PDF). These proofs are formatted as pages in the journal but will have queries for the author to check (Figure 16.1).

In this stage of publication, the author reviews the proofs, answers questions raised by the copy editor, corrects any errors in the paper as a result of the editing or formatting, and checks other details such as word divisions, accuracy of tables, and accuracy of author information. Even though the author reviewed the manuscript thoroughly prior to sending the final version, the paper has since been edited by journal staff, so the author needs to verify that the changes made during editing did not alter

was the only domain in which the score was lower postimplementation than preimplementation. The other domain percentages all increased. All but one HCAHPS domain demonstrated increases in the percentage of "always," "yes," and "9 and 10" responses during the project period, which was consistent with the evidence.

The rate of patient falls on the project unit decreased prior to implementation of structured hourly nurse rounding possibly due to a reemphasis on the Fall Prevention Program in the nursing department. When comparing falls rates from similar time periods, it appeared there was a decline in fall rates, although the trend began to decline prior to project implementation. Historically, fall rates had been highest in the October to December time period. That usual pattern did not recur during the project implementation (Figure). A reduction of 11 fall incidences between the pre- and postimplementation period reflected a cost avoidance of $46 563 ($4322 × 11) for the project implementation period.[33]

The reduction in the rate of patient falls, when comparing analogous yearly time periods, was similar to reports from other projects and studies documented in the literature. While the decline in fall rates during implementation was modest compared with preceding quarters, it was clinically significant for the winter quarter especially considering historic data and case-mix indices. Both Bourgault et al[16] and Krepper et al[21] noted no effect in patient falls with implementation of rounding following preexisting robust fall prevention programs and low rates of patient falls prior to implementation.

[AQ2]
[AQ3]

HAPU rates per 1000 patient-days had also declined in the 6 months prior to implementation on the project unit. However, a reduction of 4 HAPUs comparing pre- and postimplementation resulted in a cost avoidance of $172 720 ($43 180 × 4).[33] This reduction in HAPU rate was similar to results reported by Ellis,[19] Sherrod et al,[24] and the Studer Group.[2]

[AQ4]
[AQ5]

Limitations

This project was implemented on 1 medical-surgical unit in 1 hospital. In addition, 3 months is a short period of time to evaluate a change in nursing workflow or cultural adoption of this intervention for sustainability.

CONCLUSIONS

Change management strategies were used to influence the culture of nursing practice, so changes were not be perceived as simply additional tasks to complete. Recommendations for project sustainability include incorporating unit-based rounding champions to continue to stimulate enthusiasm and prioritize discussions so that the initial improvement changes do not drift. Periodic monitoring and public display of the data stimulate continual focus on the results of this intervention.

Evidence indicates that structured hourly nurse rounds are safe, efficient, and useful in today's practice. Performing hourly nurse rounding may be cost-effective as an intervention because it promotes cost avoidance by reducing injuries related to patient falls and pressure ulcer formation, both of which may extend hospital length of stays. The corpus of evidence suggested that structured nurse rounding demonstrated favorable trends in improving patient satisfaction and reducing patient falls, HAPUs, and call light usage. This project demonstrated overall improvement in patient satisfaction indicators and decreased patient harm through lower patient fall and HAPU rates. Reduced patient harm contributed more than $200 000 in cost avoidance of care that is not reimbursed to organizations.

FIGURE 16.1 Sample proof of journal page.

Source: From Brosey, L., & March, K. S. (2015). Effectiveness of structured hourly nurse rounding on patient satisfaction and clinical outcomes. *Journal of Nursing Care Quality, 30,* 153–159. Reprinted by permission of Wolters Kluwer Health, 2018.

the intended meaning. This is the last chance for the author to find errors in the paper prior to its publication.

Authors need to read the proofs carefully because copy editors are not nurses, and they do not have expertise in the topic; the copy editor may have altered the meaning of a sentence when grammatical errors were corrected or the paper was formatted for consistency with the journal style. In this process of editing the paper, some of the meaning may have been changed, and errors in the content may have resulted. The author is responsible for identifying these when reviewing the proofs. Authors should check carefully their tables and figures because they will be modified to conform to the journal style and formatting, and errors may have occurred as a result of this process.

There is generally a limited period of time—for some journals only 48 hours—for the author to read and correct the proofs of the manuscript. The author should adhere to this time frame. Otherwise, the article may be printed as is with any errors present. Generally, authors are emailed a link for them to access the proofs of their paper (for example, at the journal submission website), or the PDF may be emailed to them. Authors should notify the editor if there is a change in email address or if an alternate one should be used for emailing the proofs. When registering at the journal website, it is a good idea to include a backup email address; then the proofs and other correspondence will be sent to both email addresses.

Formats for Author Review

With chapters and books, authors may be emailed the edited version of the manuscript that shows the corrections made in the paper, or they will be emailed the proof pages of the chapters, which are in PDF format, and look like the final chapters will look in the book. The edited manuscript displays the original text and each revision using track changes such as in Microsoft Word or a similar program. The author should read the edited version carefully, noting any errors or revisions that are needed, because few changes can be made in the proof stage. With some edited books, the copyedited chapters or proofs are emailed to the editor rather than the individual author(s) of the chapter, and only the editor reviews them. Alternately, the copyedited chapters or proofs will be reviewed by the authors themselves and then sent to the editor to return to the production manager. With journals, however, as mentioned earlier, the author receives the edited paper in the form of proofs that incorporate the copy editor's revisions.

Proofing the Manuscript

Authors review the edited version or proofs of their chapter or journal article for two purposes: to check for errors and answer queries about it. For chapters and books, authors can use the track changes function to indicate additional revisions or modify ones made by the copy editor and can insert notes in the edited version of the text. Authors should alter the color used in track changes to a different one from the edited version; that way the author's revisions of the edited manuscript will be apparent to the copy editor.

For proofs of articles, and also of chapters, the author cannot rewrite the text except for what is necessary to correct an error. The paper was accepted as submitted in the final version, following peer review, and the author cannot rewrite it at this stage. If the content has changed since the paper was accepted, this should be discussed with the editor rather than modifying the proofs, as changes at this point in the publishing process are expensive for the publisher. Authors can print the proofs, answer queries, and note revisions in the margins and on the PDF pages. Another way is to indicate the revisions and answer the queries on the PDF pages using the Comments function, which allows authors to insert and delete text and answer queries in notes to the editor. The marked-up proofs with answers to the queries can then be emailed to the production editor or uploaded at the journal submission website.

Some journals publish papers electronically ahead of print. These articles are available on the publisher's website prior to the publication in the journal. When papers are published ahead of print, their citations are listed in PubMed as "[epub ahead of print]." These variations of the publishing process are described for authors on the journal website or in the author information page.

Answering Queries

The author must answer each query raised by the copy editor. Often this is done easily by checking a revision, inserting text, modifying a reference, and revising the table or text so they are consistent. Some queries require an explanation, which the author can add in the margin or as a note to the editor in the PDF file. If unable to answer a question, this should be noted.

Areas to Proof

What should the author check when reviewing the proofs? First, the main goal is to ensure that there are no errors in the content. There are times when a minor editorial revision changes the meaning of the sentence, and this is the author's only chance to correct the paper prior to publication. The author should confirm that the content is accurate; the changes made by the copy editor did not alter the meaning; nothing was omitted from the paper that is essential; and the correct numbers are in the text, tables, and illustrations. In proofreading the paper, the author should compare the original copy submitted against the proofs.

Second, the author should check for spelling and grammatical errors. Even though this was done in preparing the final version, a misspelled word might not have been noticed, and words correctly spelled might have been used incorrectly, such as rational for rationale. The spelling of authors' names, their credentials, their positions, and the contact information of the corresponding author should be verified. The author should check the title of the article and spelling of words in it.

The author also should pay attention to how words are divided. In aligning the right margin of the text, some words may have to be divided. The author should check that these divisions of words are correct and make sense. If not, authors can add a note for the editor to check a "bad break" in a term.

Third, the author should review the abbreviations, numerical values in the text and tables, statistical results, references, tables, and figures. Errors may have occurred when these were formatted for the style of the journal. For research articles, the author should verify that the numbers used to report the findings are the same in the abstract, text, tables, and figures, and that no data are missing. The author should check carefully numbers with decimals, P values, and statistics. The copy editor may have made changes in how the statistics are presented to conform to the journal's style, and the author needs to review these for any errors.

The names of authors cited in the text should be compared with the reference list. If numbers are used for the citations, these should match the correct reference.

For some journals, tables require substantial reformatting; for this reason, tables in the proofs should be checked carefully. Each column and row should be examined, paying attention to whether the numbers are accurate and aligned properly. Notes on the original copy may be changed to the symbols used by the journal; the author should verify that these are correct. The proofs of figures such as flowcharts, guidelines, and other illustrations should be examined carefully to ensure that they are clear and can be read when published in the journal. Titles of the tables and figures also should be reviewed.

Exhibit 16.1 is a checklist authors can use when reading proofs. Authors should not take this step lightly, because the author is responsible for identifying and correcting errors before the paper is printed.

Citing In-Press Papers

Manuscripts accepted for publication by the journal can be cited as "in press" (American Medical Association [AMA], 2007; American Psychological Association [APA], 2010). Some publications require authors to verify that the paper has been accepted (AMA, 2007). Manuscripts that have been submitted to journals and are in review cannot be listed with the references. Instead, the

EXHIBIT 16.1

Proofing Checklist

Use this checklist to review your manuscript before submitting it for publication and again to check the proofs.

Check

- That the author information is accurate and all coauthor names are spelled correctly
- That all content is accurate, including any numbers, medication names and dosages, names of instruments and measures, statistical symbols and results, information in the tables and figures, and other content
- Line by line for grammatical, punctuation, and other errors
- That acronyms are spelled out the first time cited in the paper and that only the acronym is used from that point on
- That all author names cited in the paper have a reference to the source
- That citations and references are accurate and formatted per journal style
- That the level of headings is correct based on how the content is organized and per journal style
- That each table, figure, and other illustration is correct
- That individuals and hospitals cited in the acknowledgment, text, or elsewhere in the paper have given written permission, which was sent to the editor
- That written permission for using or adapting copyrighted material was received and the appropriate credit line was added

author should cite the work in the text as "unpublished data" or an "unpublished paper." For example:

> Similar findings have been reported in a rural health clinic
> (J. A. Smith, DNP, unpublished data, June 2014).

If the "in press" paper is published by the time the author receives the proofs in which it was cited, the proofs can be updated; similarly, if a submitted manuscript is accepted, the proofs can be changed to "in press."

Ordering Reprints

After reviewing and correcting the proofs, the author has some assurance that the manuscript will be printed without errors and in the issue indicated by the editor. A form for ordering reprints is usually available at the time the author receives the proofs. If the author is interested in having reprints to distribute to colleagues, students, and others, they should be ordered when the proofs are reviewed or whenever the author receives the information about reprints. After the journal is published, reprints may be more expensive or may not be available. Thus, authors should decide early if they want reprints. Generally, the more reprints that are ordered, the less expensive they are for the author.

After the article is published, the author will receive a limited number of complimentary copies of the journal or a final PDF of the paper, depending on the publisher. Complimentary copies are not mailed to coauthors; the corresponding author is responsible for distributing copies to them.

CORRECTIONS AND RETRACTIONS

If the author discovers after an article is published that there were errors in the data reported or the conclusions reached, the author should contact the editor and email a letter correcting the information. A correction or erratum of part of the work will be published in a later issue of the journal. The corrections will appear on an electronic or numbered print page and be listed in the table of contents to ensure proper indexing (International Committee of Medical Journal Editors [ICMJE], 2017). The ICMJE recommends that the journal post the new version of the article with details about the changes, including the relevant date.

If there is scientific fraud, however, the paper should be retracted (ICMJE, 2017). The author should submit a letter, signed by coauthors, to the editor requesting a retraction and indicating the reasons. The retraction will be published in a subsequent issue of the journal. If the paper is not yet published, the editor more than likely will allow the author to withdraw it. Along the same line, if the author determines later that a coauthor published the same data in another paper, without indicating this in the current article, a letter is sent to the editor, who will note this as a repetitive publication. If issues about the conduct of the research or questions are raised about the integrity of the work described in the article, the ICMJE recommends that the editor follow the guidelines of the Committee on Publication Ethics (COPE; publicationethics .org/resources/flowcharts) or a similar body.

COPYRIGHT

Copyright is a form of legal protection to the authors of "original works of authorship," including literary, dramatic, musical, artistic, and other intellectual works, preventing others from copying them (U.S. Copyright Office, 2017). U.S. copyright law is defined by the Copyright Act of 1976. Copyright provides protection for any original material created by the author, including both published and unpublished works. Coauthors of papers written collaboratively have equal rights to the copyright.

The copyright law gives authors, or whomever holds the copyright, six exclusive rights: (a) to reproduce the work, (b) to prepare derivative works, (c) to distribute copies of the work to the public, (d) to perform the work publicly, (e) to display it, and (f) for sound recordings to perform the work by means of digital audio transmission (U.S. Copyright Office, 2017, p. 2). The owner of the copyright is the only person allowed to exercise these rights;

anyone else who wants to reproduce, modify, publish, perform, or display the work must get permission from the copyright owner.

Protected Works

Copyright protects original works "that are fixed in a tangible form of expression" (U.S. Copyright Office, 2017, p. 3). These protected works are listed here.

1. Literary works (e.g., articles, books, journals, software, and digital formats)
2. Musical works, including the accompanying words
3. Dramatic works, including the accompanying music
4. Pantomimes and choreographic works
5. Pictorial, graphic, and sculptural works
6. Motion pictures and other audiovisual works
7. Sound recordings
8. Architectural works (U.S. Copyright Office, 2017, p. 1)

For works created from 1978 to the present, the term of protection for copyright is the life of the author plus 70 years. For works created between 1964 and 1977, the protection for copyright is 28 years for the original term plus an automatic 67-year renewal; for materials created between 1923 and 1963, the protection extends for the original 28-year term with an additional 67 years if the copyright was renewed. Works created before 1923 are in the public domain.

Unprotected Works

Several categories of materials, though, are not protected by copyright. These include, among others:

- Ideas, procedures, methods, systems, processes, concepts, principles, or discoveries
- Works that have not been fixed in a tangible form of expression, such as speeches or performances that have not been notated, written down, or recorded
- Titles, names, short phrases, and slogans
- Familiar symbols or designs
- Mere variations of typographic ornamentation, lettering, or coloring
- Mere listings of ingredients or content (U.S. Copyright Office, 2017, p. 2)

U.S. Copyright Office

Information about copyright, frequently requested circulars, copyright application forms, and related materials are available to authors through the U.S.

Copyright Office on its website (www.copyright.gov), as well as by email from that website, by telephone, and at the following address:

Library of Congress
U.S. Copyright Office
Publications Section
101 Independence Avenue, SE #6304
Washington, DC 20559-6304

Transfer of Copyright

The copyright is held initially by the author, or coauthors, of the manuscript. When a manuscript is being considered for publication by a journal, each author contributing to the paper typically transfers the copyright to the publisher either at the time the manuscript is submitted or when it is accepted, unless the journal is open access, as described in Chapter 17. Publishers usually require assignment of the copyright to them so that they in turn may publish the article and distribute it in different forms. If the copyright transfer form is submitted with the manuscript, prior to its acceptance by the journal, the copyright reverts to the author, or coauthors, if the manuscript is not published.

Publishers have their own copyright transfer forms that are signed by each author. When the copyright is transferred, the publisher becomes the legal owner of the published paper (Nicoll, 2016). Neither the author nor others may reproduce the paper without written approval of the copyright holder—the publisher. Authors who want to reproduce any figure, table, or text from the copyrighted material must receive permission from the copyright holder. This is true even for the author's own article because the copyright was transferred to and is then held by the publisher. The situation is different, however, for open-access journals.

This is an important principle for all manuscripts but especially for papers that include forms, tools, and other materials from clinical agencies, schools of nursing, and other institutions. The institution must grant permission for authors to include the material with their manuscripts; the credit line should indicate that the materials were reprinted by permission of that institution; and a statement should be added that the institution retains the copyright to them. Otherwise the form, tool, guideline, or other document in the manuscript will be included in the transfer of the copyright to the publisher, and the institution will no longer be able to use it without the publisher's permission. Authors should check with the journal editor about how best to handle materials such as these in a manuscript.

Copying and Reproducing Copyrighted Material

The fair use provisions of the copyright law, contained in Title 17 of the United States Code, Section 107, allow the author to quote, copy, or reproduce a small amount of text from a copyrighted work without permission of the publisher or other holder of the copyright (U.S. Copyright Office, 2016). Fair use of copyrighted materials for purposes such as teaching, scholarship, and research, among others, is not considered an infringement of copyright. If it is more than a small section of copyrighted work, though, the author needs to get written permission from the copyright holder to use the material. Fair use does not give authors permission to reproduce complete articles nor to republish an article they wrote in a different journal.

In determining fair use, four factors are considered:

1. Purpose of the use, including whether it is for commercial purposes or for nonprofit educational purposes
2. The nature of the copyrighted work
3. The amount of the material copied and how substantial it is in relation to the copyrighted work as a whole
4. The effect of the use on the potential market for or value of the copyrighted work (U.S. Copyright Office, 2016, p. 19)

The amount of text subject to fair use is based on the proportion to the whole, but this proportion is not determined by number of words (AMA, 2007). There is no specific word length in the copyright law that is acceptable. For this reason, the author needs to consider the preceding four factors when questioning whether permission should be obtained from the copyright holder. Some publishers may specify the number of words that are allowed to be reproduced without written permission. For example, the APA provides guidelines for authors as to the extent of text and number of tables and figures published in an APA journal that may be reproduced without written permission from the journal (APA, 2010).

The author should be careful to include the reference to the original source. Any direct quotes should be placed in quotation marks, or indented to set off the quoted material, again with a reference to the original source.

Permission should be obtained for quotes that extend for a few paragraphs. The length of the quoted material should not diminish the "value of the original work" (AMA, 2007, p. 198). Entire tables, figures, and illustrations may not be reproduced without permission. This includes use of a table, figure, or other type of graphic in a paper prepared for a course. Using one or two sentences from a table is acceptable if the original source is referenced, but reprinting the entire table is not. As discussed earlier, authors should obtain permission to adapt and reproduce tables, figures, and illustrations for a manuscript and for other types of writing projects.

The decision to reproduce text, tables, figures, and other illustrations in a paper is made early in the writing process. Authors need to allow sufficient time to receive these permissions to avoid delays in the submission and later publication of the manuscript. Although a paper can be submitted for review pending the permissions to reprint, it cannot be published without them. How to obtain permissions was described in Chapter 4; that chapter also included sample letters and credit lines. It is best for authors to have these permissions in hand prior to submitting the manuscript because if permission is denied or not received in time for publication, the paper will have to be rewritten to avoid the use of the quoted material, table, figure, and other illustration. For some manuscripts, this might require a significant amount of revision. Editors will likely ask authors for the permission from the copyright holder to reproduce the material.

Materials on the Internet and in Electronic Format

These same principles apply for materials published on the Internet and in electronic format. Works published on the Internet are not automatically in the public domain, and it cannot be assumed that they can be used in a manuscript. The fair use considerations identified earlier apply to websites, electronic documents, and digital works such as photographs, slides, and audio and video files. These materials are protected under copyright law and cannot be used in a publication without permission from the copyright holder (AMA, 2007). If there is any question about whether permission is needed, authors should seek permission to reproduce materials they did not develop themselves.

SUMMARY

The publication stage provides an opportunity for the author to review the proofs of publications, answer questions raised by the copy editor, correct any errors in the proofs as a result of the editing or formatting, and check other details, such as accuracy of tables and author information. Even though the author reviewed the manuscript thoroughly before submitting the final copy, the paper has since been edited, so the author needs to verify that the changes made during editing did not alter the intended meaning. This is the last chance for the author to find errors in the paper prior to its publication. There also may be questions or queries about the text, references, or tables and figures that the author needs to answer.

There is generally a limited period of time for the author to read and correct the proofs of the manuscript, and the author should adhere to this time frame. Otherwise the article may be printed as is with errors present. Authors should notify the editor if there is a change in the email address for receiving the proofs or make this change at the journal website.

With chapters and books, the author or book editor may be sent electronically the edited version of the manuscript that shows the corrections or the proofs (in PDF format) to check. With journals, the author receives the proofs of the article.

The proofs are sent to the author to identify errors, not for rewriting. After correcting them, the author has some assurance that the manuscript will be printed without errors. When the article is published, the author receives either complimentary copies of the journal or a PDF of the paper.

Copyright is a form of legal protection for the authors of "original works of authorship." Authors own their manuscripts until they sign a copyright transfer, which then transfers the ownership to the publisher. This then gives the publisher the right to reproduce, modify, publish, perform, and publicly display the work. Authors who want to reproduce any figure, table, or text from the copyrighted material must receive permission from the copyright holder. This is true even for the author's own article because the copyright was transferred to and is then held by the publisher. This process varies, however, with open-access journals, discussed in Chapter 17.

REFERENCES

American Medical Association. (2007). *AMA manual of style: A guide for authors and editors* (10th ed.). New York, NY: Oxford University Press.

American Psychological Association. (2010). *Publication manual of the American Psychological Association* (6th ed.). Washington, DC: Author.

Brosey, L., & March, K. S. (2015). Effectiveness of structured hourly nurse rounding on patient satisfaction and clinical outcomes. *Journal of Nursing Care Quality, 30*, 153–159. doi: 10.1097/NCQ.0000000000000086

International Committee of Medical Journal Editors. (2017). Recommendations for the conduct, reporting, editing, and publication of scholarly work in medical journals. Retrieved from http://www.icmje.org/urm_main.html

Nicoll, L. H. (2016). A primer on the copyright transfer form. *Nurse Author & Editor, 26*(3), 5. Retrieved from http://naepub.com/publishing/2016-26-3-5

Orchard, L., Jackson, C., & Bishop, P. (2016). Behind the scenes of JAC: The publisher's role. *Journal of Antimicrobial Chemotherapy, 71*, 3321–3326. doi:10.1093/jac/dkw413

U.S. Copyright Office. (2016). *Copyright law of the United States and related laws contained in Title 17 of the United States Code. Circular 92*. Washington, DC: U.S. Copyright Office, Library of Congress. Retrieved from https://www.copyright.gov/title17/title17.pdf

U.S. Copyright Office. (2017). *Copyright basics*. Retrieved from http://www.copyright.gov/circs/circ01.pdf

OPEN ACCESS AND AVOIDING PREDATORY JOURNALS

Communication among and between scholars and clinicians can be both informal and formal, unpublished and published. Some informal types of scholarly communication include personal communication and email. Some formal types include presentations at conferences and articles in peer-reviewed journals, for which the scholarly publishing industry is largely responsible. This industry includes commercial publishers such as Springer Publishing, Elsevier, and Wiley, but it also includes nonprofit scholarly societies, such as Sigma, which publishes books, scholarly journals, and an online newsletter.

The advent of the Internet in the 1990s greatly changed many information-based industries and practices, and scholarly communication is no exception. Years ago journals and books were available only in print form, but now both are published in print and electronic formats, and some are online only. Nurses and other health professionals need to keep abreast of changes in scholarly communication, selecting the best models and practices for disseminating, communicating, and promoting the results of their research and practice changes.

TRADITIONAL MODEL

A few online journals preceded the appearance of the World Wide Web, but for the most part, electronic journals started to appear in the late 1990s and early 2000s. As e-journals became immediately popular, publishers had to deal with what was called "flipping their model"; this meant changing from being a print journal that also offered an online version to an online journal that offered an optional print version. Then, after making this change, the question for some publishers became when to eliminate their print versions altogether. Most scholarly journals are now published online as well as in print, but many readers still prefer the print version of the journal and to print out individual articles.

In the third edition, this chapter was written by Jeffrey Beall.

Despite being published online, traditional journals are generally not open access. Traditional journals by definition use the subscription model, requiring libraries or individuals to subscribe to the journal to access the content. *Scholarly open-access content* refers to scholarly content that is freely available to everyone via the Internet. One innovation to the subscription model that the Internet has enabled is the ability to access articles individually, paying a one-time fee for an article instead of having to subscribe to all issues of the journal. In the print-only world, the option to purchase individual articles was rarely offered, was difficult to arrange, or was expensive.

THE OPEN-ACCESS MOVEMENT

In the early 2000s, several meetings were held around the world to organize what has become known as the open-access movement. Organizers sought to create alternative distribution models for scholarly journals, because the subscription model had become too expensive for many libraries, forcing them in many cases to cancel subscriptions. The goals of the open-access movement have been twofold. The first was to make scholarly content freely available over the Internet, and the second was to promote the use of free licenses for open-access content, enabling the free copying and even redistribution of scholarly papers on the Internet by anyone.

Open-Access Distribution Models

Open-access articles are freely available on the Internet: they do not require users to pay a subscription to a journal or to pay a fee to access an article. The definition of *open access* has expanded over time. Some consider open access to mean that access to the content is free and in a repository; others would expand this definition to include the immediate deposit of content; and still others add specifics about the type of Creative Commons license required (Anderson, 2017b).

Several models are in place for distributing scholarly content published using the open-access model, and these are often designated by the colors gold, platinum, and green (Exhibit 17.1). The predominant open-access model is *gold open access*. In this model, authors are charged a fee upon acceptance of a paper in a scholarly journal. The fee, referred to as an *article processing charge* or APC, supports the publishing process and expenses. These fees can range from a low of $200 to more than $5,000, especially in top journals. For researchers performing grant-funded research, money to pay the APCs can be taken from grant funds, but this ultimately means that less of the allocated grant money can be devoted to the actual research. In other cases, organizations may cover the costs of the APC. Increasingly, universities or academic libraries have funds that faculty can use to pay the APC.

The *platinum open-access* model is similar to the gold model, with the difference being that no fees are charged to the author. Thus, this model represents true open access, free to both authors and readers. In platinum open access, the

EXHIBIT 17.1

Open-Access Models

Gold: Authors are charged a fee on acceptance of paper. Fee is called an article processing charge or APC. Fees can range from $200 to more than $5,000.

Platinum: Similar to the gold model, but no fees are charged to the author. This model represents true open access, free to both authors and readers. Publishing costs are generally covered by publisher itself, and in most cases publishers are nonprofit organizations.

Green: Involves authors archiving postprints of their articles in open-access repositories. Postprints are final Word versions of manuscripts after all recommended changes from peer review have been incorporated (i.e., final copy the author sends to publisher).

Hybrid: Traditional subscription journals offer authors of accepted articles an option to pay for their article to be open access.

publishing costs are generally covered by the publishing company itself, and in most cases the publishers are nonprofit organizations.

The *green open-access* model involves authors archiving postprints of their articles in open-access repositories. *Postprints* are the final Word version of a scholarly manuscript after all the recommended changes from peer review have been incorporated—in other words, it is the final copy the author submits to the publisher. Open-access repositories include those set up by universities (either individually or in groups) and within specific disciplines. PubMed Central (PMC) is a repository for journal articles in biomedical and life sciences prior to their final publication (U.S. National Library of Medicine, 2015). Articles are deposited by participating journals or authors to be in compliance with the public-access policies of funding bodies such as the U.S. National Institutes of Health. PMC does not publish journal articles but provides public access to them. The green open-access model is a way to make the text of articles published in subscription journals available freely on the Internet. Authors submit papers to a subscription journal but make the postprint open access via an online repository.

Authors also should be aware of the hybrid model. This model, sometimes called *hybrid open access*, involves subscription journals that offer an open-access option at the individual article level. When a paper is accepted for publication in a traditional subscription journal, authors have an option to make their papers open access by paying the APC. If the author is not interested in this option, the paper will be published in the journal at no cost to the author.

Advantages and Disadvantages of Open Access

It helps to examine scholarly content in the context of consumers and producers. Consumers (or readers) of scholarly content include most nurses, students, and faculty. For these consumers, the advantages of open access are many. Open access completely eliminates price barriers in the acquisition of and access to scholarly content. This is a radical change from the subscription model and enables essentially everyone, including the general public, to access articles, which previously were more limited in their distribution.

For the producers of scholarly content, there are also some advantages. Because scholarship published using the open-access model is free, it is distributed widely. Authors engage in scholarly communication because they want to share the results of their research, their clinical and educational practices, and other information, and open access dovetails perfectly with this: open access enables a broader sharing or communication than was previously possible. Increasingly, scholarly output is subject to analysis, measurement, and assessment. With open access, study findings are more readily available for analysis by others.

Another advantage of open access is that the reuse of graphs, figures, and data published in earlier open-access works is much easier to retrieve, provided that they were published under a liberal Creative Commons license, which is generally the case in scholarly open-access journals. Creative Commons is a nonprofit organization that provides six main types of copyright licenses to share documents and creative works and allow them to be reused by others (Creative Commons, 2017). For example, a CC BY license lets others distribute and modify an author's work, even commercially; this license provides the widest dissemination. Another type of license, CC BY-NC (noncommercial)-ND (nonderivative) is the most restrictive license. With this license, which is common for open-access articles, others can download the article (or another work) and share it as long as the original author is given credit. The article cannot be modified or used commercially (Creative Commons, 2017). Authors reproducing work published under Creative Commons licenses do not need to get permission to republish text, figures, and the like; the permission is already given via the license. Researchers traditionally did not share the datasets they generated in the course of their research, but this practice is now changing. Scholarly authors can publish their research datasets in institutional and disciplinary repositories and license them with Creative Commons licenses, making them freely available for other researchers to reuse. There are also repositories that specialize in the publishing of scholarly datasets that accompany published articles.

One disadvantage of open access for authors is the cost. The gold open-access model requires payments from authors. Some universities have funds that their faculty can use to cover these payments, but in most cases these funds are limited. Funding to cover the APC for open access is likely not provided for clinicians. For most nurse authors, the traditional model, with no costs to the author for publishing in the journal, is preferred.

PREDATORY PUBLISHERS

By far the most negative effect of scholarly open-access publishing has been the proliferation of "predatory publishers" (Beall, 2017; Shen & Björk, 2015). These are publishers that operate using the gold model, in which authors are charged a fee—the APC—on acceptance of a paper. Unfortunately, many questionable publishing operations have been set up just to earn the fees, publishing low-quality papers with little value added to them. Predatory journals conduct questionable peer reviews of articles, if any, catering to the needs of authors to publish quickly and easily. Of concern, in addition to the lack of peer review and publication of low-quality papers, is that articles in predatory journals are not indexed in bibliographic databases such as PubMed/MEDLINE and the Cumulative Index to Nursing and Allied Health Literature (CINAHL). As a result, the articles in predatory journals will not be found by others when searching for information in one of these commonly used databases in nursing and other healthcare fields.

Few studies of predatory publishing in nursing have been done. Oermann et al. (2016) found that 140 predatory nursing journals were published as of 2016. That number is likely higher today. A study of those journals found questionable peer-review processes, inaccurate and deceptive information (e.g., statements about the journal's indexing and impact factor scores) on the journal website, many journals without editors, and poor quality of content being published (Oermann et al., 2016, 2017).

Predatory publishers rely on spam email to solicit article submissions. These spam emails can be clever and appeal to the needs of authors. Some are personalized spam emails that praise an author's earlier work and invite another. They often fail to mention the APC, and it is possible for an author to submit a paper, only to have it quickly accepted and then receive an invoice for the APC. Predatory publishers may be transitory, appearing for a time and then disappearing from nursing journals (Oermann et al., 2016). Publications are meant to be permanent, and authors should not submit to publishers whose content is not backed up and digitally preserved.

Predatory publishers produce low-quality publications. They offer a fast publication process, an easy temptation for authors who are often bewildered by the complex scholarly publishing process that involves a robust peer review, multiple revisions, copyediting, and eventually publication. The work of nurses deserves the highest possible publication options. Authors should avoid the temptation to publish quickly and easily in low-quality journals and should seek out and publish in only the best possible journals. A vigorous peer-review process, though difficult and long, can greatly improve the quality of a paper; it can remove errors and misjudgments that would otherwise get published. Scholarly publishing, done correctly, is not always easy, but the benefits to the profession and to science are of critical importance.

With open-access journals, it is conventional for authors to release their articles under a Creative Commons license, giving the publisher a nonexclusive right to publish the works. This means that the authors retain the copyright on their works. Therefore, authors should be wary when an open-access publisher demands that they transfer copyright of their works to the organization, especially since they are paying an APC to the publisher. Nurses are cautioned to avoid submitting manuscripts to predatory journals and abstracts to predatory conferences.

DIRECTORIES OF OPEN-ACCESS JOURNALS AND RESOURCES FOR AUTHORS

Scholarly journals are listed in many directories and bibliographic databases, and are covered in online repositories, as discussed in Chapter 2. Directories aim to be comprehensive and may not screen for quality. Some predatory publishers feign legitimacy by boasting about being included in certain journal directories. Some may falsely state that they are "indexed" in journal directories or other resources. In the context of scholarly journals, there is an important distinction between indexing and being included in a directory. Directories list at the journal level; indexing is done at the article level. One popular journal directory is Cabells (www2.cabells.com). This is a proprietary resource, meaning that one's library must have a subscription for authors to access it. Cabells is a comprehensive directory, and much of the information it contains is self-reported. Cabells includes a journal whitelist (trustworthy academic journals) and a journal blacklist (journals that were screened using more than 60 indicators and should be avoided (Silver, 2017).

Before the advent of the Internet, bibliographic databases were the chief means of finding desired information in scholarly journals. Databases such as MEDLINE and CINAHL are selective and only include journals that are evaluated prior to indexing. Fortunately, many of the high-quality databases such as these exclude predatory journals. However, some predatory journals are being inadvertently indexed in PubMed, which provides access to the MEDLINE database. These journals are not in MEDLINE because they do not meet the criteria for inclusion. If authors search for potential journals for their manuscripts in PubMed (using the link "Journals in NCBI Databases"), it is important to avoid a journal with this statement "Not currently indexed for MEDLINE" (Anderson, 2017a).

In academic libraries, technology has enabled the merging of abstracting and indexing services with the actual content they index. In the past, authors would first search a database such as PubMed or CINAHL and then perform a second search for each of the relevant items turned up by their previous searches. Now, academic libraries have technology that connects their users directly to the full text, right from the database they searched.

The most popular academic index is Google Scholar. This resource has the advantage of being comprehensive, but has the disadvantage of including many low-quality and predatory journals in its central index. Thus, it must be used with caution.

There are a few online directories of scholarly open-access journals worth noting. One of these is the Directory of Open Access Journals (DOAJ), found at doaj.org. The DOAJ is an online directory that indexes and provides access to nearly 11,000 open-access, peer-reviewed journals. Like most directories, the DOAJ should not be used as a measure or guarantee of quality; it is only a directory.

The Open Access Scholarly Publishers Association (OASPA) is a trade association for scholarly open-access publishers (oaspa.org). Those seeking a whitelist (trustworthy open-access journals) may find the association's membership list to be a useful tool. The organization does not give memberships to all publishers that apply, and applicants undergo an extensive review process prior to being included.

RESOURCES FOR IDENTIFYING PREDATORY JOURNALS

Authors need to review carefully potential journals for submission of a manuscript. Nicoll and Chinn (2015) referred to this as *journal due diligence*. Authors should confirm qualities of the journal such as peer review, indexing in bibliographic databases (e.g., MEDLINE and CINAHL), and accuracy of information on the journal website. A checklist is available at the "Think. Check. Submit" website (thinkchecksubmit.org) for use in reviewing potential journals.

Authors can search for possible journals using the Directory of Nursing Journals at the International Academy of Nursing Editors website (nursingeditors.com/journals-directory). This directory of about 250 nursing journals includes only journals that have been evaluated based on the Committee on Publication Ethics (COPE) Principles of Transparency and Best Practice in Scholarly Publishing (COPE, 2014). By using this directory, authors avoid predatory nursing journals. This is the best place to start to find a potential journal for a manuscript. Guidelines for searching for and selecting a journal were discussed in Chapter 2.

Authors can also search for possible journals using the Journal/Author Name Estimator (JANE) at jane.biosemantics.org (The Biosemantics Group, 2017). The JANE website uses data from PubMed. To avoid selecting a predatory or low-quality journal inadvertently included in PubMed, JANE tags journals that are indexed in the MEDLINE database; only those journals should be used. JANE also indicates open-access journals in the DOAJ (The Biosemantics Group, 2017). JANE and the Directory of Nursing Journals at the International Academy of Nursing Editors website were described in Chapter 2.

Another strategy for identifying possible journals and avoiding predatory publications is to search bibliographic databases such as PubMed/MEDLINE and CINAHL for journals that publish papers in the topical area. For example, if the manuscript is on preventing ventilator-associated pneumonia, the author can search for journals in one of these databases that publish articles on critical care nursing. To be included in these databases, journals are evaluated to ensure they meet certain criteria. New journals may not have had time to be added to them, assuming they meet the criteria. Authors considering submitting an article to a new journal that is not listed in any of these resources should be cautious. Learning about the top journals in one's field comes with reading the scholarly literature and consulting with colleagues. The challenge lies in evaluating new or recently launched journals, publications that may not yet be included in standard databases.

Examples of Legitimate Open-Access Publishers and Megajournals

Although predatory publishers have exploited open-access publishing for their own benefits and profits (McCann & Polacsek, 2017), this does not mean that all open-access journals should be avoided. Many publishers operate ethically using the gold open-access model. For example, BioMed Central is an example of an ethical open-access publisher using the gold model. Many of its journals have high-impact factors, enjoy a high download rate, and are among the top journals in their respective fields.

NursingOpen is a peer-reviewed open-access journal that also uses the gold model. It publishes articles on nursing practice, research, education, and policy under a Creative Commons license CC BY 4.0 (Wiley Online Library, 2018). With that license, others can share the article and adapt it (for any purpose, even commercially) as long as the original author is given credit, there is a link to the license, and there is a statement about the changes made. The APC is stated on the journal website and is easy to find, in contrast to the APCs in predatory nursing journals, which are often difficult to locate on the journal websites (Oermann et al., 2016). Authors need to evaluate the quality of open-access nursing journals just as they would do for traditional subscription journals. In one of the few studies done in nursing, Crowe and Carlyle (2015) examined the quality of open-access nursing journals in the DOAJ that published articles in 2013, were in English, and were freely accessible. There were 19 journals included in the study; those journals were judged to have lower quality than most traditional subscription journals.

Megajournals, such as PLoS One, are scholarly open-access journals that accept articles from all scientific fields, but do not necessarily review for novelty or importance. Most scholarly journals use peer review to filter out articles that offer little or no new information or that reviewers see as unimportant. Megajournals generally ignore these filters, and the peer review focuses on assessing papers to ensure that they are methodologically and statistically sound. Because the peer review is simpler, megajournals tend to have a shorter time to acceptance of the paper for publication. A study of 11 open-access megajournals found wide variations in terms of their size, disciplinary area, author characteristics, and citation profiles (Wakeling et al., 2016). Megajournals use a gold open-access model.

SUMMARY

The Internet has brought many changes to scholarly publishing, and authors need to keep up with these changes so they can select the best venue for sharing their work. Open-access publishing has the advantage of making research freely available for everyone, and research released under certain Creative Commons licenses can be copied and redistributed, a condition that promotes cumulative research and the sharing of research. Open-access publishing is not likely to disappear, but neither is subscription publishing. There are currently several scholarly publishing distribution models in place, and this diversity will likely continue to exist.

Unfortunately, the gold or author-pays model of open-access publishing has led to the creation of numerous low-quality publishers. These entities, often referred to as predatory publishers, offer authors a quick and easy acceptance and dissemination of their manuscripts. Although this process may promise a short-term gain, publishing in a low-quality journal can hurt authors over the long-term course of their careers.

To avoid predatory journals, nurses can use resources such as the Directory of Nursing Journals at the International Academy of Nursing Editors website. This chapter included other strategies to avoid submitting to a predatory journal. Authors should be familiar with the main journals in their fields or specializations through a wide reading of pertinent sources.

No one knows for sure how scholarly communication and scholarly publishing will continue to evolve. It is likely that numerous publishing models will continue to exist. Authors not only have to be experts in their fields, they should also gain expertise in scholarly communication. The key to success for authors in the next decade will be keeping on top of the changes in scholarly publishing and making publishing decisions based on what is best for each individual author over the long term. Open-access publishing has created new opportunities for authors, opportunities that are there for the taking.

REFERENCES

Anderson, K. (2017a). A confusion of journals–What is PubMed now? *The Scholarly Kitchen*. Retrieved from https://scholarlykitchen.sspnet.org/2017/09/07/confusion-journals-pubmed-now

Anderson, K. (2017b). Diversity in the open access movement, Part 1: Differing definitions. *The Scholarly Kitchen*. Retrieved from https://scholarlykitchen.sspnet.org/2017/01/23/diversity-open-access-movement-part-1-differing-definitions

Beall, J. (2017). What I learned from predatory publishers. *Biochemia Medica, 27*, 273–278. doi:10.11613/bm.2017.029

The Biosemantics Group. (2017). Jane: Journal/author name estimator. Retrieved from http://jane.biosemantics.org/faq.php

Committee on Publication Ethics. (2014). Principles of transparency and best practice in scholarly publishing. Retrieved from https://publicationethics.org/files/Principles_of_Transparency_and_Best_Practice_in_Scholarly_Publishingv2.pdf

Creative Commons. (2017). *About the licenses*. Retrieved from https://creativecommons.org/licenses

Crowe, M., & Carlyle, D. (2015). Is open access sufficient? A review of the quality of open-access nursing journals. *International Journal of Mental Health Nursing, 24*(1), 59–64. doi:10.1111/inm.12098

McCann, T. V., & Polacsek, M. (2017). False gold: Safely navigating open access publishing to avoid predatory publishers and journals. *Journal of Advanced Nursing, 74*, 809–817. doi:10.1111/jan.13483

Nicoll, L. H., & Chinn, P. L. (2015). Caught in the trap: The allure of deceptive publishers. *Nurse Author & Editor, 25*(4), 4. Retrieved from http://naepub.com/predatorypublishing/2015-25-4-4

NursingOpen. (2018). Website. Retrieved from http://onlinelibrary.wiley.com/journal/10.1002/(ISSN)2054-1058

Oermann, M. H., Conklin, J. L., Nicoll, L. H., Chinn, P. L., Ashton, K. S., Edie, A. H., … Budinger, S. C. (2016). Study of predatory open access nursing journals. *Journal of Nursing Scholarship*, *48*, 624–632. doi:10.1111/jnu.12248

Oermann, M. H., Nicoll, L. H., Chinn, P. L., Ashton, K. S., Conklin, J. L., Edie, A. H., … Williams, B. L. (2017). Quality of articles published in predatory nursing journals. *Nursing Outlook*, *66*, 4–10. doi:10.1016/j.outlook.2017.05.005

Shen, C., & Björk, B. C. (2015). 'Predatory' open access: A longitudinal study of article volumes and market characteristics. *BMC Medicine*, *13*(1), 1–15. doi:10.1186/s12916-015-0469-2

Silver, A. (2017, May 31). Pay-to-view blacklist of predatory journals set to launch. *Nature*. Retrieved from https://www.nature.com/news/pay-to-view-blacklist-of-predatory-journals-set-to-launch-1.22090

U.S. National Library of Medicine. (2015). *PMC FAQs*. Retrieved from https://www.ncbi.nlm.nih.gov/pmc/about/faq/#q14

Wakeling, S., Willett, P., Creaser, C., Fry, J., Pinfield, S., & Spezi, V. (2016). Open-access mega-journals: A bibliometric profile. *PLoS One*, *11*(11), e0165359. https://doi.org/10.1371/journal.pone.0165359

APPENDICES

APPENDIX A

SELECTED STATISTICAL SYMBOLS AND ABBREVIATIONS

Symbol or Abbreviation	Definition
$>$	Greater than
$\geq$	Greater than or equal to
$<$	Less than
$\leq$	Less than or equal to
α	Greek alpha, probability of Type I error; also reliability coefficient
ANCOVA	Analysis of covariance
ANOVA	Analysis of variance
β	Greek beta, probability of Type II error; also standardized regression coefficient (beta weight)
b	Regression coefficient
χ^2	Chi-square test
CI	Confidence interval
d	Cohen's measure of effect size for comparing two sample means
df	Degrees of freedom
ES	Effect size
f	Frequency
F	F distribution, Fisher's F ratio
$F_{(v1, v2)}$	F with v1 and v2 degrees of freedom
H_0	Null hypothesis
H_1	Alternate hypothesis
HSD	Tukey's (honestly significantly different) test
k	Kappa statistic

(continued)

SELECTED STATISTICAL SYMBOLS AND ABBREVIATIONS (*continued*)

Symbol or Abbreviation	Definition
KR20	Kuder–Richardson reliability index
LR	Likelihood ratio
LSD	Least significant difference
M(X)	Mean of sample (arithmetic average)
MANCOVA	Multivariate analysis of covariance
MANOVA	Multivariate analysis of variance
Mdn	Median
MS	Mean square
MSE	Mean square error
n	Number of cases (size of subsample)
N	Total number of cases (total sample size)
ns	Not statistically significant
OR	Odds ratio
p	Probability
r	Pearson product–moment correlation coefficient
r^2	Coefficient of determination; estimate of Pearson product–moment correlation squared
R	Multiple correlation
SD	Standard deviation of sample
SE	Standard error
SEM	Standard error of measurement
Σ	Sum
SS	Sum of squares
t	Student *t* (include *p* value, 1- versus 2-tailed)
U	Mann–Whitney test
z	Z score; value of a statistic divided by its standard error

APPENDIX B

UNNECESSARY WORDS IN WRITING

Unnecessary Words	More Concise
a decreased amount (number) of	less (fewer)
a number of	many, several
accounted for by the fact	because
along the lines of	similar, like
an adequate amount of	enough
as a consequence of	because of
as of this date	today
at a period of time when	when
at this point in time	now
by means of	with, by
consensus of opinion	consensus
due to the fact that	because
during the course of	during, while
fewer in number	fewer
for the purpose of	for, to
for the reason that	since, because
give an account of	describe
has been engaged in the study of	has studied
has the capability of	can
in a position to	can
in an effort to	to
in all cases	all, always
in close proximity to	near
in excess of	more than

(continued)

UNNECESSARY WORDS IN WRITING (*continued*)

Unnecessary Words	More Concise
in my opinion, I think	I think
in order to	to
in regard to	about
in the event that	if
in view of, in view of the fact that	because
it has been reported by Smith	Smith reported
it would appear that	apparently
make reference to	refer to
many in number	many
of great benefit	beneficial
on account of	because
on the basis of	because, from
prior to (in time)	before
regardless of the fact that	even though
subsequent to	after
take into consideration	consider
the majority of, the vast majority of	most
with reference to	about
X-year period of time	X years

Sources: Adapted from Day, R. A. (1998). *How to write and publish a scientific paper* (5th ed., pp. 238–243). Phoenix, AZ: Oryx Press; Huth, E. J. (1999). *Writing and publishing in medicine* (3rd ed., pp. 189–190). Baltimore, MD: Lippincott Williams & Wilkins.

APPENDIX C

GUIDELINES AND RESOURCES FOR PREPARING MANUSCRIPTS

CONSORT (Consolidated Standards of Reporting Trials)	CONSORT Statement is intended for use in reporting a randomized controlled trial. It includes a checklist and flow diagram. Available at www.consort-statement.org CONSORT Explanation and Elaboration Document enhances use and understanding of CONSORT Statement. It includes examples and explanations for each item in checklist. Available at www.consort-statement.org/extensions
COPE (Committee on Publication Ethics)	COPE is concerned with integrity of peer-reviewed publications in biomedicine. Its Code of Conduct has defined best practice in ethics of scientific publishing to assist authors, editors, and others. Available at publicationethics.org/resources/code-conduct. COPE has developed flowcharts that provide algorithms for editors if they suspect publication misconduct. Flowcharts and many other useful materials are available at publicationethics.org
COREQ (Consolidated Criteria for Reporting Qualitative Research)	COREQ includes a 32-item checklist for explicit and comprehensive reporting of qualitative studies (in-depth interviews and focus groups). Available at www.equator-network.org/reporting-guidelines/coreq
ENTREQ (Enhancing Transparency in Reporting the Synthesis of Qualitative Research)	ENTREQ statement includes 21 items grouped into five domains: introduction, methods and methodology, literature search and selection, appraisal, and synthesis of findings (see www.equator-network.org/reporting-guidelines/entreq)

(continued)

GUIDELINES AND RESOURCES FOR PREPARING MANUSCRIPTS (*continued*)

EQUATOR Network	The EQUATOR initiative promotes accurate and transparent reporting of healthcare research. Includes a comprehensive list of hundreds of reporting guidelines organized by study type (www.equator-network.org)
ICMJE (International Committee of Medical Journal Editors) Recommendations	ICMJE is a group of medical journal editors who developed and update the *Recommendations for the Conduct, Reporting, Editing, and Publication of Scholarly Work in Medical Journals.* This document includes guidelines on ethical considerations, publishing and editorial issues, manuscript preparation, references, and other information relevant to writing for publication. Available at www.icmje.org/recommendations
PRISMA (Preferred Reporting Items for Systematic Reviews and Meta-Analyses)	PRISMA Statement guides authors in reporting systematic reviews and meta-analyses; was referred to earlier as QUORUM (QUality Of Reporting Of Meta-analyses). PRISMA Statement is a checklist for reporting these reviews and a flow diagram for identifying the process used for the review and studies included at different phases. Provides Word templates that can be downloaded for authors' use, including a flow diagram, and other resources that can be accessed at PRISMA website. Available at www.prisma-statement.org
SQUIRE (Standards for QUality Improvement Reporting Excellence)	SQUIRE guidelines are for use when preparing manuscripts on quality improvement (QI) studies and projects. Available at squire-statement.org
STROBE (STrengthening the Reporting of OBservational studies in Epidemiology)	STROBE is a checklist for reporting items that should be included in articles describing observational research (case-control, cohort, and cross-sectional studies). Available at www.strobe-statement.org/index.php?id=strobe-home
WAME (World Association of Medical Editors)	WAME is a nonprofit, voluntary, international association of editors of peer-reviewed medical journals. *Principles of Transparency and Best Practice in Scholarly Publishing* is available at the website. Available at www.wame.org

INDEX

Printed in the United States
by Baker & Taylor Publisher Services